THE
IMMORTAL
MITOCHONDRIA

Our Electronic Life, Longevity, and Health

Triveni P. Shukla

Library of Congress Control Number: 2019913178
ISBN-13:   Paperback: 978-1-64398-828-3
            Epub: 978-1-64674-015-4
            Kindle: 978-1-64674-016-1
            PDF: 978-1-64674-017-8

Printed in the United States of America

LitFire
PUBLISHING

LitFire LLC
1-800-511-9787
www.litfirepublishing.com
order@litfirepublishing.com

Contents

List of Tables

List of Figures

FOOTERS

Chapter 1: Introduction
Mitochondria help us breath protons and produce enegy molecule ATP.

Chapter 2: Food for Mitochondria
A low calories methylation diet with antioxidants, essential amino acids, omega-3 fatty acids, vitamins, and trace minerals is a must for functional mitochondria.

Chapter 3: Vital Signs and Vital Organs
Number of mitochondria in a cell is a response to a cell's energy demand.

Chapter 4: Mitochondrial Diseases
Mitochondrial gene therapy by editing and rewriting the genes will soon become a routine medical practice..

Chapter 5: Summation
Longevity requires plentiful undamaged and healthy mitochondria.

DEDICATION

I dedicate this book to my wife, Girija Shukla, whose story of vital signs during her stem cell transplant as a cure for Multiple myeloma inspired me to learn and write about our vital organelle behind vital signs.

FOREWORD

All begins with water and the sun light
(यौ॒ऽपां॒ पुष्पं॒ वेद....)

Mantrapushpam (Krishna Yayurveda, 29)

We have known Triveni Shukla as a food scientist with a bent on learning Eastern Hindu philosophy and theology. His recent book "our Genes Our foods Our Choices" let us in on his expertise in nutritional biochemistry. Now in exploring the mitochondria of our 200 type varied cells as master organelle that manage routine energetics, signals, and connections of food with daily metabolism he positions himself as a good advocate of molecular dynamics as it relates to a long disease and pain free life. He convincingly connects daily nutrients with DNA tooling and repair, epigenetics and gene expression, cellular bioenergetics, energy transformation, and management of free radical signaling and body wide communication. There is a revolution taking place in quantum biology that may lay a firmer foundation for our daily nutrition, he says. We would like to give a summary of what Triveni advocates in his Immortal Mitochondria.

Photosystem II is the only biological molecule capable of splitting water into protons, electrons, and oxygen and so begins the making of foods we eat. Water is essential for a plant's ability to make foods for human life. The sun, the star of our galaxy, is the source of our daily energy. Sun light impinges on chlorophyll, electrons get excited, hydrogen ion protons are produced by oxidation of water, electrons are accepted by NADP (Nucleotide Adenine Dinucleotide Phosphate), and resulting NADPH is processed though electron transport chain in order to make ATP, the energy molecule adenosin triphosphate for all that lives. Finally ATP and NADPH are used by plants to make electron rich foods for animals including humans. Animal cells are endowed with the capacity to reverse the process and extract energy for day to day living. In order to complete electron extraction from foods of carbohydrates, proteins, and fat humans need an optimum daily dose of vitamins and minerals and this book identifies and names such a food as methylation diet. It describes the biochemistry and bioenergetics of ATP production by mitochondria in chapter one, design of methylation diet for optimal mitochondrial function in chapter two, vital signs as measures of function of vital organs of mitochondria in chapter three, mitochondrial diseases in chapter 4, and summation as an epilogue describing good eating and good living over a long life span. In its entirety, albeit a bit technical, "Immortal Mitochondria" maintains that the life and work of mitochondria for human health and well being depends largely on a well designed antioxidant rich daily methylation diet. This book makes a good case for DNA methylation as an evolutionary tool for managing human chronobiology and daily circadian rythm. It clarifies that whereas production of reactive oxygen species (free radicals) is a necessity for body wide communication and signaling, excessive free radicals must be quenched successfully each day by antioxidants present in our properly designed methylation diet based on fruits, vegetables, whole grains, legumes, lentils, and dietary fiber. Probiotic foods add to human microbiome for immunity.

"Immortal Mitochondria" reveals that upon it depends our electronic life and life span, daily extraction of food energy, and functional optimization of physiology by life style choices we make in terms of puntuated mobility, restricted calorie and oxygen intake, and conditioned mind-body interaction by meditation, mindfulness, and most important of all, the spiritual practice.

The main message in this book is that mitochondria are central to human life and longevity. They are present in all cells of our body except red blood cells. Their function is to extract, concentrate, and manage electrons and protons for energy production from foods and beverages we consume and for body wide signaling, communication, and control. They enhance longevity by optimizing production of reactive oxygen species and regulating stress respone while doing their own quality assurance.

Too many calories simply means overloading mitochondria. The overload by way of excess electron is worse in case of high fat diets. Life style issues of aerobic exercise and physical activity including deep breathing and restricted oxygen intake modulate and enhance the health of mitochondrial in our cells and, therefore, our own health and well being.

Dying it appears is integral to living. Our 10 trillion cells divide 2 million times each day and 2 billion red blood cells in our blood die each day. There will be no energy by glycolysis if there is no NAD^+ and our heart and brain shall cease to function in absence of oxygen. Behind the works of NAD^+ is electron and energy. Each mole of glucose produces 12 moles of electrons. Since one mole of green electron equates to 216 KJ and since 1 Kcalorie equals 4.184 KJ, a 2000 Kcalorie diet provides 38.4 moles of electrons for running our life. The electrons help translocate protons uphill and then downhill for making 10^9 ATP molecules in each cell of a mere 300 nm^3 volume. Each cell then functions with 3 X 10^{-10} Watts. Even a cursury reading of this book highlights the power of coding events by our DNA and the power of nutrients in our diet that modify our DNA and help direct gene expressions associated with each and everyone of our activities. When in trouble, our body cells can make up to 2000 identical antibodies or immunoglulins per second failing which we can die. But all this depends, describes this book, on what we eat, when we eat, and how optimally we eat.

Meal timing affects circadian rythm and weight, overnight fasting burns fat, NAD^+ drives the circadian rythm, and almost all depends on mitochondria with its 800 nm long inner membrane, 37 nm long cristae, and **25 nm long electron transport chain**. ATP synthase of complex V revolves 47 times per second and each molecule of this enzyme makes 100 ATP by processing 300- 564 protons.

Our life is run by 32-38 moles of electrons each day meaning that humans are an 83.3 Kcal per hour nano-machine, a mere 90.99 Watts/hr that is. This book is rarely rich with human body statistics and quantitative logistics on eating and living well.

A very old bacterium became our mitochondria in our ten trillion cells. There are 100 trillion of them in our colon in orde for managing and building our immune system, talking to our brain, and for giving us 10 tmes more potential gene power for an optimal proteome and metabolome. Let us call it the power of the COLONIC PROBIOTICS. Obviously probiotic foods must be part of methylation diet. No wonder why "To live well by methylation diet" is the major emphasis in this book. "To eat well" means eating a lot of fruits, vegetables, nuts, seeds, chocolate, and animal products for essential nutrients that can provide an optimum of omega-3 fatty acids, folic acid, acetyl-L-carnitine, lycopene, leutin, B vitamins in general and vitamins A, C, D, E, and K, enough of coenzyme Q_{10} and Niacin or vitamin B_3 for NAD^+ along with trace minerals of copper, manganese, magnessium, selenium, and Zinc. Such diets must deliver enough antioxidants in order to keep free radicals in balance for good immune function and signaling with least mutative effects on our DNA.

That eating well in a punctuated manner can keep our vital organs running free of pain, ailments, and chronic diseases for a longer span of time is the simple truth we should follow in our day to day living. Our telomers will not shorten, our cells will make enough of enzyme telomerase, and methylation diet will help maintain cellular polarity and plasticity for an ideal immune and nervous system interaction. The readers will live long and stay healthy by adapting to what this book teaches.

Govindjee
Rajani Govindjee
Professor Emeritus
University of Illinois

ACKNOWLEDGEMENT

I express my deep appreciation for edits, reads, and review by three very dear friends, Drs Ila Misra, Anil Dwiedi, and Dr. Abdul Waheed. It is very lucky for me to get to know these friends. Drs. Misra and Waheed used their biochemical eyes to help me probe the workings of "Mitochondria" and Dr Dwivedi helped me, I must say, physicise the grand biology of "immortal Mitochindria."

I shought Dr. Govindji's and his life long consort Dr. Rajani Govind Ji for their expertise in photosynthesis. Plants use the photosynthetic apparatus to capture sun's energy and synthesize foods for us and mitochondria help us break foods down and use the stored energy.

The list of associates and friend who gave me insight by their questions is too long to mention. I should simply acknowledge by saying that my ability to think through "powers of our daily foods" woul have been unbearably incomplete without their probing.

PREFACE

I should like to state upfront that proton gradient is as universal in biology as is genetic code and that all life breaths protons. Life transcends though proton gradient and genetic code.. Electrons push protons uphill and protons travel through a molecular motor (ATP synthase) that churns out energy molecule ATP. The powers of electrons and protons are coupled in every mitochondria of our cells. Paramagnetic oxygen is necessary at the end as the spent electron acceptor.

Our mitochondria must function well In order to breath protons for ATP production for an energetic and predicable health. Our genome and its DNA must be stabilized and preserved. Much of this preservation can be accomplished by diets that help methylate our DNA and modify our chromatin sheath that envelops the DNA. This is more true for the circular mitochondrial genome. Methylation, I must emphasize, is directed to DNA repair and control.

Life as we know it shall be impossible without paramagnetic oxygen as final spent electron acceptor. Other life supporting molecules are omega-3 DHA (docosahexanoic acid), water, and even free radicals with unpaired electrons. However, the original source of energy is sun's light. Photosynthesis traps it in the bonds of food molecules present we eat. Water is an ionic plasma. It is comprised of the lightest atom of hydrogen (without nucleus and with a single electron and a single proton) and oxygen. It is present in our body in the largest (58%) amount. Water serves as a coherent medium for superconducting electrons and for transfer of energy and information. Hydrogen bonds of water between hydrogen and oxygen serve as the mechanism for memory and proton conduction.

Every cell in our body is a system of interwoven nano-scale molecular and atomic events and a lot happens in it within a distance of less than 10 nanometers or 100 Angstroms. Coupling of electron transfer in mitochondria over a distance of 7 nanometers and proton translocation over 4 nanometers (across the inner mitochondrial membrane) rules our life. An equilibrium of pro and anti oxidant states is part of cell's intelligence system based on signaling based in turn on molecules of B vitamins, N-Acety Cysteine, and vitamin D, and complexes of magnesium and zinc. Nutrients in foods and activity and exercise including meditation and yoga assist signaling. Amazingly, all this is consistent with thermodynamic law of conservation of energy and all life is electronic and ionic.

The electronic power produced in human body is merely 200 milliVolt, a sum of 140 milliVolt of mitochondrial transmembrane potential and 60 milliVolt due to difference of 1 pH unit between inside of mitochondria and the rest of the cell. Although this is a very low voltage battery but 7.5×10^{13} mitochondria functioning together permit us to function well and to stay live. Just think of the mitochondrial power packed in the muscle of a 10 cm long humming bird as she flaps and hums 50 times a minute. Every flap and every hum typifies a Quantum operations.

Biology has conserved life sustaining power of electrons and protons. Down deep on the ocean floors live bacteria that eat and excrete pure electrons. Our cells are dedicated to triggering electrons for making a living by power of hydrogen ion, hydrogen being the smallest and plentiful 1 proton-1 electron light atom in our body. We live by electrons in the bonds of glucose, amino acid, and fat present in our daily food. Unlike electric bacteria, human cells use middlemen for extracting and shuttling electrons directed to making Adenosine Triphosphate(ATP) by enzyme ATP synthase. ATP is the molecule of chemical energy stored in its terminal high energy phosphate bond.

Actually, the story of electrons as they travel on and through enzyme complexes of inner mitochondrial membrane is an outcome of a 1.45 - 2.00 billion years old merger of a bacterium with some other not yet known human cell. I call this semi-autonomous **endosymbiont,** the "Immortal Mitochondria". Amazingly, the merger has kept its terms and tenure in transcendence throughout the eukaryotic world most likely by rules of quantum mechanics. No doubt! The living organisms are electromagnetic manifestations.

Excluding 2.5 trillion red blood cells, there are 10 trillion cells in human body and every cell on average has 500 mitochondria. Thus energy in our body comes from at least 3,750 trillion mitochondria each capable of producing 36 energy molecules of ATP from the bond energy of each glucose molecules it processes. Mitochondria use co-enzymes Nicotinamide Adenine Dinucleotide (NADH) and Flavin Adenine Dinucleotide (FADH$_2$) as electron carriers from Kreb's cycle to electron transport chain. The cariers, in a sense, extract and carry electrons during glycolysis, acetyl CoA production, and operation of the Krebs cycle and deposit them to the Flavin Mononucleotide centers of enzyme complexes of the electron transport chain. The glucose molecule, I just reffered to, is the mother molecule made during photosynthesis in the leaves of plants by sun's energy. All else is made from glucose which is produced from carbon dioxide and water, both being plentyful on planet earth.

Some 3.75 million trillion (3,750 trillion X1000 DNA copies) mitochondrial DNA$_s$ work in everyone of our cells. This exceeds all DNA in the nucleus of our cells. The role of mitochondrial DNA, therefore, is much more dominant in determining our daily health and life than the nuclear DNA. Although mitochondria's main job is to produce chemical energy molecule ATP and manage energy metabolism but it does much more. Folks around the world in various cultures call it life "energy" without which we will cease to exist. They have given it names like prana in India, , Qi (chee) in China, and ruah in Israel.

Human mitochondria have their own circular genome of 37 genes that make molecular machinery for processing of electrons and protons. The electrons dance through five enzyme complexes in the inner mitochondrial membrane with a nanoscopic precision. **Mitochondrial DNA no doubt takes a little help from the nuclear DNA but bothers them the least in doing their life supporting high voltage job.** This high voltage job needs a very critical balance and regulation or else we die. The job involves quantum effects like electron tunneling throughout electron transport chain and proton tunneling in hydrolysis of ATP by enzyme ATPase. Enzymes in general are great examples of proton tunneling effects. Quantum physics, it appears, met biology eons ago. Too bad! it is a bit spooky and difficult to understand but it has enormous power. Just imagine that 150 millivolt across 4.5 billionth of a meter inner membrane of mitochondria translates to 30 million volts per meter in macroscopic world. That is the power of a thunderbolt.

I must talk of one more universal secret.To say that we live by our mitochondria is to say that we live by our mother because the inherited homology of mitochondria DNA is an exclusive gift to us from our mother. This exclusivity has a lot to do with not only our daily health and well being but also with health of our subsequent generations. John Kendrew's "Thread of Life" or what I call immortal mitochondria, although prone to mutation, have preserved its capacity and character for millions of years. Our mitochondrial DNA is strictly maternal because sperm mitochondria are all destroyed during zygote formation. The egg mitochondria out number and more or less help dissolve the sperm mitochondria. The poor sperms had just enough power to seek union for perpetuating the next life and die in the process. The mitochondria from mom perpetuate life and remain immortal.

Mitochondria help make 13 essential polypeptides for electron transport chain, 2 RNA_s and 22 $mRNA_s$. The guanine-rich heavy strand of mitochondria makes 28 genes and the cytosine-rich light strand makes 9 genes. Mitochondrial DNA affect our weight and height and thus health. Height-weight combinations have been known for a long time to determine mortality. About 18 genes are involved in weight as it relates to use of calories. The simple fact is that the health of all 7.5×10^{13} mitochondria in our body is the basis for vital signs, good metabolism, high energy and fatigue free living, longevity, and cognition. Therefore, the health of mitochondria simply means health of our body and mind.

That our biology has been physicized remains unnoticed by our health service providers and fitness gurus on television and social media. To my dismay, I find little or no mention of mitochondria in the majority of texts on health, nutrition, mood modification, weight control, and molecular gastronomy. I list a few of these books just to make the point: Dr. Andrew Weil's Spontaneous Healing, Dr. Phil Mcgraw's The Ultimate Weight Solution, Dr. Michael Rosen's The Real Age Makeover, Drs. Michael Rosen and M.C Oz's You on a Diet, Drs. William Evans and Irwin H. Rosenberg's Biomarker, Dr. Dean Ornish's The Spectrum, and Dr, David L. Katz's Flavor point Diet. A rare exception is Dr, Candice B. Pert's book on Molecules of Emotion which has a short four line brief on mitochondria. How could these experts ever talk about our health and well being without talking about the mitochondria, an organelle that is life itself by its functional association with other essential organelles and vesicles. They rarely mention that our daily food is largely a supply of electrons that (1) translocate protons uphill for making ATP and (2) orchestrate the electromagnetics of mitochondria.

No doubt that the DNA in the nuclear genome of our cells, the brain of our cells, is the commander-in-chief. There are 23 pairs of chromosomes comprising the genome which has 25,000 to 35,000 genes, all fully sequenced for 3 billion base pairs. Humans differ in their genetic makeup very little. The author of this book and the readers are different by no more than 3 million base pairs or just by 0.085%. This difference manifests in many ways in terms of appearance, weight, height, efficiency of therapeutic drugs, and propensity to cancer and chronic diseases.

Preponderance of mitochondrial genes is behind cell's power to live, to communicate, and even its vulnerability to die. No doubt! Our health and life depend on enormous power of mitochondria. Mitochondria can separate electrons and protons from hydrogen atom, transport them, translocate protons across the inner membrane, and reroute protons back through enzyme ATP synthase, and thus make energy molecule of life, ATP. They can produce biophotons, the infra-red light. We can think of mitochondria as a **spintronic transistor** because of their ability to use spin of electrons for inter and intra-cellular communications.

No more than 0.5 to 1 micrometer in diameter, mitochondria are capable of changing their shape and size by fusing and dividing. High energy electrons managed by mitochondria produce net 32 energy molecules of ATP per glucose molecule, almost 90% of all energy we use daily. Mitochondria use electron shuttling molecules for transferring electrons around. A familiar electron shuttling molecule is Coenzyme Q_{10} , marketed today as a major anti-aging food supplement. It is part of the electron transport chain of mitochondria. Q_{10} helps our nerve cells or neurons in our brain operate by the power of electrons, ions, and protons.

The middlemen molecules that carry electrons are dinucleotides made of basic structures common to DNA and RNA. NADH donates electrons and NAD+ accepts electrons. NAD+ can be synthesized in our body from tryptophan and aspartic acid present in protein foods we consume or more directly from vitamin niacin . Our body cells may have up to 2 gram of NAD+ at a given time for maintaining proper reserve of life energy, ATP. We also depend on special proteins like hemoglobin and myoglobin that help move and store oxygen by rearrangements of electrons. And then there is non-protein ubiquinone that shuttles electrons to the electron transfer chain and there are hemoglobin like proteins that act like rungs of electron transfer ultimately for reducing oxygen to water.

Hydrogen, the unlimited and long lived proton source, makes life possible in a cooperative quantum dance, Hydrogen bonds in our DNA, enzymes, receptors, and key functional proteins are great quantum measuring devices. Mitochondria, with a lot of hydrogen cations in its matrix, are nanomagnets and life in essence is semi conductive electronics where hydrogen bonds of water help coherent transfer of energy and information. They can act as capacitors for storing charge also.

Electrons and protons move around in our body over hydrogen bonds. Our cells have hydrogen and oxygen in order to uncondense or unfold protein polymers, a process necessary for modulating electron flow while we are active and awake. The middlemen molecules like NADH matter a lot in matters of electron flow in our multicellular body. The motion of hydrogen bonds in biomolecules provides for memory (thousand beats per second) of the entangled pair of electrons of free radicals. Mitochondria use entangled free radicals for magnetic memory. Also, entanglement happens right at the cytochrome sites with light or other magnetic fields of very specific monochromatic frequencies. Much of information is tied to actions of light with water. Water is the source of superconducting protons for rapid communication. Coherent domains allow H^+ to move through hydrogen bonds. Also, coherent domains trap electromagnetic frequencies for biochemical reactions and precise mechanism for gene function.

As a matter of fact mitochondria communicate (signal) with the environment because of the hydrogen bonding network and free radicals. Mitochondria produce free radicals, the spinning electrons off iron-sulfur clusters of electron transfer chain complexes (proteins) and send then all over the body in their signaling processes. They use free radicals to change their shape and size and even to code information when we are asleep, a quantum mechanical state of maximum coherence.

Mitochondria in our cells not only produce and conserve energy but they also serve as signal, memory, and general information transfer system using hydrogen bonds and free radicals. Our life depends on the spin of electrons. Unlike continuous flow in a copper wire in the household electrical circuit, electrons ride in steps on enzyme proteins, coenzyme Q and cytochrome C and couple the very act of proton movement across the membrane for energy production as ATP. ATP synthase, a huge lollipop like enzyme molecule, is a molecular motor that extrudes protons for making ATP. This process of proton propulsion by ATP synthase across the membrane is coupled to electrons movement in steps from one protein molecule to another for finally reducing oxygen to water at the end of electron transfer chain.

The 16.6 kilo byte mitochondrial genome is fully sequenced and we are beginning to understand the health problems due to their more frequent mutations. An average human cell may have 1000 copies of mitochondrial DNA. They are very prone to damage by free radicals produced both as an unintended byproduct of the electron transport process operating just next to them or produced on purpose for (1) functioning of our immune system, (2) biogenesis of mitochondria, (3) signaling in general, and (4) programmed death of our cells. Although great at self-quality control and editing, mitochondrial DNA is less capable of repairing itself. Mutations in mitochondrial DNA can and do cause diseases and physiological havoc in our lives.

Photosynthesis makes human foods and liberates oxygen while directly harvesting sun's energy. On planet earth it fixes 10 billion tons of carbon per year, part of which is our daily food, the repository of hydrogen that provides electrons and protons to our mitochondria for making ATP.

We are largely aerobic beings. This book explores foods for mitochondria. Mitochondria and their 37 genes relate to our vital signs, daily health, and physical performance. More importantly, it examines the central role of mitochondria in aerobic energy production by managing the dance of electrons in its inner membrane including cell signaling and death and birth our cells. Mitochondria oscillate and so does enzyme ATP synthase making 3 ATP per revolution. Neurons work at 60 gigabits or seven order of magnitude faster than our computers. Imagine that human brain can intensify an image at an incredible speed in 13 milliseconds and human thought speeds up infinitely.

Human, the most advanced multicellular organism lives by mitochondria whose function is tied to quantity and quality of our daily food. We live by electrons and their spins, mini magnets of protons, and the free radicals. It appears that we can't live totally divored from earths magnetism, electrons around it, and its temporal rhythms in relation to the sun and the moon. This book then is about how electrons, protons, and ions run our life. It offers biochemical reasoning and logic behind daily consumption of not only the electron rich foods and beverages but also the electron donating antioxidants, other essential molecules, and even free radicals for signaling.

As such this book is about high antioxidant methylation diet containing coenzyme Q_{10}, PQQ, Carnitine, lipoic acid, conjugated linoleic acid, and omega-3 fatty, vitamins B complex, C, D, E, and K for efficient mitochondria. DASH diet, mind diet, Mediterrnean diet, and Redox diets are varieties of methylation diets. This book seeks to describe the epigenetic switch like effect of nutrients we eat along with our caloric foods of proteins, carbohydrates, and fats.

The good works on vitamins, glycolysis or glucose splitting, making acetyl CoA, the electron mill we call Krebs cycle, and various aspects of electron transport chain have been rewarded with Nobel Prizes. Embedded in these discoveries is the knowledge about the structures of electron carriers, isoprenoid antioxidants, and hemoglobin like heme proteins of electron transfer. All of it depends on daily nutrition. As a matter of fact, biochemistry, medicine, and nutrition co-developed side by side during the last 100 years. We must probe into the essence of this knowledge and put it to practice for maintaining our health and wellness. To select good foods as methylation diet is to respect and obey mitochondria, an organelle that manages our vital organs by purposeful use and mediation of electrons, protons, and ions from foods we eat.

1

Chemical energy that runs our lives is made in mitochondria from major caloric nutrients of carbohydrate, proteins, fat and even soluble dietary fiber. The scheme of energy production by mitochondria is complex and considerably technical. This chapter is designed to illustrate an understandable story of energy production in human body cells.

We use 54.41 Kg of ATP each day. The first assumption for simplicity is that a 70 Kg person needs every day (1) 70 gram protein, same calories as that of 70 gram carbohydrate, (2) at least 60 gram energy packed good fat which is an equivalent of 135g carbohydrate, and (3) 332 gram carbohydrate per se, and (4) 30 gram dietary fiber. Let us assume that our daily energy source is this sum of 70 + 135 + 332 = 537 g glucose equivalent. A chemist or food scientist calculates it as 2.98 moles of glucose by deviding the sum by by 180.1559, the molecular weight of glucose. Since oxidation of each molecule of glucose yields 36 molecules of ATP, mitochondria in our cells produce 2.98 X 36 = 107.28 moles or 54.41 Kg of ATP every day given the molecular weight of ATP of 507.18 g.

We produce energy with 39% efficeiency. In theory consumption of 2.98 moles of glucose provides 2.98 X 686 Kcalories per mole, a total of 2,044 Kcalories. Since 36 ATP from each glucose molecule account for only 36 X 7.5 Kcalories per mole of ATP hydrolysis or 270 kcalories the efficiency is 270/686 = 39%. The following prevails as our mitochondria processes 2.98 moles of glucose per day.

We use 29.8 Moles of NADH. NADH helps translocate 298 moles of protons. At the rate of 3 protons per ATP 298 moles of protons can producef 99.33 moles of ATP. Plus 5.2 moles of $FADH_2$ produce additional 10.4 moles *of ATP giving a total of 109.73 moles of ATP. This is very close to 107.28 moles arrived at in the previous paragraph. NADH and FADH$_2$ combined transfer a total of 31.2 moles of electrons that can potentially translocate about 310 moles of protons. This too is in close agreement with 298 moles arrived at earlier in this paragraph. Thus ATP is the result of proton power. Since 4 protons reduce oxygen to water at the end of electron transfer chain, 310/4 or 77.5 moles of oxygen is reduced. So saying that we breathe protons translocated up across inner mitochondrial membrane into intermediate space and then passed through ATP synthase is very accurate. This happens by the power of electrons from foods we eat. Oxygen is a paramagnetic agent that accepts low energy spent electrons away and reduces itself to water.*

Plants and animals including human beings convert photon power to ATP with only 4.29% efficiency. During photosynthesis 2.98 moles glucose is created at the expense of 14 moles of photons or a total of 8,409 kcalories. Since 2.98 moles of glucose have only 2,044 Kcalories, the efficiency of photosynthesis is relatively low at 1,783/8409 = 21.20 %. Another way to calculate efficiency is divide 114 Kcalories needed to reduce 1 mole of carbon dioxide with 381 Kcalories energy of 8 moles of 600 nm wavelength. This calculates to 114/381 = 29.92%. But photosynthesis is known to proceed with even lower energy photons and since only 45% of incident light is in photosynthetic range, the photosynthetic efficiency is variously reported to be only 11%. From sun to our cells, the overall efficiency of conversion of photon power to ATP for human use is only 4.29%.

Glucose at daily consumption of 2.98 moles produces 107.28 moles of ATP with a maximum energy value of 13.6 Kcalories/mole under cellular condition. The total is only 1462.90 Kcalories. This energy is produced as NADH (Niacin or vitamin B$_3$ based molecule) and FADH$_2$ (riboflavin or vitamin B$_2$ based molecule) carry electrons from the bonds of food molecules and deliver them to the electron transport chain of inner membrane of mitochondria for eventual production of energy molecule ATP.

Mitochondria are omnipotent and transition metals are critical to electron transfer . Mitochondria produce energy, manage ions and free radicals for communications, communicate to nuclear DNA and other organelles in our cells, and conduct routine quality control of our cell's manufacturing processes. We are healthy, therefore, only when mitochondria are healthy and to live well is to consume methylation diet complete in nutrients, antioxidants, omega-3 type essential fatty acids, and precursors for essential nutrients such as Coenzyme Q_{10} and transition minerals iron, copper, molybdenum, sulfur, and zinc. Let us never forget that transition metals are key to electron transfer in our body.

We need energy to make mighty proteins- enzymes, receptors, strucyural, and mass transfer proteins. Energy is needed to make proteins that run every thing in our body including metabolism, transport across cell membrane, nerve firing, proton pumping, homeostasis, and basic functioning of our vital organs. It is the proteins that help make electron transfer complexes, energy, hormones, and neurotransmitters. More than 2500 genes code for 10 billion proteins made after decoding the genes at a rate of 80 base pairs a second. Much of our life is all about manufacturing proteins and peptides. Good health depends on manufacturing these on time without loss of quality and quantity, a process whose management is molecularly orchestrated both by genome and epigenome. Epigenome directs gene expression and both, the genome and epigenome, are rendered stable and functional by methylation diet whose nutrients function as epigenetic switches.

Health of a given tissue may depend on 37 genes and every tissue in our body is different in this regard. What defines a tissue's function is the mix of proteins in its cells. All 10 billion proteins are tweaked and modified a bit after their manufacturing by 10 million strong army of nano-scale ribosomes, themselves an assembly of some 30 proteins. The assembly line of ribosome proteins may take up to 3 hours to make a large protein even though they can line up 200 amino acids per minute. Mitochondria do it all for us. Therefore, the maintenance of mitochondrial health by methylation diet is critical. I strongly suggest that, for full enjoyment, the readers should go through chapter 5 first. They will find that repetition of the concept of Methylation Diet concept by concept in all chapters is necessary for emphasis due to the concept.

Chapter 1
Introduction

Thirty seven genes of 5 billion mitochondria in our cells are closely tied to our daily health.

Triveni P. Shukla

This universe is made of matter and energy. Matter is comprized of electrons and protons present as atoms and molecules. Atoms and molecules can exist in living systems as ions also. The hydrogen ion (H^+) is prevalent in all living systems. Electrons, protons, atoms, and molecules are governed by the forces of both electromagnetism and gravitation. **In particular, electromagnetism is our life support**. We live by electrons, protons (Hydrogen$^+$ ion), and ionic forms of atoms and molecules. Cells are building blocks of life but atoms are the basic building blocks of all living and non-living matter. Cells routinely deal with large molecules of DNA (deoxyribonucleic acid), RNA (ribonucleic acid), and many kinds of proteins including enzymes, receptors, and neurotransmitters. Life is possible only with nucleotide polymers like DNA and RNA, energy molecule adenosine triphosphate or ATP which is a protein complex with nucleotide sites of enzyme activity, and proteins as polymers of amino acids. Atoms make molecules or constituent groups of molecules when they bond. The bond of phosphorus and oxygen, the phosphate group, is very special in biology of foods. This bond is present as a *diester bond* in DNA, nucleoside diphosphate in adenosine diphosphate, adenosine triphosphate in ATP, and diphosphate bond in nicitinamide adinine dinucleotide present in life molecules of NAD$^+$ and NADH that help shuttle food electrons for making life energy. The phosphate bond of DNA is central to life as we know it. ATP is life energy and enzyme ATP synthase is truly the molecule of life. Chemistry of life is chemistry of these molecules and electrons and protons in and around them.

Methylation Diet is The Electromagnetic Fuel of Life

Biochemistry of life centers around biochemistry of mitochondria including those of water, hydrogen bonds in DNA and proteins, DHA (docahexanoic acid), electrons, protons, and spins of electrons and free radicals. Biochemistry of transition metals, what we call trace minerals, is very critical to functioning of enzyme protein complexes of the electron transport chain of the inner membrane of mitochondria. The robustness of biochemical events in mitochondria depends on the quality and quantity of our daily food which is the basic source of electron, proton, free radicals, and ions. All health and wellness involves control, communication, balance, and homeostasis. We know that much of human biology is about electron and free radical transfer and about shape and size of molecules through and on which electrons and free radicals move randomly and rather chaotically. The movements depend on creating and organizing redox potential controlled by electromagnetic processes in and around our cells. Such, it appears, has been the grand evolutionary scheme which includes minimagnets and magnetization, paramagnetism, resonance, spins of electrons, spins of free radicals, and polarization. Our daily foods in optimal quantity and quality must serve the following functions.

I.   Provide for 90% usable energy from the electronic bond energy of reduced molecules of carbohydrate, protein, and fat.
II.   Provide for essential amino acids and fatty acids that human body is incapable of making.
III. Provide for vitamins and minerals for effective metabolism.
IV.   Provide for precursors for hormones and neuro transmitters.
V.   Provide for a large battery of antioxidants for quenching excess free radicals.
VI.   Provide for trace transition metals.
VII. Provide for antimicrobial, antiinflammatory, and anticarcinogenic functions for good health and well being.

VIII. Provide for beneficial bacteria for building gut microbiome for health and immunity.

Nature, Human Life, and Magnetic Mitochondria

The evolution has had to be in tune with planet earth, moon, and sun. It appears that gravitation, magnetism, electricity and electrons, protons, free radicals, and ions have played there part in making who we are. This is readily evident from the apparent effects of solar and lunar cycles on the life of all living organisms of planet earth. Just think of human chronobiology and circadian rhythm in terms of puberty, and up and downs of homones in time and their variations among us. Also just think of the lone electrons on free radicals that help our cells signal, communicate, and even fight bacteria and viruses. *These paramagnetic free radicals as oxygen species of O_2^-, H_2O_2, OH, ROOH, RO, ROO, and ONOO⁻ have foot prints in cells of our body and they can be aligned in a magnetic field. Mitochondria, by way of being a magnet, use their space orientation very skillfully.* This happens in water, the dipolar and dielectric molecule within our cells by which we have evolved and by which we live. We can isolate mitochondria magnetically [1]. Molecules in mitochondria can create magnetization transfer [2], [3],[4]. Magnetism comes about when electrons dance and swirl on and around life supporting biopolymers of proteins and polynucleotites like RNA and DNA. Our life, it appears, is governed by spins of electrons, spins of free radicals, magnetism, and polarization. *Hormone sensing pineal gland, the soul of our brain, is influenced by the earth's magnetic field*[5]. We now know that a few picotelsa of magnetic field cures migraine headache [6]. No wonder why mitochondria always stay in touch with nuclear DNA and other organelles within the cell.

Oxygen helps oxidize glucose for energy and its transduction, killing of cells and killing of mitochondria, and participates in signaling activities. Its reactive species called free radicals are necessary for immune performance, calcium signaling, and metabolism. But too many of them force us to age

---

1   http://www.miltenyibiotec.com/~/media/Files/Navigation/Molecular/Mitochondria_isolation_bro-chure.ashx
2   http://cds.ismrm.org/ismrm-1999/PDF5/1309.pdf
3   http://www.ncbi.nlm.nih.gov/pubmed/22389629
4   http://diabetes.diabetesjournals.org/content/61/11/2669.full
5   http://www.psi-researchcentre.co.uk/article_10.htm
6   http://www.ncbi.nlm.nih.gov/pubmed/1305631

faster. Unlike ions, free radicals can be positive, negative, or even neutral. Antioxidants in our daily foods are necessary nutrients that quench or subdue free radicals.

Planet earth, with its central core of molten iron flowing like a river and thus creating magnetic field, has effects on ATP production in our cell's mtochondria[7] . Most likely the living systems evolved by an elaborate organic molecular construct guided by natural electric and magnetic fields. We know that electrons have varying speeds depending on where they are and that they create magnetic field by spinning up and down in our mitochondria. *It is important to know that they move along at a rate that depends on the rate at which we consume energy.* Also, we know for sure that they are affected by the solar and lunar rhythms and by our 24 hour circadian cycle. Any effect on electrons affects our physiology and metabolism. This is true because we can isolate mitochondria in the laboratory by magnetic means and watch its electrical components: a voltage of 0.25 mVolt and a current in a range of milliamperes per square centimeter.

The Electrical Power from Daily Food

We are a 2,377 watts per day or 99.04 watts per hour machine. Most relevant is the energy in the orbitals of electrons that join bonds in the food molecules. Bonds of food molecules are broken, molecules are rearranged and interconverted in glycolysis and Krebs cycle, electrons are removed and carried by special redox carriers like NADH to the electron transport chain, electrons travel on the redox ladder of protein complexes, and protons are moved out and then in for making energy molecule ATP. Such is the function of the veritable miochondria in our cells. Myriads of reaction take place and we live by Gibbs free energy from a kind of infinite battery. Myriads of molecules are transformed and made for our daily living.

Assume that we consume 60 gram fat (546 kilocalories), 70 gram protein (260 Kilocalories), and 332 gram glucose from carbohydrate (1240 Kilocalories) present in a 2000 kilocalorie per day diet. All in terms of concentration of glucose equals [70 g protein + 135 g (fat equivalent) +332 g carbohydrate]/180.16, the molecular weight of glucose = 2.98 moles of glucose that yields 2,044 Kilocalories upon oxidation, *2,046 Kilocalories to be exact. This equals 2046 X 3.9656 = 8,113.67 BTU. Close to seventy*

---

7   http://www.pnas.org/content/109/5/1357.full

percent of this energy is used to keep us alive by functions of heart, lung, brain, and other vital organs. Converting this to watts we find that an average human being has a power of no more than a 2,377 watts per day or 99.04 watts per hour.

Nutrients in Foods We Eat Talk to Our Cells by Resonance

Wherever and whenever possible we depend on *resonance* because in essence we are vibrational beings. **Energy itself comes from vibration and our senses of perception work by vibration.** We are made of atoms and molecules with their covalent bonds held by electrons that cause them to vibrate all the time, **We are a vibrating being. Like a blade of grass our DNA resonates at 528 Hz** [8]. Our muscle vibrates in a range of 10-80 Hz during during activities of twitching fingers and using our arm to lift things. A developing fruit acts like a electromagnetic dielectric resonator [9]. Nutrients we eat have their characteristic resonance and so do each of our cells [10]. **In a way cells and nutrients talk by resonance** [11]. Imagine a singer's voice which when in resonance with vibrations in a wine glass, can literally shatter it and a bunch of soldiers walking in synchrony over a bridge can destroy it. A good example is 1940 Tacoma Narrows **Bridge collapse** in Washington, USA. **The power of resonance in our body is unlimited and we understand it only poorly.** The activity of an enzyme protein regulating a gene can be enhanced by change in its shape by ultrasound. Enzyme activity can be destroyed also by destroying the protein complexes in cancer cells by resonance.

Mitochondria deals with charge transport associated with immortal electrons that can neither be created nor destroyed. Mitochondrial electron transport system reduces oxygen to water during the process of energy transformation. Although miniscule in mass (1.783×10^{-35}Kg) and charge of (1.602×10^{-19}J), most everything happens in our body by 2.4×10^{27} electrons associated with various atoms and big and small molecules. They are integral to the scheme of resonance.

Our current environment meets us at the surfaces of our cells that *work by collecting magnetic resonance and induction.* The cell surface can absorb mechanical vibration which is coupled with piezoelectric transducers for

8   http://altered-states.net/barry/update205/
9   http://www.ncbi.nlm.nih.gov/pubmed/22326259
10   http://www.pemf.com/en/resonance.html
11   http://blogs.mcgill.ca/oss/2013/05/11/nutrients-with-the-right-%E2%80%9Cresonance-frequen-cy%E2%80%9D/

converting mechanical energy to DC current. *We should remind ourselves of mitochondrial works underlying message therapy.* Nature's old molecule, Omega-3 fatty acid, can rearrange our muscles and their metabolic state.

Genes, Proteins, Electrons, and Intermittant Eating

We eat foods containing electrons intermittently and there is a need for hormones insulin and glucagon to regulate glucose, the major source of electrons. *Insulin gene that helps glucose enter our cells is on chromosome 11 and glucagon gene that helps store glucose in liver is on chromosome 2. Also hunger hormone ghrelin has its gene on chromosome 6 and appetite control hormone leptin has its gene on chromosome 7. Beyond dealing with glucose, there is a critical need of controlling 60% of water in our body. This is done by a only 9 amino acid long arginine vasopressin. Vassopressin gene is on chromosome 20.* Why are these genes scattered all over the genome? Why do ghrelin and leptin work by same receptotrs? Why does every fat cell secrete its own leptin? Whatever the reasons for this apparent disparity, all these hormones, receptors, and transmitters control homeostasis by controlling mitochondrial function.

Electrons in our foods or elsewhere in our body belong to the quantum world. It is a bit clearer today that life organizes itself at the edge of quantum world simply in order to remain metastable amidst excited electrons and to keep electron and proton entangled in our cells as a whole.

> **Let entanglement be defined as closely tied and localized electrons such that the state of one is similar to the state of the other.** *We must sleep and we must take rest if we want to prolong this state of entangled electrons.*

Electrons and protons move in our body. Our cells have liquid crystalline semiconductors for this purpose and movements happen best in water, in hydrogen bonds of water, DNA, and proteins. The process is metastable (longed lived excited state stable except for minor disturbances) by design for the entanglement of electrons and protons. **It appears that sunlight, earth's movement, solar and lunar rhythms, and electron transport chain in mitochondria with its hydrogen ions or protons and magnetism are somehow connected.** Electrons as inputs to mitochondria, the organelle that produces energy and signals, monitors events, and communicates through out the body are part of the grand scheme of connection. Cold and heat matter. Semi conductive currents work faster in cooler environments. Cold increases dielectric constant of water so it can condense and support changes in our daily biology.

Living beings evolved via genetic engineering of water. DNA came some 3.5 billion years ago and a few very old molecules like DHA (docosahexanoic omega-3 fatty acid) came a little later. Light and Omega-3 DHA make infrared light right in the mitochondria. Let us make note of some more common features.

- Ultimate digestion or conversion of electrons of food into energy involves reduction of oxygen to water for purposeful disposal of spent electrons.

- Light decreases magnetic strength of mitochondria, infra-red photons in our cells uncondense matter and release energy (Einstein's photoelectric effect). Light, a signaling metric, pretty much destroys melatonin at sunrise. Certain frequencies in IR and UV zone have specific effects. For example infra-red in particular changes the hydrogen bonds in water of our cells.

- Proteins know how to respond to light signals. Actually, we now have the evolving discipline of optogenetics[12]. Just think of the photon handling power of our retina! For every photon that impinges on it, the mitochondria have to manage 10,000 ions. Electrons create bimolecular oxygen in mitochondria and oxygen creates changes in its electric and magnetic field.

- We evolved in water and we still live in water. A good night sleep and 24 hour circadian rhythm are also part of our evolution. It affects electron and proton tunneling and entanglement or their controlled moving around within a molecule or from molecule to molecule. Just imagine that SCN (suprachiasmatic nucleus) has 20,000 nerve cells controlling night hormone and a powerful antioxidant melatonin. We must sleep to entangle electrons and protons. We are in a coherent quantum state when we sleep so our brain can recycle. Electron transport chain

---

12   http://optogenetics.weebly.com/what-is-it.html

is uncoupled and less ATP produced. Fe-S redox clusters of enzyme complexes of electron transport chain produce monochromatic IR at the expense of free fatty acids. IR light as heat condenses water making it possible for iron-sulfur clusters to shoot free radicals into water.

A good sleep equates to good mitochondrial function. Actually, obesity in human biology is a story of circadian signaling for effective use of electrons gone wrong.

- Magnetic field of mitochondria shrinks when electrons flow and dance on their axes over electron transport chain complexes. Groups like FAD (flavine adenine dinucleotide, a redox cofactor) know all about this spin necessary for magnetism. FAD needs higher power photon in order to produce superoxide when electrons slow down[13]. Cells detect signals via the water molecules, an ionic plasma like non-homogeneous fluid capable of imprinting energy and information.

- We are learning now that just like skin, cell membranes are connected to mitochondria by proteins actin and integrin [14]. They act like wireless charging systems fed by magnetic field and photons of the sun. Lipid bilayers in membranes and the proteins sandwiched between them are loaded with DHA on purpose. They are connected to cytoskeleton and always stay in communication with mitochondria and nuclear DNA. It is now more clear than before that magnetism connected to electrons matters in human biology and mitochondria act as magnets.

- Sandwiched proteins in our cell membranes have the 5th dimension of electrochemical profile and the sixth dimension of time [15]. Both are important in maintaining our health because the quantum processes function by electrochemistry of these proteins.

- Food and hormones are proxies to subtraction or addition of electrons in our cell systems. The proteins, **the best and most vital condensed matter in our body,** work under a bit unfolded configuration by works of electrons and at the expense of ATP.

13   http://jasn.asnjournals.org/content/20/6/1293.full
14   http://www.ncbi.nlm.nih.gov/books/NBK26867/
15   http://people.umass.edu/bioch623/623/Second.Section/11.%20vonheijne.pdf

Mitochondria, Free Radicals, and Electrons

We hear from the media and learn from published works that free radicals are all bad. Not really. There shall be no signals in our body and no metastability if there is no superoxide free radical production. **Our cells wouldn't be able to read the environment within or around them.** There shall be no DHA effects and no hydrogen bond chaos created on purpose. A few well known examples: 1. D shell electron of transition metal molybdenum balances quantized motion of Iron-Sulfur clusters in cytochromes of mitochondrial electron transport chain. 2. Xanthine oxidase makes a lot of superoxide because of *molybdenum's resonant coupling*. 3. Chromium helps glucose metabolism in case of diabetics. *Mitochondria use paramagnetic DHA, oxygen, and free radicals and they have the ability to sense frequencies wider than we hear and see* [16], [17]. *This is the only way they can monitor 10,000 reactions per second .* The triple helix of collagen, highest amount of protein in our body, helps us do much of sensing in cooperation with molecules of water.

Foods donate electrons. Electronic energy translocates protons across the inner membrane of mitochondria. ATP molecule is produced by mitochondria moving 10^3 proton per second through a miraculous protein called ATP synthase, a protein enzyme that acts like both a motor and generator. **Let us remember that pH relates to protons and temperature, magnetic fields, and protons move by tunneling when simple diffusion can't move enough of them. Our cells know how to manage electron flow.** Cells lose electrons in catabolism or breaking down of molecules and they transfer electrons during the night when we are asleep. Melatonin released in the night increases electron flow by uncoupling electron transport chain and loosing energy as heat of infra-red radiation.

Food, Energy, Vital Proteins, and Our Existence

Living is much more than simply eating. What matters for good health is synergy among water, light, sunlight, sleep, and the hormonal proxies. This synergy makes our mitochondria tick. All life is driven by energy, enegy from electrons that mitochondria know how to manage and use.

---

16   http://www.ncbi.nlm.nih.gov/pmc/articles/PMC2692514/
17   http://journals.cambridge.org/action/displayAbstract?fromPage=online&aid=7972220

How does food become energy in the mitochondria of our cells is the central theme of this introductory chapter. We eat foods to digest them in our gastro-intestinal system which transfers nutrients to our blood which carries them to our cells. All major nutrients of carbohydrate, protein, and fat can and do donate electrons for energy production. Real digestion is not yet complete though. The story of energy from foods further involves (1) carbohydrate breakdown to glucose that can enter blood and then to management for a constant supply of glucose by joint actions of insulin and glucagon for its storage and mobilization, (2) controlled breakdown of fats to fatty acids and glycerol and then diffusion of fatty acids to the cells where β-oxidation makes acetyl CoA that can enter Krebs cycle, and (3) controlled breakdown of proteins to small peptides and amino acids that can be actively transported to our cells by membrane proteins under electrochemical gradient of sodium. Using glucose from carbohydrates, fatty acids from fat, and amino acids from ptoteins, the ultimate ATP energy is produced via electron transport chain in mitochondria in three steps.

- First high energy electrons are carried away from carbon-hydrogen bonds of food molecules by a combination of processes involving electron carrier molecules.

- Second the electron on the backs of carrier molecules are transferred to and through a chain of enzyme complexes and non-enzyme Coenzyme Q_{10}.

- The most important third step involves use of part of the energy of electrons to move hydrogen ions and simultaneously use them to make chemical energy as ATP, our power to live, move, think, and stay conscious.

Mitochondria make usable energy molecule ATP from food molecules of glucose, fat, and protein. Sometimes molecules of amino acids stripped of nitrogenous amide groups are just as good energy producers as glucose. An average highly reduced triglyceride or fat molecule loaded with carbon-hydrogen bonds is most energy intensive. It can yield up to 500 ATP molecules.

Six moles of carbon dioxide become one mole of glucose with the help of 48 moles of photons during photosynthesis. Every mole of glucose has

686 Kcal. Only about 60% of it is routinely stored as ATP. **One ATP molecules is produced at the expense of three to four protons.** All 36 ATP molecules produced per glucose molecule consume 108-144 protons. The energy of electrons translocates protons in steps and creates a proton gradient for producing ATP. Hydrogen ions (H^+) are important protons in our cells; they carry and releases energy for making ATP. Actually, the so called electron carriers often carry both electrons and protons as an atom of hydrogen. The power, we will read later, resides with electron donor-acceptor pair NADH: NAD^+.

Genes encode proteins that run the life of our cells. There are thousands of protein encoding events per second taking place in our cells but only a fraction are expressed as proteins at a given time.

What is decoded off DNA, expressed, and translated as protein is very well regulated for our cell's function in a given environment. The control comes via constant and continuous communication between mitochondrial and nuclear DNA and the wonder of nano-scale biology lies in this control.

Electrons relate to magnetic field and protons to magnetic resonance. Electrons resonate with higher frequency at fixed magnetic field. MRI diagnostics in our hospitals today works by the power of resonance. We may soon be able to learn more about our daily physiology by use of Nano-thermal IR cameras. We have magnetic resonance finger printing and magnetic contrast reagent for diagnosing the vascularity of central nervous system. **Soon we may have a device that measures the memory of water in our body by measuring empidence by a Monitor).** This may help us gain understanding of the electrochemical mystery behind other molecules that come in contact with water.

Our cells are timed. The biological clock is the driver of our 24 hour circadian cycle, a response to light and darkness via a gene regulated system of interacting molecules in our body and brain. The process is affected by light. Melatonin is released by pineal gland when the thermostat in hypothalamus is reset when we sleep on a cold night. Therefore, we must control circadian biology for good health by letting mitochondria manage electron flow; we should mind our circadian rhythm and use appropriate day light time. Morning light decreases magnetic sense. Water stretches our neurons when we get up in the morning. Proteins get unfolded for specific purposes. This is when environment and epigenetics exert more effect. Behind it all are mitochondria as an engine fueled by our daily food.

Our Cells

Each cell in our body has its own mitochondrion and it is an independent unit in doing its energy conversion by managing the quantum dance of electrons and protons. I personally learned about mitochondria during my Ph.D. Degree curricula at the University of Illinois, Urbana-Champaign, IL but its science was only in its infancy then. Today the biophysical story of this electromagnetic nano-apparatus is much more complete.

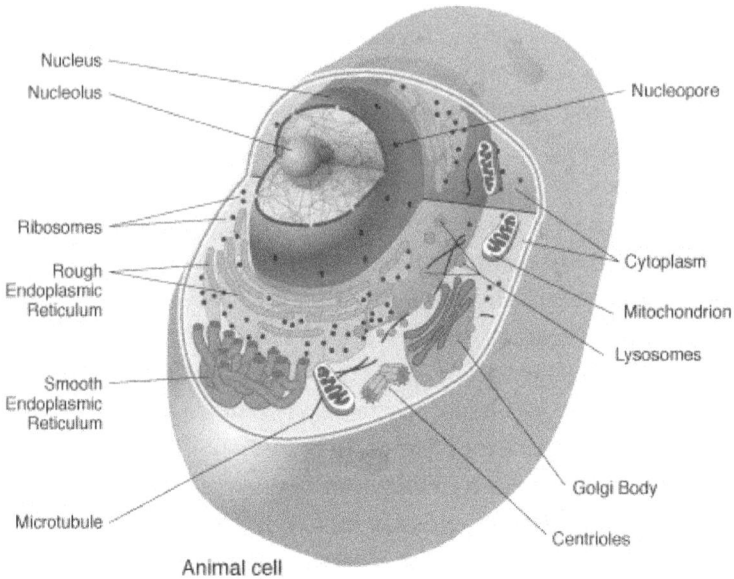

Figure 1.01 An Animal cell.
Source: National Institute of Health.

Let's begin with the picture of a typical cell in Fig. 1.01. Mitochondria take less than 20% of cell's volume which may vary depending on demand for energy production. The epigenome of the cell, combination and variety of gene expression, goes beyond its nuclear DNA because daily nutrients that we consume interact with the epigenome of individual cells, all 200 types of them; nutrients confer upon them the selective power of gene expression. Each type can modify its DNA and DNA package to facilitate type and timing of special genes for specific functions. Gene expression has to do with mRNA (messenger RNA) and signaling directed to making of proteins including gene regulating proteins called ***transcription factors***. Table 1.01 has a detailed list of various structure in our cells and their relationship and dependence on mitochondria.

Imagine that we have magnified an average size of 30 micron cell by a factor of 20 million. Now the nucleus in it will be 33 feet in diameter, mitochondria will be 12 -18 feet, and the lysosome will be around 18 feet. The 18 feet mitochondria will be packed with 500 enzymes in their matrices surrounded by 75 feet inner membrane with cristae. Some twelve criastae, 4 feet a piece, may have at least one but often more electron transport chains for power production. So mighty mitochondria are a very busy and crowded place (Fig. 1.02 and 1.03). They dominate other organelles by their critical life supporting functions of energy production, control, signaling, and a cell's external communication in which it lives in. Whereas electrons flow through the enzyme complexes for ATP production in the inner membrane of mitochondria, DNA and the electron mill called Krebs cycle, are situated in the matrix. It is the Krebs cycle that loads electron on to NAD^+ and helps reduce it to NADH.

Mitochondria (Fig. 1.02, Fig. 1.03a, and 1.03b) are membrane bound organelle with a circular double stranded DNA of a single chromosome with 37 genes. They are present in the matrix. These genes, all 10,000 copies in up to 500 mitochondria per cell, are very prone to free radical damage and mutation because of being close to electron transport chain where free radicals are produced.

Table 1.01 Functions of major human cell components	
Components	**Function**
Cell Wall	Securitized boundary of the cell.
Cell Membrane	Control movement ions and molecules disallowing intruders; strict border control
Nucleus	Central command center that holds DNA, the code of life
Nucleolus	Assembly line of construction workers
Mitochondria	Power house and center of ultimate digestion for energy.
Golgi Apparatus	Packaging and transporting of proteins and other products.
Rough Endoplasmic Reticulum	Hallway and the passage around work place
Smooth Endoplasmic Reticulum	Protein traffic and detoxification.
Ribosomes	The protein factory that can make 70 of them.
Lysosome	Disposal center for the old, dead, and useless.
Centriole	Organelle near the nucleus that makes spindle fibers.
Vacuoles	Food bank and the warehouse
Vesicles	A fluid filled pouch

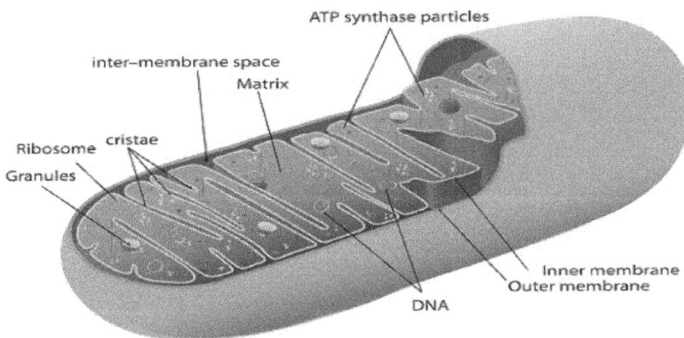

Figure 1.02 The Morphology and Structure of Mitochondria

Source: National Institute of Health.

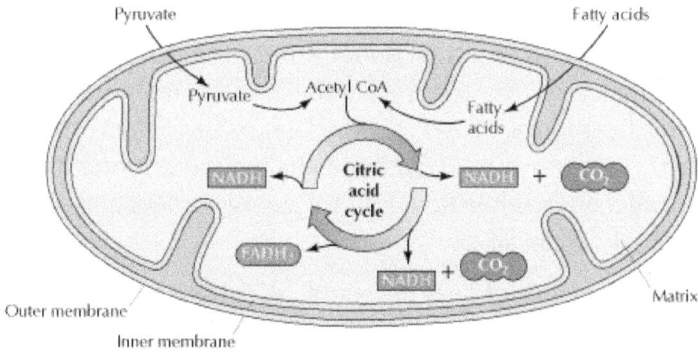

Fig. 1.03a The details of Mitochondrial inner membrane's cristae.

Source: National Institute of Health

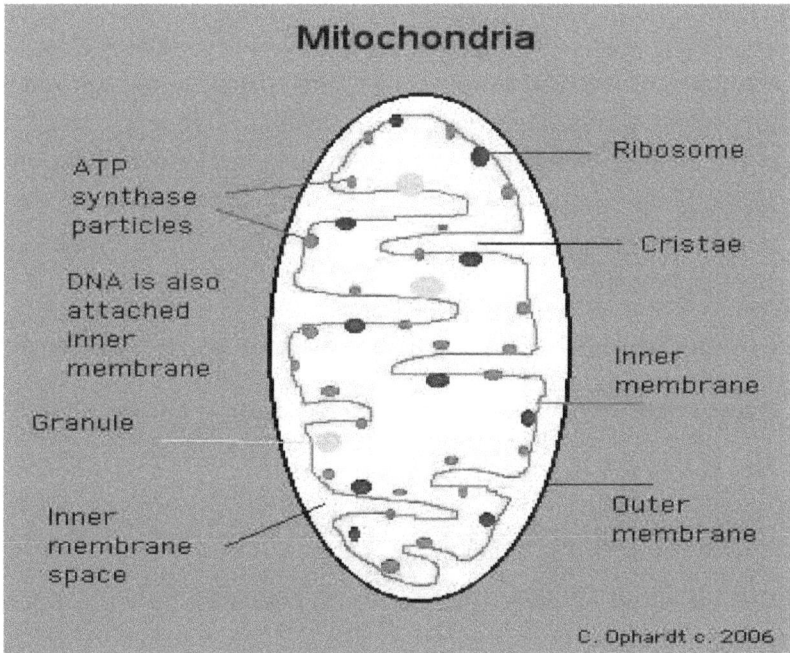

Fig. 1.03b The expanded details of mitochondrial inner membrane

Source: http://www.elmhurst.edu/~chm/vchembook/images/591mitochondria.jpg

Seven and a half trillion cells with 500 mitochondria each with 10,000 copies may on an average have a total of 37.5 thousand trillion of circular mitochondrial DNA. So mitochondria have much larger crowd of DNA molecues than the nuclear DNA . These genes are semi-autonomous and critical to cell's life. Five major Nobel Prizes have been awarded in the areas of Krebs cycle, respiratory enzymes, inner membrane structure, chemoosmotic theory of ATP production with respiratory coupling, coenzyme Q_{10}, and enzyme ATP synthase, the molecular motor that extrudes protons. Mitochondrial functions beyond energy production nclude many others. Let us list them all.

- Production of 90% of daily life energy, ATP. Mitochondria can increase their number for extra energy production on demand.

- Cellular metabolism and routine cross-talking with the cellular enzymes systems and acting as detox center. Actually, they manage more than 500 proteins at a given instant.

- Creation of vesicles for communication and control. Taming of vesicles, assembly of fat and fat like molecules, that change their shape and size, total surface area, movement, recombination frequency, transitions in the inner membrane, and space of operation for effective transfer of molecular cargo to lysosomes. Self-degradation and suicide via vesicle processing in brain where neurons talk to their synapses using electrical signals.

- Control of cell cycle (death, birth, and growth), longevity, and health.

- Quality control of cellular processes in general.

- Cellular differentiation.

- Balance of electron leakage.

- Cell signaling by free radicals. Form networks for long distance transmission. Act as a transmission grid and communications network.

- Cell cycle control, growth, division, and control of environment

- Storage of calcium and manage clotting

- Regulation of membrane potential.

- Control of metabolism and heme and steroid synthesis.

- Maintenance of ion gradient and ion channel regulation.

- Oxygen sensing and neurotransmission

- Insulin and other hormone secretion.

Mitochondria move and manage direction of their movement while doing all the above. Nutrition and food science research interest today is targeted to prolonging age without neurological disorders by preventing injury to mitochondria [18], [19], [20],[21],[22],[23]. The focus in this book is on energy production, vital organs, vital signs, mitochondrial diseases, and aging and longevity. All depends on well designed and methylation foods for ensuring health and well being.

Electron Processing by Immortal Mitochondria

Electrons from foods are processed by Krebs cycle and the electron transport chain which is is embedded in inner mitochondrial membrane. Enzyme proteins of electron transport chain in the cristae of inner membrane of mitochondria unfold, hydrate, and change their geometry and topology. Energy molecule ATP is produced by proton transfer through enzyme ATP synthase. Electron leakage off the chain is purposefully designed for (1) mitochondrial biogenesis and death and rebirth our cells and (2) cellular communication, signaling, and control. All this takes place inside the immortal mitochondria with strict quality control that can go wrong when we do not eat well, do not sleep well, and do not willfully manage oxygen intake and our body's motion by exercise. Foods we eat matter to our health which depends on the health of mitochondria in cells of not only our vital organs but cells elsewhere in the body. Let us think of our cells as glucose factories. Electrons from around 0.14% glucose in our blood are extracted continuously on demand on the backs of NADH and $FADH_2$ and transported through a chain of multiunit enzyme proteins containing FMN

18   http://www.ncbi.nlm.nih.gov/pubmed/22399429
19   http://www.jci.org/articles/view/64125
20   http://hms.harvard.edu/news/genetics/new-reversible-cause-aging-12-19-13
21   http://www.lef.org/magazine/mag2013/aug2013_Three-Step-Strategy-to-Reverse-Mitochondri-al-Aging_01.htm
22   http://www.ellisonfoundation.org/research/mitochondrial-damage
23   http://www.hindawi.com/journals/jar/2012/194821/

(Flavin Mononucleotide) centers. NADH binds to FMN and oxidises to NAD$^+$ which recycles continuously. We call this assembly line of enzymes Electron transport Chain.

Electron Transport Chain.

Let us take glucose as source of energy for discussion in this section. Two ATP are produced from glucose during anaerobic glycolysis in the cytoplasm that breaks glucose to 2 pyruvic acid molecules, 2 ATP during conversion of pyruvate to acetyl-coA, and 32 during acetyl CoA processing through Krebs cycle.

On an average a molecule of glucose or protein produces 32 ATP and that of a fat molecule may produce 150 ATP molecules. This book uses a value of 36 ATP per glucose molecule. There are 9.1 kilocalories per per gram of fat compared to only 4 from glucose and protein. The average fat molecule produces only 72 ATP molecules. NAD$^+$ is a two electron carrier. It receives two electrons and delivers two electrons.

Ten protons are produced by a pair of electrons and 3-4 protons are required to produce 1 ATP molecule. Each NADH carrier is responsible for 3 ATP and each FAD carrier for 2 ATP meaning each electron pair can produce 3 ATP molecules. At the end four electrons are required to reduce oxygen to water.

Lower energy spent electrons have got to be removed. That is where supply of oxygen becomes necessary. Diatomic xygen is activated, the bond broken, and two electrons and to protons are added to make H_2O. Electrons come from water by splitting hydrogen during photosynthesis and electrons go back to water when oxygen is reduced by spent electrons at the end of the electron transport chain.

The energy from electrons in 10 NADH and 2 FADH$_2$, excluding glycolysis and counting Kreb cycle alone (34 ATP) can be up to 130 watts. minute/kg body weight. A 90 Kg cyclist may produce 350 Watts.minutes/Kg body weight.

At a given time mitochondria produce about 200 mv energy. This is what makes us tick and our cells alive and conscious. The tiny 200 mv of energy across a few nanometer wide inner mitochondrial membrane translated to per meter basis is millions of volts like a thunderbolt in the sky. *Life is about the use of this thunderbolt of energy but in innumerable nanoscale steps.* As a whole we are no more than a 100 watts per hour light bulb.

Quantum Biology and Mitochondria

We are made of atoms, molecules, and electron and proton particles that are part of them. Electromagnetic actions in our our body have got to be Quantum mechanical in the order of the Planck's constant, 6.626 X 10^{-34} Joules/second, which is the ratio between the energy in a quantum of radiation and its frequency. It now appears that quantum phenomena are involved in biology of DNA replication, decoding of DNA via transcription, recombination, gene expression, differentiation, and development [24].

Our daily nutrients talk to cell surface and and they can either inhibit or sometimes activate transcription and gene expression[25], [26]. Heavily damaged DNA can be healed by enzymes that methylate our DNA. Cancer is now known to be largely epigenomic due to aberrant DNA methylation [27]. A photon can travel Planck's length of 1.6 X 10^{-35} meters in Planck's time of 10^{-43}seconds. May be photon travel in our brain cells relates to consciousness?

Functioning of our mind, our olfactory receptors, our cell's electron transport chain, and of enzyme reactions in general is understood a bit more today than even 10 years ago. Nanoscale biology and nano-scale quantum physics meet right in the mitochondria in our cells [28]. Modern research suggests that mitochondria exhibit quantum effects of electron tunneling in complex I [29], hydrogen bonded DNA exhibits proton tunneling[30], and it is very likely that our brain works by quantum bits [31]. The mighty mitochondria, visible even under light microscope, faithfully follow nature's dictate of energy conservation in line with the laws of Thermodynamics. Many nano-scale processes are bound to mitochondrial membrane. For most of us, including this author, the quantum conundrum is rather abstract, esoteric, and spooky. We will not dwell any deeper about it but we must respect it for its universality and implications in our daily physiology.

Mitochondria function as quantum bodies by maintaing an electromagnetic field. Whatever the mechanism, we do need to understand the morphology and energy producing power of mitochondria, their ability to control and regulate themselves and the cells they live in, and their

24   https://www.newscientist.com/article/mg22429950-700-are-we-ready-for-quantum-biology/
25   http://www.ncbi.nlm.nih.gov/pubmed/26122708
26   http://www.ncbi.nlm.nih.gov/pmc/articles/PMC359396/
27   http://www.ncbi.nlm.nih.gov/pubmed/15822191
28   http://www.ncbi.nlm.nih.gov/pmc/articles/PMC2839811/
29   http://www.sciencedirect.com/science/article/pii/S0005272806001083
30   http://journals.aps.org/rmp/abstract/10.1103/RevModPhys.35.724
31   http://www.quantumconsciousness.org/overview.html

central role in giving us a long and disease free life. We now know that their functions deal with stress, aging, and our very survival but only when aided by a good methylation diet[32].

The topic of mitochondria is multidisciplinary and as such it requires an understanding of physics, biochemistry, and physiology deep at the level of ions, electrons, protons, atoms, and molecules. The demonstrable fact amidst it all is that we live by the power of special enzyme protein complexes for transfer of high energy electrons at less than 14 Angstrom distance. Slow electrons, however, may span more than 14 Angstrom. The dynamic morphology of inner membrane and its cristae is regulated by different energy states[33] (Figures 1.01, 1.02, and 1.03) precisely for this purpose. The life of mitochondria is electronic and it depends on light, electromagnetic field, electrons, and protons. Our life is tied to mitochondrial transfer of electrons from foods we eat and the protons that the electron transport chain translocates out of inner membrane to intermediate space and then back into the matrix.

The cells of a 10 days old fetus, a new born baby, you, and I all function by gycolysis, Krebs cycle, and the electron transfer chain. This chapter includes references for additional reading on basic human anatomy, biochemistry, molecular biology, physiology, and applied physics for readers who want to expand their knowledge about the immortal mitochondria within our cells.

Electron Processing Power of Mitochondria

The biological power no doubt is based on electrons, protons, free radicals, and ions. **As a matter of fact, mitochondria act like a battery for "life energy".** This bio-battery sandwiched between two electrodes, say the scientists at the St. Louis University, can create up to a few milliamp current for tomorrow's consumer electronics [34]. We need to understand the implications of this mitochondrial current that flows in our bodies and brains. **It may soon power our pacemakers, nanobots, cell phones, and tablet computers.** We may be able to connect our day to day biology with our environment. Let us learn the potential of this power from the humming bird and the firefly.

---

32   http://www.michmontreal.com/quantum-biology/
33   http://journals.aps.org/pre/abstract/10.1103/PhysRevE.88.062723
34   http://www.rsc.org/chemistryworld/News/2010/August/27081001.asp

The Humming Bird

A humming bird is a powerful energy generating bio-machine. This small 10 centimeter long creature has wing muscles that can flap 80 times per minute and consume twice its weight of 20% sugar solution of nectar, digest it all in less than an hour, and fly 500 miles nonstop at a speed of 34 miles an hour. A high glycemic index diet poses no problem to the humming bird. *Humming bird's heart, assisted by a very high metabolic rate, beats 1,260 times per minute to meet the double demand of oxygen compared to other locomotive animals.* **No wonder why about 35% of her fight muscle volume is mitochondria whose inner membrane has more surface area and volume than other mammals in general**[35]. Humming birds have the highest aerobic metabolic rate of all vertebrates [36]. The bird's mitochondria, with a preference to sugar consumption, produce more ATP/molecule of oxygen in long migratory flights than you and I do in a fast running mode [37]. Such can be the mighty power of mitochondria. This power comes from 7-10 ml oxygen consumption per cm^3 of mitochondria/minute [38] and equates to a power of 100-120 Watts/kg weight at 9-10% mechanochemical efficiency [39].

The Firefly

Another example is light production by mitochondria of fireflies [40], [41]. Luciferin binds to ATP and the combined molecules bind to a 61,000 Daltons enzyme luciferase. When in contact with oxygen, oxyluciferin glows with a wavelength of 510-670 nm. ***Almost 100% energy is emitted as light without any heat loss.*** Firefly needs nitric oxide for light production, the same chemical that is produced by Viagra in humans. Certain fungi and marine animals also have light on their fingertips by the power of their mitochondria. That insect, snail, and slug eating fireflies and beetles have mitochondria that can complete a proton to photon cycle, just like what happens in our brain cells is another wonder in biology. The primordial

---

35   http://www.ncbi.nlm.nih.gov/pmc/articles/PMC51768/
36   http://www.pnas.org/content/87/23/9207.full.pdf
37   http://jeb.biologists.org/content/214/2/172.full.pdf
38   http://link.springer.com/article/10.1007/BF01920240#
39   http://jeb.biologists.org/content/178/1/39.full.pdf
40   https://www.google.com/?gws_rd=ssl#q=scientific+american+fireflies+light+up
41   http://www.piercenet.com/method/luciferase-reporters

process that happens in stars and our sun happens in photosynthesis in plant cells and oxidative phosphorylation in human cells.

The running powers of a cheeta and a tiger, weight bearing capacity of an elephant, shear strength of a bear, and 1 ampere and up to 600 volt electricity producing power of an electric yeal[42] are testimony to the biological miracles of mitochondria with a single circular genome in a sise range of 16,000 to 18,705 base pairs. Same ATP that powers human heart gives an electric eel power to produce rather high voltage electricity through ion channels. What matters is their structural organization for power production in parallel.

1.01 Human Mitochondria

Human mitochondria can be traced to a single woman ancestor living about 150,000 to 200,000 years ago [43]. As things stand today in human biology, mobile and continuously transforming mitochondria are capable of changing their shape and size [44] and dividing or fusing for efficiency and extra functionality. Although observed during late forties, we learned about mitochondrial details only less than 28 years ago in 1988. Mitochondrial genome got fully sequenced by late nineties and we now know that mitochondria decide not only the birth and death of our cells but also gene expressions of nuclear genome by what we call **retrograde signaling**. Their malfunction can cause heart diseases, type 2 diabetes, autism, depression, learning disabilities, and many neurological disorders. The problems get out of control when mutated DNA copies exceed 60% of the total of mutated and unmutated wild types. **The biggest culprit behind many chronic diseases is oxidative stress, a product of mitochondrial malfunction.**

Size matters and we should begin with sizes we are familiar with. Coffee bean is 12 X 8 millimeter, rice grain is 8 X 2.5 millimeter, and sesame seed is 1.5 X 0.75 millimeter. In comparison, a bacteria is 0.0015 millimeter, a virus is 20-100 nanometer, *mitochondria is 1500 to 2000 nanometers*, protein manufacturing ribosome is 25 nanometers, a single protein molecule is around 5-10 nanometer, and DNA is 2 nanometer. In comparison an atom is - 0.2 nm, water- 0.1 nanometer; amino acid- 0.8 nm; and red blood cell is 9 nm. DNA, mitochondria, and ribosome are inside a human cell whose size

---

42   http://www.ncbi.nlm.nih.gov/pubmed/11343127
43   http://www.britannica.com/EBchecked/topic/386130/mitochondrion
44   http://www.ncbi.nlm.nih.gov/books/NBK26894/

varies from 10,000 to 100,000 nanometers. On an average mitochondria are 10% pf the size of the cell, very analogous to size of a bacterium.

Mitochondrial matrix bound by its inner membrane is a very crowded place in terms of number of molecules that control operations of the electron mill known as **Krebs cycle**. Ribosomes, matrix granules, and mitochondrial DNA exist in the matrix also and so do more than 500 enzyme proteins that run Krebs cycle. We should add to the list recyclable intermediates that shuttle energy, oxygen, water, and carbon dioxide (Fig. 1.03 and 1.04).

Mitochondria depicted in Figures 1.02 and 1.03 can be visualized as a wrinkled bag inside another unwrinkled bag. Its 20 nanometer wide outer membrane is made out of phospholipids and proteins in 1:1 ratio with around 3 nanometer pores for moving proteins across. The inner membrane of mitochondria is much more complex. Its cristae can be up to 27 nanometer and their cross-junctions around 18 nanometers [45]. Although freely permeable to water, carbon dioxide and oxygen, it manages large molecules by active transport assisted by enzymes. Mitochondria accommodate life sustaining enzyme protein complexes I through IV and ATP synthase- the Vth complex. The central liquid core of the wrinkled bag, matrix, is loaded with enzymes for Krebs cycle, DNA, tRNA, ribosome, oxygen, water, and carbon dioxide. Electrons from NADH and $FADH_2$ transfer through complexes I through IV only after translocation of protons across the inner membrane to the intermediate space. **Complex IV transfers up to 10^3 protons per second to the intermediate space across the inner membrane.** Protons produce ATP as they attempt to travel back into the matrix from the intermediate space by a molecular motor enzyme called ATP synthase. Electron transfer is same as hydrogen atom (with only one electron) transfer. *By design, electron transfer stops when energy to push protons out to intermediate space exceeds 69.5 KJ/mole.* This rarely happens though because protons are concomitantly fed back into the matrix. Please see protons being pushed out in the intermediate space (Fig. 1.04).

The number of mitochondria is highest in our brain cells followed in descending order by retina in the eyes, liver, heart, tongue, and muscles [46]. Our eyes have 10,000 mitochondria because there are a lot of energy based activities of photoreception, imaging, and neurotransmission [47]. Muscles have close to 5000 mitochondria per cell. On the other hand skin cells, that require least energy, have only a few hundred mitochondria. Sperm cells

---

45   http://www.ruf.rice.edu/~bioslabs/studies/mitochondria/mitotheory.html
46   http://www.ivy-rose.co.uk/Biology/Organelles/Structure-of-Mitochondria.php
47   file:///C:/Users/Owner/Downloads/Funk4162014ARRB9550_1.pdf

have only 16 mitochondria but the human egg cell has 1000 of them. Liver and muscles cells can have up to 10,000 of them also. *Actually, 20% of liver volume is mitochondria.*

Mitochondria provide up to 90% of body's energy from conversion of potential energy of foods we eat to ATP for growth, work, building of blood and bones, moving, and thinking. . *In simple terms mitochondria are nanomagnets that act like a solid state nano-scale spintronic heat pump [48]. Let us imagine them as an organelle that controls its transistor like property by managing the spin of free radicals for signaling and communication. .* Also, they control cell cycle and death. They talk to nuclear genome and can even change gene expression. The number of mitochondria in cells of our vital organs depends on instantaneous energy demand.

The foods we consume produce electrons (as NADH) via glycolysis and Krabs cycle as input to electron transport chain, protons are pushed outside the inner membrane at various complexes, and complex IV reduces oxygen to water. Iron-Sulfur clusters on complex IV play a big role. They have magnetic sense and are source of direct current.

Sunlight began it all. From sunlight came organized molecules and then human body and mind. In a sense we have a water based sun (IR light) within us in the name of mitochondria which uses free radicals for many vital functions. It is the medium where electric and magnetic fields make energy. Mitochondria are in constant communication with multimembrane endoplasmic reticula that communicate in turn with the nucleus and the cell membrane[49]. List of their Overall functions includes

- Mitochondria as semiautonomous organelle within our cells are the powerhouse of energy production as ATP.

- Mitochondria use magnetic memory to generate **entangled** free radicals as particles, the source of information and energy.

- Free radicals as reactive oxygen and nitrogen species are yoked and coupled for body wide communication [50]. Proteins and water together power quantum information and energy. Mitochondria are the centers of cellular communication.

---

48   http://themedicalbiochemistrypage.org/oxidative-phosphorylation.php
49   http://www.ncbi.nlm.nih.gov/pubmed/22435828
50   http://www.sciencedirect.com/science/article/pii/S0005272810000435

- Magnetic sense is built into mitochondria, a sensor that can hold electrons, protons, and photons.

- Infra-red light and DHA (docosahexanoic acid) make DC current which is a key signal in the brain mitochondria[51]. This light changes H-bonding and associated electron, proton, and waves.

- Protons serve as energy source. Mitochondria simply release kinetic energy and produce wave like protons that can tunnel and produce IR light [52].

- As an electromagnet with significant current, mitochondria have means to control flow of information. *We know that hydrogen ion have a half life of 10^{36} years [53].* Thus the electromagnetic mitochondria never die, they have been passing themselves with some selectivity from mother to another mothers throughout most of human evolution as a multicellular organism.

- Mitochondria produce factors for decoding DNA and expressing genes for functional proteins, regulate and maintain quality control, control birth and death of the cell and of their own, control DNA, RNA, and protein synthesis, and generating, maintaining, and using their inner membrane potential.

- Mitochondria manage homeostasis.

- The spatial and temporal organization of mitochondria is complex.

Both oxygen and DHA have quantum features of paramagnetism. DHA couples sunlight as electrons flow in and through water-collagen network. The truth is that water is life's battery power. Light and magnetism start mitochondrion and oxygen is coupled with magnetic field in mitochondrial electron transport chain.

Movement of electrons and protons in protein complexes of mitochondria's electron transport chain makes them more **elastic semiconductors**. Electrons reduce oxygen and increase electric and

51   http://arxiv.org/ftp/arxiv/papers/1012/1012.3371.pdf
52   http://www.hindawi.com/journals/tswj/2013/195028/
53   http://jcs.biologists.org/content/125/4/801.full

magnetic fields of mitochondria. Amazing! Mitochondria separates electrons and protons and even makes them act like one. Iron-sulfur redox clusters in these complexes are sensitive to small magnetic field. Even more amazing is the fact that mitochondria can entangle electrons by their spin state and release monochromatic infra-red light [54]. Transition metals, all mineral micronutrients including iron and sulfur, have special function in quantum biology. There is evidence that biophotons (IR) are produced in microtubules of neurons [55].

EAs highlighted earlier, energy molecule ATP is produced via electron transfer and proton translocation while we are awake. There is low ATP production during our REM (Rapid Eye Movement) sleep because electron transport is uncoupled. Yet ATP can be produced by free fatty acids. **This is when IR light is produced as heat when electrons and protons are quantum coherent .**

Cytochrome, common to all biology that uses light and magnetism, has FAD for magneto reception. It absorbs only IR blue light. FAD entangles electrons with unpaired spin. Protons tunnel during tautomerization or making of constitutional isomers involving just a single proton movement in forming a single bond. *We must have paramagnetic oxygen and DHA for efficient mitochondrial works [56].*

Dehydration reduces metabolic rate. Mitochondrial output is positive protons and more protons mean poor redox system. More electrons simply means better redox system. Inflammation that causes health problems is positive. Light and water start mitochondria because there will be no charge separation in absence of water.

Spin of electrons relates to momentum and mitochondria are the masters of using the momentum of electron spin. Same spin electron to MINOS **(mitochondrial inner-membrane organizing system)** tell mitochondroa how much IR to produce. Iron-Sulfur clusters in electron transport chain enzyme complexes have a lot to do with Spin [57]. They shoot free radicals into water and oxygen in order to keep the system coherent during our sleep via water's density and icosahedron (a solid figure with twenty plane faces, especially equilateral triangular ones) form.

Infra-red light entangles free radicals [58]. Density of water, shape, and temperature are the key factors in the process. *Electron transport is spin*

54   file:///C:/Users/Owner/Downloads/MitochondrionEellsWongWhelan.pdf
55   http://arxiv.org/ftp/arxiv/papers/1012/1012.3371.pdf
56   http://www.ncbi.nlm.nih.gov/pubmed/22248591
57   http://www.pnas.org/content/108/15/6097.full
58   http://www.neuroquantology.com/index.php/journal/user/viewPublicProfile/1060

dependent and spin states are manipulated by electric and magnetic fields that creates spin momentum. The mitochondrion makes use of directional dependence (anisotropy) of magnetic field [59].

Free radicals are single electron redox system. ***Good health is out of the question for us, if we can't make free radicals,.*** Too much of superoxide free radical production by iron-sulfur clusters is a problem though for type II diabetics [60]. True! Free radicals do cause oxidative stress but we must understand that mitochondria produces them on purpose for signaling, communication, and immune response. What good nutrition needs to offer is a balance by quenching of free radicals by antioxidants..

Here high dielectric constant of water keeps charges separated so cells can decipher signals. **Blue light has more high energy photons and summer light has more of blue light.** It hits FAD (Flavin Adenine Dinucleotide)and there is enough energy in it to knock an electron off for generating quantum signal in Iron-sulfur Cluster. This seems to be the basis of communication with SCN (suprachiasmatic nucleus in brain) that controls our 24 hour circadian rhythm [61].

Food is source of electrons and our digestive system and metabolism pool electrons for running our mitochondria. Electrons are coupled, coordinated, controlled and rendered coherent. **The faster they get to oxygen, the quicker is the setting up of electrical and magnetic fields.** That makes better electromagnet and mitochondria act as spintronic semiconductor. We need electrons to change proteins and their work habits. Also, we need to remember that electrons add elasticity and protons add stiffness. Cold slows electrons down, increases electron tunneling, and increases electron flow to oxygen. Let us also keep in mind that oxygen tension, magnetic field, and magnetic sense increases under cold conditions due to high dielectric constant of water [62].

National Institute of Health offers a condensed picture (Figure 1.04 below) of the outer cell and the matrix bound by the inner mitochondrial membrane. Various enzyme complexes including ATP synthase are shown along the inner membrane and Krebs cycle in the matrix which has high pH or low hydrogen ion concentration. The space between the two membranes is shown as having low pH or high hydrogen ion concentration because of outward hydrogen ion (proton) translocation from the matrix. *Proton motive*

---

59   http://www.ncbi.nlm.nih.gov/pmc/articles/PMC2697599/
60   http://circres.ahajournals.org/content/107/9/1058.full
61   http://www.hhmi.org/biointeractive/human-suprachiasmatic-nucleus
62   http://www.google.com/patents/EP2739353A1?cl=en

force in our cells is 21.80 KJ/mole of proton and that is enough to support our living. For a 70 Kg person who uses 70 Kg or 127 moles of ATP per day, this translates to 381 moles of protons energy per day. The Free energy of 3 moles of protons associated with each mole of ATP is 50 KJ/mole. Transfer of a mole of proton from cytoplasm to the matrix is negative - 21.5 KJ/mole. Thus 50- 3 (-21.5) or -3.4 Kj/mole is energy by proton transferred makes ATP synthesis rather spontaneous.

The inner membrane of mitochondria have four enzyme complexes for electron transfer and enzyme ATP sunthase. There are ten protons translocated by the electron transport chain for each NADH: Complex I translocates 4, complex III translocates 4, and complex IV translocates 2. Complex II serves as a second entry point.

Enzyme complexes that translocate the protons are bound to the inner membrane, a lot of them in the cristae as shown earlier in Figure 1.03a.

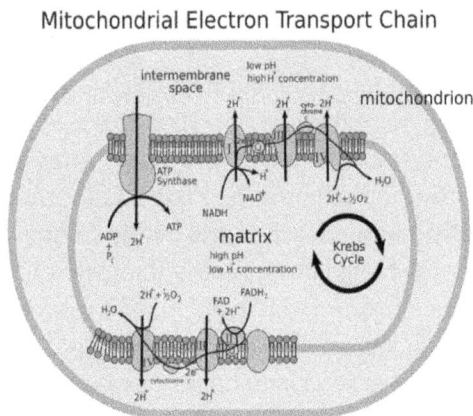

Mitochondrial Electron Transport Chain

Figure 1.04 Electron Transport Chain of Inner Mitochondrial Membrane.
Source: National Institute Of Health

Fifty micron in size, the liver cell mitochondria serves as a good example. Whereas the cell's membrane is about 7 nanometers (7 billionth of a meter) in thickness, outer and inner mitochondrial membranes within are only 3-4 nanometer thick with a length of about 7 micron [63]. The inner membrane of mitochondria creates enormous surface area because of numerous cristae

---

63   https://answers.yahoo.com/question/index?qid=20081106150416AAblyta

or lamellae protruding into the matrix . Each cristae can have more than one electron transport chain and ATP generating system for increased efficiency.

Outer Membrane

The outer membrane of mitochondria is a kind of a molecular sieve permitting free diffusion of molecules smaller than 10,000 Daltons. Ions and minerals, nutrients, ADP, and ATP can pass through outer mitochondrial membrane made of bilayer of phospholipids and proteins integrated into phospholipids in a ratio of 1:1. Relatively open diffusion makes intermediate space of mitochondria equivalent to cytoplasm with respect to all small molecules of life. It has porin channels for small proteins to enter in and ways by way of TOM (Translocase for the outer membrane made by nuclear DNA) to let protein complexes in by special signaling as outlined and depicted pictorially below [64], [65].

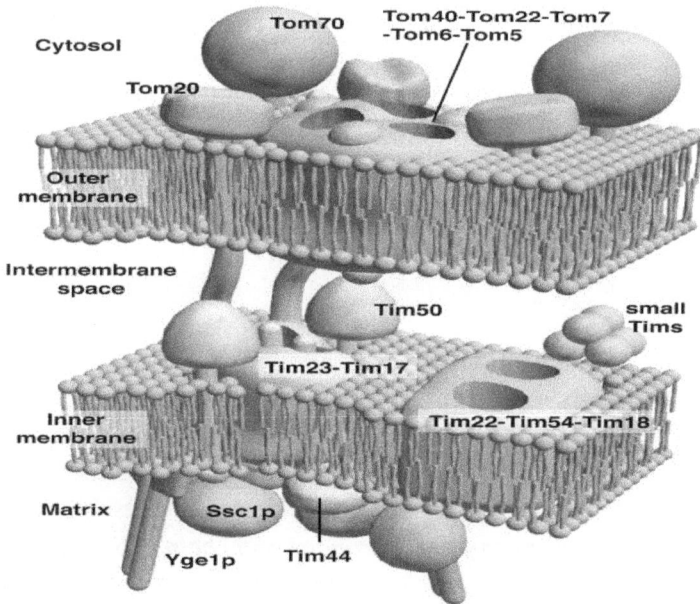

64   h http://jcs.biologists.org/content/125/4/807.full.pdf
65   ttp://www.ncbi.nlm.nih.gov/pmc/articles/PMC2172422/

Outer membrane interacts with the inner membranes to expedite protein transfer[66]. It is 6 nm in thickness and functions very much like the cell membrane.

Inner Membrane

The inner mitochondrial membrane (800 nm long, 200 nm wide and 25 nm high with a surface of 20,000 square nm) is very structured and five times longer than the outer membrane. It may contain up to 150 different polypeptides. As a matter of fact it may contain almost 1/3 of total mitochondrial proteins. Eighty percent of the inner mitochondrial is made up of proteins. **Impermeable to ions and molecules, it is a protein-lipid bilayer permeable only to water, oxygen, and carbon dioxide.** *Metabolites cross across only with the help of transport proteins.* It has all electron transport complexes and enzyme structures, transfer proteins, and ATP synthase (Fig. 1.05a and 1.05b) including fusion and fission proteins, protein import machinery, and a total of other 15 protein or polypeptides. The energy molecule ATP is made as hydrogen ions (protons) attempt to move back to matrix through enzyme ATP synthase[67] (Fig. 105b). There is a 10 nm wide intermediate space between the two membranes. The inner membrane is also 6 nm thick with a transmembrane potential of 200-225 mVolt.

Matrix

Enclosed by the inner membrane is the matrix where various enzymes perform their life supporting functions. The key ones are enzymes that work on pyruvic acid, run Krebs cycle, and enzymes that break down fatty acids. Also, the matrix contains circular mitochondrial genome of 37 genes, ribosomes, and messenger RNA. *Mitochondrial DNA is present in the matrix and because of its proximity to electron transfer chain, it is subject to seven times faster mutations than nuclear DNA [68].* The matrix contains almost 2/3 of the total proteins.

Heart muscle mitochondria with 615 proteins is a great example. The cristae as wrinkled folds or extensions of inner membrane providing high

---

66   http://www.sciencedirect.com/science/article/pii/S016748890200263X
67   http://www.uta.edu/biology/wilk/classnotes/cellphys/oxidative%20phosphorylation.pdf
68   http://www.ncbi.nlm.nih.gov/pubmed/16895436

surface area and often accommodating more than one set of complete electron transport chain while staying close to the inner membrane.

Understanding of disorders caused by mutations of mitochondrial DNA today is only in its infancy. Just to reiterate mitochondrial disease was first discovered in 1962. There can be low energy production in case of diseases such as hyperthyroidism, hypothyroidism, and high cholesterol and triglycerides. Sir John Cowdery Kendrew's television series came out on British Broadcasting Corporation when this author was in graduate school. The series published in 1966 has fascinated him ever since. Mutations of mitochondrial DNA are many with major feature of inadequate energy production resulting from coagulation of electron transfer enzyme complexes, uncoupled reduction and oxidation, and excessive accumulation of abnormal mitochondria say light microscopic ragged fibers that cause paralysis of eye muscles. Other consequences are cardiac conduction defect and hearing loss. **Point mutations and deletions in mitochondrial genes are now identified to be the cause of many diseases affecting central and peripheral nervous system.** Cells of brain, muscle, nerves, retina, and kidneys that can't proliferate well are more vulnerable because of the organ's high energy demand and because they are non-renewable. Inadequate energy production because of mismanagement of electron flow by mitochondria causes many inherited and acquired disorders due to inheritable and somatic mutations, exposure to toxins, and old age.

Poorly nourished mitochondria with respect to vitamins, Coenzyme Q_{10}, and minerals fail to follow orders from nuclear DNA and malfunction. *We talk a lot about fixing our cardiovascular problems due to fat and cholesterol but very little about our mitochondria that becomes sick for lack of methylation diet.* Sick and faulty mitochondria lose control of metabolic reactions and detoxification processes. *Cell to cell communications degrades, cells don't die as expected and immortal cells become cancerous tumors.* **This is often the case when production of free radicals exceeds over 3% of total oxygen intake, DNA and proteins get damaged, aging accelerates, and energy production as ATP suffers.** We quickly succumb to diseases of central nervous system and muscles when electron flow as depicted in Fig. 1.05a suffers and ATP production shown in Fig. 1.05b is hampered [69]. Ideal free radical concentration is less than 1%. Chemical mechanics of mitochondrial biobattery in our cells is complex but a discussion here and later in chapter 5 on summation seems necessary in order to understand various roles

---

69   http://jeb.biologists.org/content/208/9/1717.full

of mitochondria in maintenance of vital signs, health of vital organs, and prevention of chronic diseases. Mitochondrial performance, it goes without saying, depends on vitamin, mineral, and phytonutrient rich methylation diet. Both good health and longevity depend on mitochondrial performance.

The Electron Transport, Proton translocation, and ATP Production

Evolution began with electrons and protons and therefore it is instructive to trace the power of these particles in routine biology of foods we eat. Earth is 4.5 billion years old, photosynthetic organism came on earth some 3.5 billion years ago, plants populated the earth, and oxygen became abudant 3 billion years ago. Mitochondria are belived to be no more than 2 billion old. The scheme of managing electrons and protons by mitochondria had to begin in water, an atom with a single proton and electron. This is the most abundant source of proton or hydrogen ion in our body, in our foods and beverages, and on planet earth. Also, protons are mobile and they can associate, dissociate, jump or move over long hydrogen bond structures. *The biological story of electrons and protons transcends evolution [70], [71]* and the scheme of managing electrons and moving protons around in, on, and over small and large carrier and transfer molecules is rather old and common to bacteria , plants, animals, and humans. It includes a major carrier pair of NADH/NAD$^+$ with a redox potential of minus 320 milliVolt, a water-oxygen redox pair with a redox potential of plus 820 milliVolt, and four other enzyme proteins for step wise electron transfer where steps really mean manageable release of free energy. The difference of 1,140 milliVolt is managed by four major enzyme systems of redox molecules identified as complex I, II, III, and IV. *The fifth complex is the enzyme ATP synthase that produces energy molecule ATP loaded with minus 7.3 Kcal/Mole or almost a third of the energy of one electron transfer that happens in no more than 5-20 milliseconds.* The four complexes are orange heme proteins designed with numerous iron-sulfur clusters so electron can jump over a a 2 nm gap. Genes that encode these complexes are genetically conserved [72].

---

70   http://www.ncbi.nlm.nih.gov/books/NBK26849/
71   http://www.bmb.leeds.ac.uk/illingworth/oxphos/evolve.htm
72   http://www.sciencedirect.com/science/article/pii/S0168952504002513

Electricity japs through our body and the journey of electrons can be described as

- Twenty four electrons are used to make a glucose molecule during photosynthesis.

- The bonds of glucose are broken down in our cell to extract 12 pairs of 2 or 24 electrons during respiration.

- Electrons are carried to the entry point of electron transport, transported by the chain of special proteins, and finally used to reduce oxygen. The process is coupled to proton translocation across the inner membrane to the intermediate space.

The electric current in mitochondria runs through a set of electromagnetic molecules made out of enzyme proteins of varying size, depth, and geometric conformation. We call them complex. *The complexes act like electromagnetic compass designed to tell mitochondria how to respond to the environment.* They even know how much infra-red radiation should go to MINOS (mitochondrial inner membrane organizing system) surrounded by water layer whose dielectric constant shields positive and negative charges during energy extraction by redox reactions [73], [74].

Current research describes a close relationship between foods we eat and our mitochondrial apparatus in that (1) *composition of our daily foods dictates the rate of energy extraction by molecular machines of electron transport chain via the relative* abundance of NADH and $FADH_2$, the electron energy carriers [75]. Often electron tunneling suffers in complex I (NADH-ubiquinone oxidoreductase) [76], (2) **ATP molecule itself is a proton acceptor** when it comes to energy release by its hydrolysis[77], [78], (3) mitochondria in our brain cells produce weak biophotons by conversion of electrical signals to light [79], (4) a single mitochondria can be extracted out of the cell and its genetic makeup examined by

---

73   http://www.ncbi.nlm.nih.gov/pubmed/22918945
74   http://www.molbiolcell.org/content/23/20/3948.full.pdf
75   http://www.sciencedaily.com/releases/2013/06/130627142404.htm
76   http://www.pnas.org/content/107/45/19157.full
77   http://www.ncbi.nlm.nih.gov/pubmed/23320924
78   http://pubs.acs.org/doi/abs/10.1021/bi301109x
79   http://arxiv.org/ftp/arxiv/papers/1012/1012.3371.pdf

sophisticated lasers[80], [81]. *(5) mitochondria power our life and death* and
(6) *mitochondria play a central role in converting a normal cell into a cancer cell.* We live and die by our mitochondria that transfer themselves from one generation to the other by mother's ovum. *Most important of all is the finding that mitochondrial function depends on varieties and amount of foods we eat. Values reside in their composition with respect to vitamins, minerals, essential amino and fatty acids, and antioxidants.* Our cells get energy by breaking the bonds of carbon and hydrogen in glucose molecules and there are three steps to it (Table 1.03.01).

- Splitting of glucose into two pyruvic acid molecules.

- Conveting of pyruvate to acetyl-CoA.

- Acetyl CoA can also come from proteins and fats.

- Processing of Acetyl CoA through the electron mill called Krebs cycle after Dr. Hans Kreb.

The second and third take place in mitochondrial matrix where *high potential energy electrons from breaking of bonds* take a ride on carrier molecules NADH and $FADH_2$ and enter the electron transport chain in the inner membrane of mitochondria. NADH from glucose splitting that happens in cytoplasm outside mitochondria can't enter in directly but there are alternate reduction-oxidation reactions that do let them in. All energy as electrons from all 10 NADH and 2 $FADH_2$ carriers (Table 1.03.01) per molecule of glucose accumulate in the matrix; finally the electrons are fed to the electron transport chain in steps as shown in Fig. 1.05a for proton translocation and ATP production.

An examination of the details in table 1.03.01 tells us that the electrons via bond breaking concentrate in carrier molecules NADH and $FADH_2$. The energy of electrons is transferred in steps to oxygen reducing it to water [82]. **Part of the energy as electrons transfer from one complex to the other is used to push protons from matrix to the intermediate space.** The differential in proton concentration sets up a gradient across the inner membrane. It is this gradient that drives protons through ATP making molecular machine back to the matrix through rotations of

---

80   http://phys.org/news/2011-01-cellular-aid-mitochondrial-diseases.html
81
82   http://biochem.siu.edu/bmb_courses/mbmb451b/lectures/mbmb451b_electransoxphos.pdf

the enzyme ATP synthase. This rotor-stator enzyme molecule in effect produces ATP. NADH and $FADH_2$ can donate two electrons to complex I. Other enzymes complexes of the chain transfer only one electron at a time. *The oxygen in the matrix picks up 4 electrons from the chain and 4 protons from the matrix reducing itself to two molecules of water. What a wonder! Water that was split in electron and proton during photosynthesis becomes water again in our cells.*

Table 1.04.01 is a technical summary of steps and the structural features of complexes I through IV. There are four complexes.

- NADH dehydrogenase (I): transfers 4 hydrogen ions (H^+ or protons) and 2 electrons. NADH binds to complex I, reduces coenzyme Q through FMN and a series of Fe-S clusters.

- Succinate dehydrogenase or oxidoreductase or complex II serves as a second entry point.

- Complex III is a Coenzyme Q cytochrome C reductase: Complex III, buried 38 A^0 in the inner membrane and extending out in the matrix some 75 A^0, it reduces ubiquinol and two molecules of citochrome c, and translocates 4 hydrogen ions (protons) to intermediate space.

- Cytochrome C oxidase (IV): Cytochrome oxidase translocates 2 protons and abstracts 4 protons from the matrix.

Table 1.03.01: Summary of Production of ATP and NADH and $FADH_2$				
	ATP Produced	Electron Carriers	ATP Produced	Total
Glycolysis	2	2 NADH	4-6	6-8
Pyruvate to Acetyl CoA	-----	2NADH	6	6
Krebs cycle	2	6 NADH	18 ATP	
		2 $FADH_2$	4 ATP	24
TOTAL				36-38

Note1 : Glycolysis happens in the cytoplasm. 36 ATP is an accepted figure for ATP produced per glucose molecule. Two electrons and 1 proton (hydrogen ion) go to NAD^+ to make NADH. Glucose to pyruvate is a 10 step process. Both NADH and $FADH_2$ can split hydrogen into electrons and protons.

Note 2: Acetyl CoA enters Krebs cycle, an energy mill that produces 2 carbon dioxide, 3 NADH, 1 $FADH_2$, and 1 ATP. The cycle runs twice to process one glucose molecule. ectron and proton. There can be 320 chains for 1280 electron transfer in a millisecond.

Note 3: There can be 320 electron transport chains with 60 electron carriers.

Note 4: Each NADH can pump 10 protons and produce 3 ATP and each $FADH_2$ can pump 6 protons and produce 2 ATP. On an average 4 protons are needed to make an ATP.

Ubiquinone and citochrome c are electron carriers also. Coenzyme Q is the only non-protein mobile carrier with its own electron cycle called Q-cycle. Iron-Sulfur clusters in cytochrome structures can produce free radicals and IR radiation and mitochondria have mastery over managing electron spin [83]. *The iron-sulfur clusters are spread over the heme protein complexes and spaced so they can act almost like wires.* Complex I has nine of them, complex II has 3, complex III has one iron-Riske cluster, and complex IV has copper clusters. **In a sense electrons participate in a game of track hurdle. Spacing of clusters and ability of electrons to jump depends on their energies.** Fig. 1.05a quantifies the oxidation-reduction potential and free energy associated with enzyme complexes graphically with energy range of electron conversion spanning from -315 MilliVolt to +815 milliVolt. The organization of these complexes is unique in that I, III, and IV are incessantly pumping out protons to the intermediate space. **The energy of electrons thus flows to molecule of ATP synthase via protons. H^+ ions are plentiful in our body as part of water. They are very mobile and flicker through hydrogen bonds. That is exactly how protons move across proton pumps. ATP synthase is a very large enzyme complex made up of F_o as a proton channel and F_1 as an enzyme with nucleotide active sites that acts as a generator.**

---

83   http://jcs.biologists.org/content/125/21/4963.full

In contrast to photosynthesis mitochondria oxidize glucose and reduce oxygen to water. Thus the energy in the bonds of food molecules converts to electrons, electrons move across the electron transport chain releasing part of their energy for translocating protons and finally reducing oxygen to water. Translocated protons across the inner mitochondrial membrane to the intermediate space come back into the matrix through enzyme ATP synthase that produces energy molecule ATP. **Electron transfer and proton translocation are thus coupled and simultaneous.** Thiese processes can be uncoupled during cold thermogenesis but only under strict mitochondrial control though. As we shall see later, electron transfer and chemo osmotic production of ATP, although tandem and coupled, are two different phenomena. The science of step wise electron transfer, proton translocation, and ATP production shall be described in greater detail in chapter 5.

Table 1. 04.01 Summary of Enzyme Complexes of the Electron transport chain	
NADH + 2 H$^{\pm}$ + 2 e^{-} **NADH + H$^{\pm}$, - 0.315 Volt**	NADH is a high energy electron carrying molecules.
Complex I of NADH dehydrogenase or NADH-CoenzymeQ Reductase **40 Polypeptides** **850,000 Daltons, 30 sub units** **Flavin mononucleotide Iron-Sulfur Cluster** **- 320 milliVolt Potential**	It oxidizes NADH to NAD$^+$ and transfers two electrons from NADH to CoenzymeQ. Receives hydrogen ion and two electrons. *The electrons go to the iron-sulfur cluster and the protons to intermediate space. Transfers two electrons at a time and produces 4 hydrogen ions. Hydrogen ions or protons, move from matrix to intermediate space, accumulate there and generate proton motive force.* The reduction potential equals - 320 mV or 14.8 Kcal per mole.
Complex II or Succinate dehydrogenase **140,000 Daltons, 4 sub units** **Reduction Potential = 0 volt** **Free energy= - 5.6 KJ/ mole**	Binds Flavin Adenosine Dinuleotide (FAD) via **iron-sulfur structures** as an integral membrane protein and converts succinate to fumerate. *Releases 2 hydrogen ions or protons. There are no electron transfers at this stage.* This shuttle molecule, flavoprotein-quinone oxidoreductase, transfers electrons to a pool of ubiquinones, *the only non-protein complex of the chain anchored by its isoprenoid tail in the fatty portion of the inner membrane.*

Complex III or Coen- zymeQ-Cytochrome C reductase **248,000 Daltons** **11 Subunits** **Reduction Potential = + 250 milliVolt,** **Iron-Sulfur Clusters**	Also known as cytochrome bc_1 complex, *this enzyme has 7.5 nanometer long eleven subunits that anchor 3.8 nanometer deep into the inner membrane.* **In a way it runs a electron transfer cycle of its own.** The complex is made of two units and has four cofactors: cytochrome C_1, cytochrome b-562, cytochrome b-566, and 2 iron ferrodoxins and is very critical to ATP pro- duction. Cytochrome c is a small 13,000 Dalton single unit structure. It is very soluble (100 gm /liter) in water and carriers one electron. Four electrons are transferred and six protons trans- located by complex III.
Complex IV or Cyto- chrome c Oxidase **Iron-Sulfur Clusters** **162,000 Daltons, 10 sub units** **Reduction potential = + 285 milliVolt,** **- 5.1 Kcal/mole** $O_2 + 2 H^+ + 2 e^-$ **to** H_2O **is** **+ 0.815 volt.**	Components of this complex are heme a, heme a_3, Cu a^+ and Cub^+. Two oxygen pairs and two cytochrome C oxidase are necessary to reduce oxygen to water. Complex IV takes a total of four electrons, one each from four cytochrome C, attaches to oxygen along with four H^+, and produces two molecules of water. Simultane- ously, it pumps out four H^+ to the intermediate space acting like a molecular motor. Four elec- trons, four protons, and two oxygen thus make two water molecules. Electron transfer stops at an energy need of 69 KJ/mole or 16.491 KCal/ mole; it is driven by the proximity of complex- es.
Complex V or ATP SYNTHASE	Molecular motor-generator that makes ATP from proton power.
$\Delta G = n F_o E_o$ = RTln (product/reactants) where n is number of electrons and F_o is Faraday constant of 96.5 KJ per mole per volt.	

Fig. 1.05 a is a graphic positioning complexes in terms of their redox potentials in milliVolts and Free Energies as Kcal/mole. The key feature to note is loss of electron energy in steps and finally reduction of oxygen.

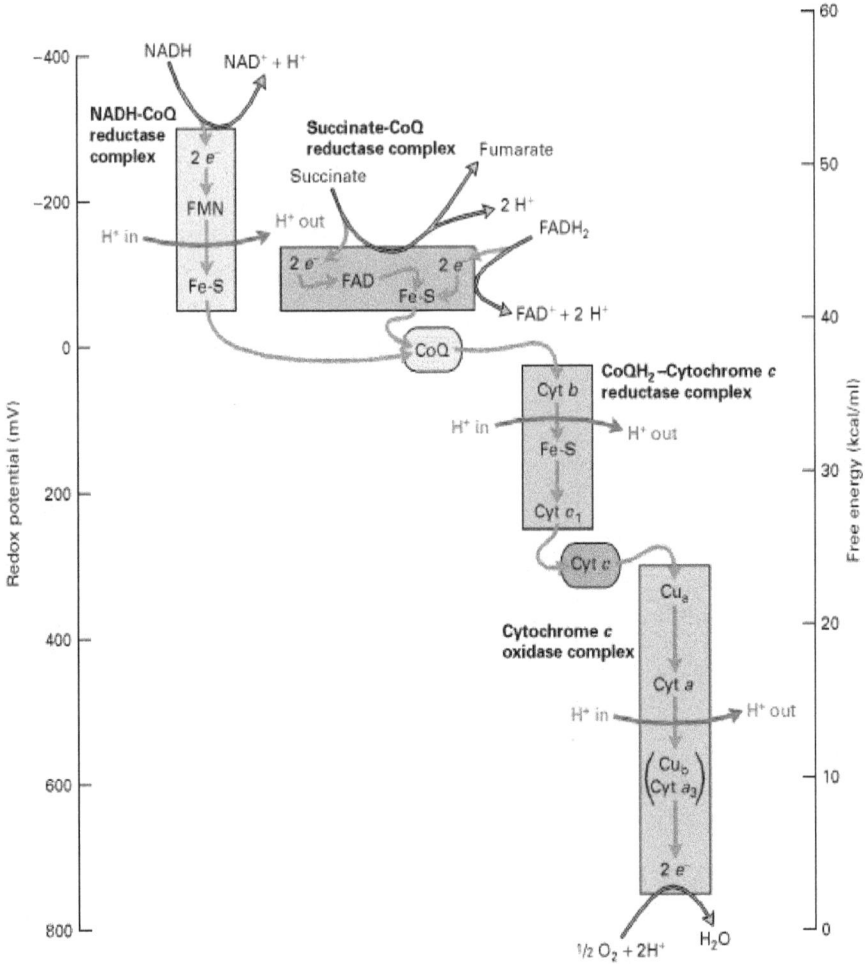

Fig. 1.05a The electron transport chain.

Source: National Institute of Health.

1.02 The Energy In the Bonds of Our Food Molecules

All energy in foods we eat comes from sunlight, Dr. Einsteine's photons. Excited electrons in plant leaves are used to produce ATP during photosynthesis within milliseconds which in turn is used to make electron and hydrogen rich (reduced) molecules of food as carbohydrate, protein, and fat. Glucose is the primary organic molecule made in photosynthesis. **With the help of sunlight plants can split water into electron and Hydrogen ion (H⁺) for their**

needs

ATP synthase is the molecule of life. Protons channel through F_0 , an 85 A^0 ball, embedded in the membrane down to matrix, ring C of F_0 rotates as the protons pass through, c ring rotates gamma within 3 layers each of alpha and beta units of 9 nanometer long F_1 , a conformational changes attends to ATP synthesis.

o f

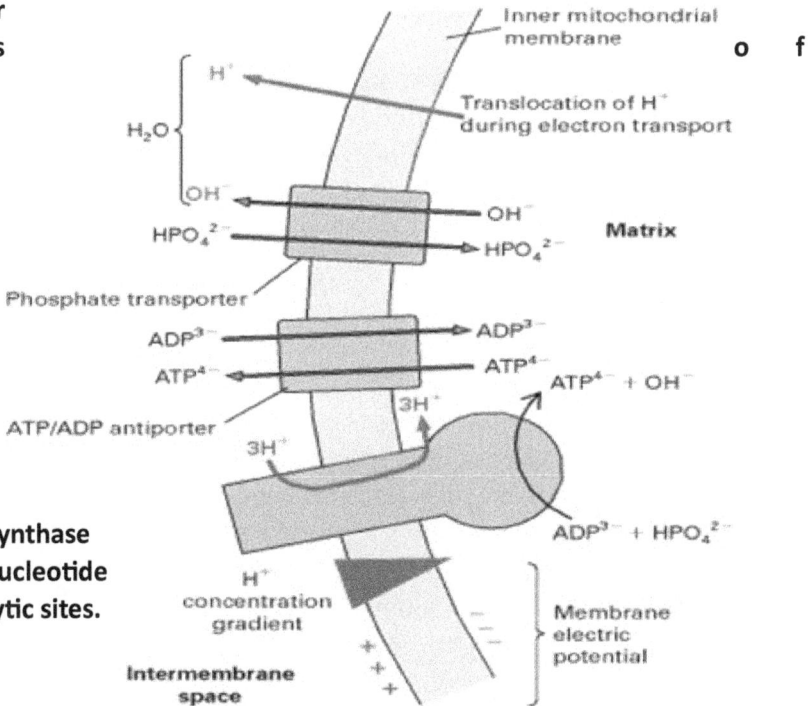

ATP synthase has nucleotide catalytic sites.

Figure 1.05b Coupling of Electron Transport and ATP Production by enzyme ATP Synthase, the Molecular Motor that runs our lives.

Source: National Institute of Health

making ATP and other vital molecules [84]. A proton motive force of 200 Millivolt is common to plant and human cells alike. Mitochondria use electrons and protons (as hydrogen ion) to reduce oxygen into water and set carbon dioxide free that we breathe out. Fig 1.05b above schematically details the production of ATP by orange ATP synthase, proton gradient, and phosphate transporter and ATP/ADP antiporter structures as part of the inner membrane . ATP synthase has reversible activity.

F_1 is like hexameric (3 units each of alpha and beta subunits) DNA helicase and F_o is analogous to flagellar motor complexes powered by H^+ protons. F_o is an electric motor powered by proton gradient. It turns the circular motor connected to chemical rotor F_1 that is powered by 100 molecules of ATP produced per second. One turns the other making it a generator and 100 anhydride phosphate bonds are added to ADP per second. Therein lies the wonder of biology at large.

Glucose with six carbon bonds is made with input of 686 Kcal or 2823 Kilo Joules/mole of glucose with carbon dioxide and water with the aid of 18 ATP and 12 reduced Nicotinamide Adenine Dinucleotide Phosphate during photosynthesis. **Photooxidation of water with 48 photons (two photons/ electron X 2 electrons per NADPH X 12 = 48) of 650 nm wavelength of 8000 KJ energy are need to make 12 NADPH.** Since the energy difference between 1 mole of glucose and one mole each of carbon dioxide and water is 2870 KJ, efficiency of photosynthesis alternatively calculates to be 2780/8000 = 35%.

The electron transport chain produces 36 ATP per glucose molecule, an average protein molecule also produces 36 ATP, and a fat molecule on an average produces 150 ATP molecules. Actually, a large energy intensive triglyceride can produce even up to 500 ATP energy molecules. The efficiency of energy extraction by mitochondria is around 38.3%%[85] based on 36 ATP produced per mole of glucose. Divide 686 KCal/mole of glucose by 36 X 7.3 Kcal present in all 36 ATP to arrive at the efficiency to be 262/686 = 38.31%.

Whereas photons translocate protons in case of photosynthesis, it is electrons from foods we consume translocate protons from in to out side of inner mitochondrial membrane in our cells for travel through enzyme ATP synthase downhill for ATP production.

84   ttp://www.physics.drexel.edu/~bob/TermPapers/Jones_QuantumPaper.pdf
85   http://www.tiem.utk.edu/~gross/bioed/webmodules/ATPEfficiency.htm

1.03 Production of High Energy Electron Carriers from Food

Human beings absorb glucose from intestine to an extent of 150 mg/min [86]. There is about 0.10 to 0.18% glucose in our blood that can reach the cytoplasm across the membranes of all cells in our body [87]. It is kept constant by works of insulin and glucagon where blood glucose from glycogen in the liver can be mobilized when needed. Endogenous glycogen and sugars like maltose, lactose, and galactose all covert to glucose, which via a total of ten reactions splits into two three carbon pyruvate molecules. **Our cells invest 2 ATP in order to create 4 ATP in this anaerobic process. The net gain is two ATP and 2 NADH.** Key metabolic reactions are about proton and electron abstraction from C-H bonds. C-C bond splitting produces carbon dioxide.

Pyruvic acid enters mitochondria and is converted into Acetyl CoA by a powerful set of enzymes with production of NADH, protons, and carbon dioxide. **Two pyruvates produce 2 NADH, 2 protons, and 2 carbon dioxide molecules.**

Carbohydrates, proteins, and fats- all end up in the mitochondrial matrix as acetylCoA which finally enter the electron mill called Krebs cycle. We should think of it as a molecular mill of Hydrogen abstraction and electron extraction. Two rounds of all acetyl CoA from glucose through this mill account for oxidation of all six carbons of glucose, the main fuel for our cells.

AcetylCoA makes a 6-carbon citric acid from 4-carbon oxaloacetic acid, citric transforms to 5-carbon α-ketoglutaric acid releasing a carbon dioxide and NADH, and 5-carbon α-ketoglutaric transforms to 4-carbon succinyl CoA with release of another carbon dioxide and NADH. All three steps of glycolysis, pyruvate to acetylCoA production and processing of acetyl CoA through Krebs cycle produce 10 NADH and 2 FADH$_2$ that finally deliver electrons to the electron transport chain for eventual production of life energy molecule of ATP and reduction of oxygen with spent electrons to water.

Carbohydrates made of glucose and proteins made of amino acids roughly have 4 Kilocalories (calories in nutrition) per gram. Fats on the other hand can on an average deliver 9 Kilocalories per gram. These numbers correspond to ATP production. The electronic energy resides in the carbon-hydrogen bonds of glucose, amino acids, and fat. As we have

---

86   http://www.pnas.org/content/98/20/11330.full
87   http://www.scientificpsychic.com/health/normal-blood-sugar.html

seen, mitochondria have the power to convert the energy of electrons into chemical energy as ATP. Fats produce high amounts of ATP because their molecules are most highly reduced or loaded with hydrogen atoms containing a proton and an electron.

All NADH and FADH$_2$, as molecules of high transfer potential, donate electrons to the electron transport chain in the inner mitochondrial membrane. **NADH is the electron donor of the first rung. Three ATP is produced from 10 protons produced for every two electrons and 36 ATP is produced per glucose molecule.** *Our cells have a way to get 360 protons from 36 pairs of electrons.* ATP is the result of proton power. As electrons move over the enzyme complexes of higher reduction potential they help translocate protons and finaly reduce oxygen. **As a matter of fact, complexes I, III, and IV release energy and pump protons incessantly from matrix to intermediate space.** Let us keep in mind that energy associated with a pair of electrons in a single covalent C-H bonds is 415 KJ [88]. It is the unpaired electrons that become free radicals of high reactivity.

Finally protons flow back through ATP synthase for making ATP. Proton motive force is transferred into ATP molecule as a terminal high energy phosphate bond. Although the terminal phosphate bond is weak, it involves high energy electrons[89]. Oxygen being most electronegative receives lowest energy spent electrons for its reduction to water. It must be replenished continuously to drain electrons from the system otherwise all of the carriers would stay reduced and the electron transport would stop. During the process of electron transfer much energy is lost as heat except for what is stored as proton gradient that helps make ATP. All this happens in the mitochondria with rigorous and meticulous control [90], [91].

1.04.01 Food Molecules as repository of Electrons and Protons

It should become more clear now that the mitochondria run cellular electronics. Our body is a sea of protons, water as ionic plasma, and submerged in it are all necessary ions and molecules essential for running

88   http://www.britannica.com/science/electron-pair
89   http://chemwiki.ucdavis.edu/Biological_Chemistry/Biochemical_Energy/ATP%2F%2FADP
90   http://ajpcell.physiology.org/content/292/1/C157
91   http://www.ncbi.nlm.nih.gov/pubmed/21742062

the chemistry of life. We eat foods containing major nutrients as molecules of carbohydrates, proteins, and fats for electrons present in their bonds.

How does the ultimate digestion in terms of electron transfer for energy needed for proton pumping across the inner mitochondrial membrane take place for our life energy is the question that, I believe, everyone who lives and intends to live well must seek an answer for. This section is a brief attempt to describe the ultimate in energy flow in the reversible biobattery called mitochondria present in cells of our body. Mighty mitochondria, with genes responsible for producing all enzyme protein complexes for electron transfer, proton translocation processes, and for running Krebs cycle, are responsible for human bioenergetics .

1.04.02 The Electron Transport Chain per se: the Biobattery

The wrinkled inner membrane of mitochondria with its cristae can be up to approximately 8000 nm long over which electron transfer and proton hydrolics take place via four enzyme complexes and ATP synthase respectively [92]. *The length of electron transport chain of four enzyme complexes, ATP synthase, and ubiquinone with a 2 nanometer gap is approximately 25 nanometers. ATP synthase alone has an approximate area of 100 nm^2. At least 320 chains with four complexes may be operating at the same time permitting 1280 electron transfers per millisecond [93].* Although complexes are independent, their precise line up in sequence is necessary. They are known to exist in different ratios in different mitochondria in order to allow transfer of close to a billion electrons per minute when we run fast. All this is rather daunting and complicated but let us look at a simpler scenario.

Glycolysis splits six carbon glucose to three carbon pyruvic acid. Pyruvic acid further converts into two carbon acetylCoA. Acetyl CoA runs twice through Krebs cycle. This completes the oxidation of glucose producing a total of 10 NADH and 2 FADH$_2$. These are the electron rich carriers that feed the electron transport chain. Our cells get electron loaded NADH from bonds of glucose. High energy electrons push protons out to intermediate space, spent electrons reduce oxygen and the process keeps going, and proton hydrolics back to matrix makes ATP. In theory each NADH can make

92   http://www.ivy-rose.co.uk/Biology/Organelles/Structure-of-Mitochondria.php
93   http://www.ncbi.nlm.nih.gov/books/NBK26904/

7 ATP but our cells make only 3ATP per NADH because close to 58% energy is used in proton translocation. What a amazing scenario of living by foods we eat that provide electrons and induce mitochondra to react !

We can say now that electron transfer over the electron transport chain is a matter of random collision over and through a number of enzyme complexes. NADH, the main source of high energy electrons, enters at complex I. Electrons pass along the chain and, although, each complex binds them rather tightly, part of potential energy is released to pump protons across the inner membrane to the intermediate space. Complex IV combines electrons, protons, and molecular oxygen to make water. **For each NADH-CoenzymeQ, there are 3 $CoQH_2$ and 7 cytochrome C oxidase systems.** These are electron shuttles. When we take Coenzyme Q_{10} as a food supplement we we take extra electron carrier molecules for the electron transport chain.

NADH transfers electron to Coenzyme Q . $FADH_2$ transfers electrons to complex II but bypassing ATP production. Complex III passes electrons to cytochrome C, a peripheral enzyme protein system, with production of 1 ATP, and finally cytochrome C passes electrons to cytochrome C oxidase and then to oxygen with production of 1 ATP.

As shown in Table 1.04.01, the reduction potential throughout the chain increases steadily from NADH to oxygen and 10 protons are translocated for every pair of electron transferred from NADH to molecular oxygen O_2. The electrons release a lot of energy and two electrons from NADH to NAD^+ move rather spontaneously. There is a huge energy gap between -52.6 Kcalories of NADH + 1/2 O_2 +H^+ to H_2O + NAD^+ and finally ADP + P_i + H^+ with a Gib's Free Energy of + 7.3 Kcalories/mole. That is why the meticulous design of step wise electron transport chain. This for sure avoids the explosion.

As electrons move from NADH to oxygen, their potential declines by 1.14 volt (26.2 Kcal) or 52 Kcal/mole for the electron pair. A direct transfer of electrons from NADH and $FADH_2$ to oxygen will cause an explosive production of heat. Step wise transfer means step wise energy release for proton translocation. Let us note that while oxygen consumption is due to electron transfer, ATP production is not. It is also true that there can be no electron transfer without simultaneous proton translocation. *Electrons are transferred one at a time via different prosthetic groups, a pair for a pair of protons translocated.* In the process our cells make 100 ATP molecules per second.

Electrons flow, release energy in steps, Chemo osmotic gradient across the inner membrane is established, and molecules of ATP are produced from ADP (adenosine Diphosphate) and inorganic phosphate. At the end, cytochrome C oxidase transfers 4 electrons to oxygen and reduces it to water. **The complexes move freely and exchange electrons** and Protons are translocated uphill from matrix to intermediate space with energy release at complexes I, III, and IV. The variety in structures of four complexes and their unique geometry is necessary for channeling electrons and protons in steps for the best energy conversion to chemical energy ATP. This change in geometry of enzyme proteins occurs as excited electrons flow through them. This is a wonder in biology.

The pH of mitochondrial matrix is higher because of low hydrogen ion concentration and the difference in hydrogen ion concentration between matrix and Intermediate space leads to Chemo- osmotic gradient. As it builds up, more energy is needed to push protons across. Proton motive force in effect is a voltage gradient. A pH difference of one unit is 59 mV and and a 160 mVolt transmembrane electric potential across the inner membrane make up the total voltage gradient of 219 milliVolt.

The 10 isoprenes of Coenzyme Q_{10} have a length a bit longer than the width of the inner mitochondrial membrane. It holds electrons rather loosely and once it has given up two electrons it becomes an antioxidant. Also, it can transfer another electron from its semiquinone state. Furthermore, Coenzyme Q_{10} is a mobile electron shuttle. Electrons from complex I and II go to Coenzyme Q_{10} shuttle and then to complex III. The electrons enter Complex IV from various cytochrome C of complex III, first to the copper center and then to the iron-copper center. **What scientist call Q-Cycle is a neat mechanism for transfer of electrons to complex III from three redox states of coenzyme Q $_{10}$.** Ubiquinol is fully reduced as QH_2 by accepting electrons from Complex I and II. QH_2 feeds the cycle as it moves around freely in the inner mitochondrial membrane. Various protein units of complex III [94] can receive electrons from three redox states of coenzyme Q_{10}. Actually, the Q-Cycle operates with complex III. Like favoproteins FAD and FMN (Flavin mononucleotide) it can transfer either one or two electrons at a time. *Cytochromes transfer only one electron at a time.* Cytochrome C carries electrons away and delivers them to cytochrome C oxidase for reducing oxygen. A total of four electrons are transferred but one at time. ATP production relates directly to the hydrogen ion gradient and not the

---

94   https://www.dartmouth.edu/~blt/Publications/11409.pdf

transfer of electrons per se. We should view enzyme protein complexes described in Table 1.04.01 as locks on electron flow. **Ten protons are pumped out to intermediate space per pair of electrons during an NADH to oxygen electron transport.** Enzymes complexes extract 2 electrons and 2 proton, transfer 2 electron and pump 1 proton in converting NADH to NAD^+. Electrons do seem to obey Laws of thermodynamics as they move around in water and among systems of molecules in water. Although calcium ions regulate this process, the inner membrane leaks protons. How much of protons it leaks is very material to our health.

Almost 70% of ATP produced is for BMR, 20% for physical activity and 10% for thermogenesis. *We should further recognize that production of protons by three molecular machines (complexes I, III, and IV) of the electron transport chain working in combination and synergy depends critically on the nature, completeness, and general composition of food we consume* [95]. A good example is hummingbird's choice of sugar over fat for fast energy production. Also, we need to remember that iron, sulfur, copper, and calcium are necessary for successful energy production by mitochondria in our cells. Biology uses transition metals as metalloproteins in order to move electrons around. Deficiency of these metallic micronutrients can be disastrous to our health.

Mitochondrial genes regulate the molecular frequency of ATP synthase. **In a sense mitochondria oscillate and three ATP are produced per revolution. This is why mitochondria are close to contractile muscles of the heart.** Also, this is why they are wrapped tightly in the motile flagellum of sperm for its arduous and rather random flight for impregnating an ovum.

A blockage of any one of electron transfer complexes can kill us. We are familiar with a few powerful poisons. Cyanide poisons works by stopping outlets for electrons needed for reduction of oxygen in complex IV. Electron transfer is reduced to zero no matter how much we breathe and how much oxygen our cells get. This is why methylene blue, of same reduction potential as oxygen, is kept in ambulances to counteract cyanide poising effects [96]. Large doses are used as an antidote against potassium cyanide poisoning. Carbon monoxide blocks complex IV. Rotenone blocks complex I and acts as poison to fish and insects. Actimycin A blocks complex III.

---

95   http://www.sciencedaily.com/releases/2013/06/130627142404.htm
96   http://jama.jamanetwork.com/article.aspx?articleid=241464

1.04.02.01 <u>Infra-red Light</u>

Mitochondrial porphyrins (cytochromes) with up to 36 conjugated bonds and heme groups emit infra-red light in pulses as they discharge ATP off ATP Synthase [97]. Thus comes the release of monochromatic infra-red radiation at the iron-sulfur clusters so electrons can tunnel [98]. Cytochromes use vitamin D and vitamin A cycle in our brain to produce electromotive force by using light. IR radiation is produced in mitochondria by electrons and protons; it entangles free radicals of same spin, which is a kind of a redox system within the redox system [99]. Infra-red radiation interacts with cytochrome c oxidase [100].

Mitochondria use magnetic memory to generate entangled particles and they use free radicals to code information by way of direction dependent magnetic anisotropy. It is now known that 48% of our circuits are dedicated to light.

1.04.02.02 <u>The Life giving and Sustaining Water</u>

Water is special case of dipole process. Positive hydrogen and negative oxygen attract each other and make a rather weak bond ($1/10_{th}$ the strength of covalent bonds). Water has high dielectric constant because of high dipole moment and as such it is easily polarizable in electric field. Water, as an ionic plasma, has memory. Electrons and protons flow through it and memory begins with H-bond by electromagnetic sensing. Mitochondria have Hydrogen ion (protons) in matrix. Water and iodine in particular make ionic plasma. When charges are separated by iodine and proteins, what results is superconducting proton cable.

Charged electron is essentially a current electron deficient hole can stop the current. This where DHA comes in because electrons move from place to place in proteins in the lipid rafts of membranes. Mitochondria use free radical as they signal by IR. Skin as a solar panel above an ionic plasma, filters light before mitochondria can use it. Collagen is a nanowire and water is a repository of solar radiation. It reacts with IR light. Water by controlling H-bond can squeeze mitochondria and create large voltage. Water and

---

97   http://arxiv.org/ftp/arxiv/papers/1012/1012.3371.pdf
98   https://www.jackkruse.com/tensegrity-9-magnetic-mitochondria-memory-creates-coherence/
99   http://www.rsc.org/chemistryworld/2014/09/does-life-play-dice-quantum-biology
100   http://www.sciencedirect.com/science/article/pii/S0005272814005799

collagen must touch each other for energy transfer. Spin information from water and its hydrogen bond network surrounding mitochondria is collected and interpreted as collagen is made coherent. Such is the importance of DHA (omega-3 fatty acids), collagen protein, and hydrogen bonded water in sustaining our lives. Life evolved in water and human brain signaling evolved with DHA, a molecule to which electrons can stick for semiconduction [101].

1.04.02.03 The Hydrogen Bonds in DNA and Proteins

Helical molecules of proteins and DNA get their spring like power from Hydrogen-Bonds responsible for the 3-D structure of springy molecules like water, DNA, and Proteins. As a matter of fact we should view Water as an energy converter. By absorbing 270 nm radiation, water separates into positive hydrogen ion and and negative electron. Dielectric constant of water alters electromagnetic fields. Water condenses when infra-red radiation hits it and cells use water to uncondense (unfold) proteins. The mystry lies in the hydrogen bonds. No life can exist without exceedingly dynamic hydrogen bond that is a quantum measuring device. It keeps memory by entangled pair of electrons in free radicals by light and electromagnetic fields. Matrix containing ionic water undergoes adaptive changes for tunneling of electrons and protons. Low pH and high hydrogen ion concentration gives rise to only low direct current. Electrons hit water always as a pair. Subsequent motion depends on the state of particles and entangled particles have their spin balanced by clock and counter-clock motion.

1.04.02.04 Hormones

Cortisol removes electrons from tissues as it opens the triple helix of collagen[102]. Melatonin is released at night when magnetic field is high but only when brain lowers the thermostat in the hypothalamus. Melatonin produced during sleep uncouples electron transport chain but only when there is ready supply of Free Fatty Acids. It tightens proteins just as a powerful antioxidant do. Blue light 450-495 nm, (606-668 T Hz, 2.5 - 2.75 eV) destroys melatonin [103].

---

101   http://coconutrevival.com/?p=1031
102   http://www.ncbi.nlm.nih.gov/pubmed/196590
103   http://www.nytimes.com/2011/07/05/health/05light.html?_r=0

1.04.02.05 Paramagnetic Materials in Mitochondria

Iron sulfur clusters are paramagnetic quantum clusters. Let us call them electromagnetic compass that tell mitochondria what the environment calls for. In a way they manage generation of IR light.

No wonder why a majority of enzyme complex systems of electron transport chain are iron-sulfur proteins. They can also have iron, transition metal molybdenum, and Flavin. These clusters can be inserted or removed from the proteins on as needed basis. **Their key role is to sense oxygen and iron.**

Iron-Sulfur cluster can have three oxidation states of different magnetic properties: Fe_2S_2, Fe_3S_3, and Fe_4S_4. These clusters are responsible for inelastic quantum tunneling and vibrational changes in blue light excited electrons, a phenomenon common to smell, the oldest mode of perception in living beings. All life forms have iron-sulfur clusters, Flavin, FMN and FAD.

Flavin Mononucleotide and Flavin Adenine dinucleotide based on vitamin riboflavin structure have triplet states whereby maximum number of electrons have paired spin. Please note that singlets have only one paired electron spin.

1.04.02.06 Role of Free Fatty Acids

Free fatty acids are essential for proton transport across inner mitochondrial membrane because proton currents need free fatty acids [104]. These molecules recognize the uncoupling protein CCP_2 and help uncouple oxygen consumption in electron transport chain. No FFA simply means no uncoupling. Thermogenin protein CCP_2 dissipates proton gradient and produce heat as IR light [105].

1.04.02.07 Cold Thermogenesis

Cold increases dielectric constant of water and water can condense or shrink when cold more than it does by IR radiation effects. Water condenses under thermal effects for more efficient mass. We sweat when there is too much

---

104   http://www.ncbi.nlm.nih.gov/pubmed/17588527
105   http://www.ncbi.nlm.nih.gov/pubmed/11850613

heat. Semi conductive current is faster in cooler environment. Noteworthy is the fact that temperature has massive effect on coherence. Cold thermogenesis increases uncoupling of energy production in mitochondria [106], [107]. It is a very ancient pathway that permits evolution to allow survial in tough environments [108].

Food molecules are not only the repository of electrons and protons but they also serve carriers and donors. The movement of electrons and protons is the basis of body and brain wide communication.

Audit and Control

1.05 Mitochondria Make Mitochondria

Every cell with mitochondria in it is an electrochemical laboratory. New mitochondria are created by other mitochondria in response to stimuli of stress and other environmental factors under control by both nuclear and mitochondrial genes [109]. PGC-1α and PGC-1β (Peroxisome-Proliferator-Activated receptor) family of master genes, the key to energy metabolism [110], are the most important players in regard to stress and environmental relationships[111]. **Peroxysome is a small organelle involved in breakdown of fat, amino acids, and branched chain fatty acids.**

1.06 Birth and Death of Our Cells

On an average 50-70 billion cells die each day [112]. So part of us dies every day and what dies needs to be replenished. Our cells die because of age, infection, and inflammation. Also, they are killed by mitochondria only to be reborn by a programmed process Our hair grows and we get it cut at the barber shop, Our nail grows beyond what defies beauty and we cut it off. We clean our tongue daily and discard a whole lot of taste buds. Inside

106   http://journals.plos.org/plosone/article?id=10.1371/journal.pone.0001777
107   http://www.jci.org/articles/view/68993
108   http://jackkruse.com/cold-thermogenesis-6-the-ancient-pathway/
109   http://www.ncbi.nlm.nih.gov/pmc/articles/PMC3883043/
110   http://advan.physiology.org/content/30/4/145
111   http://www.ncbi.nlm.nih.gov/pubmed/20533901
112   http://answers.wikia.com/wiki/On_average,_how_many_cells_die_in_your_body_per_day

the body the stomach cells die and are discarded every day. The average of 50-70 billion that die each day include all kind of different cells [113]. We begin to age when death rate exceeds the birth rate. Obvious ones are hair, nails, and skin cells that we witness being born week by week. Around 2.4 million red blood cells are replaced every second which translates to 207.3 billion per day or 1% of the total. Our neurons last almost lifelong [114]. New research does show, however, that nutrition based epigenetic switch can create new neurons [115].

Skin cells last for no more than 4 weeks and white blood cells for only a week. Overall our cells divide almost 2 trillion times each day under very rigorous control [116]. The daily food and its nutritional quality maintains this balance, in particular, the consumption of methylation diet containing antioxidant and trace minerals like selenium, copper, iron, zinc, and sulfur.

1.07 Cellular Communication and Signaling

Principles of cellular communication[117] and cross-talk are core topics of molecular biology and proteins are the keyn to cellular communication. Our cells communicate to each other via signals and protein receptors in response to another cell's command or the environment [118]. Signals pass from a protein to another protein and they can be directed to brain, to nucleus, or another part of the body. **Cells are always in contact with the brain and the genome in the nucleus.** For effective electron transport the genes are expressed all the time as a matter of housekeeping [119]. For other purposes, the cells talk to nucleus, nucleus releases DNA or genes, genes get decoded or transcribed, and new proteins are produced on demand. Cell cycle itself determines a lot. **Actually, what and when we eat something may determine this process much more than our current understanding.**

---

113   http://www.livescience.com/33179-does-human-body-replace-cells-seven-years.html
114   http://www.ninds.nih.gov/disorders/brain_basics/ninds_neuron.htm
115   http://www.hopkinsmedicine.org/news/media/releases/growth_of_new_brain_cells_requires_epi-genetic_switch
116   http://askabiologist.asu.edu/content/cells-divide
117   http://www.ncbi.nlm.nih.gov/books/NBK26813/
118   http://learn.genetics.utah.edu/content/cells/insidestory/
119   http://www.ploscompbiol.org/article/info%3Adoi%2F10.1371%2Fjournal.pcbi.1003161

1.08 Mitochondrial DNA and Genes

Mitochondria in our cells have 37 genes in their circular genome and all of these genes are of purely maternal contribution. All 13 proteins required for electron transport are mitochondrial gene products. In addition, mitochondria help make 24 essential polypeptides for electron transport, 2 RNA_s and 22 m RNA_s. **The basic metabolic rate, control of energy production, weight, and obesity are governed by mitochondrial genes [120]. Our general health depends highly on these genes [121] and new research under mitochondrial proteome initiative is revealing a lot more about their specific roles [122].** Some 200 mutations of mitochondrial DNA found to date are involved in diseases such as diabetes II, hypertension, and neurogenerative diseases like Parkinson's, Huntington's, and Alzheimer's [123], [124].

No wonder why our longevity depends greatly on mitochondrial DNA and so does cell growth, death, performance of heart and lung and daily metabolism. Our health and well being simply means health, integrity, and stability of mitochondrial genes. The entire energy production by electron transfer uses complex enzyme proteins that are made by mitochondrial DNA with help from nuclear DNA. Mutations of DNA of either origin and malproduction of enzymes they encode causes health problems.

Energy Production And DNA Damage

1.09 Energy Production

Mitochondria produce energy molecule ATP via electron transport chain a process whereby electrons are produced from bonds of glucose from carbohydrates or from fats and proteins that we consume [125]. **Our ability to do mechanical work is actually proton pumping power of ATP synthase in our cell's mitochondria.** Ten protons are used to produce three molecule of ATP [126]. Since one pair of electron translocates 10 protons, an ATP molecule

---

120   http://www.ncbi.nlm.nih.gov/pmc/articles/PMC2880836/
121   http://www.ncbi.nlm.nih.gov/books/NBK7587/
122   http://acceleratingscience.com/proteomics/the-mitochondrial-human-proteome-initiative/
123   http://www.mitoaction.org/living-well-mitochondrial-disease?gclid=COPM44Kykr0CFZJj7A-odDg8ASg
124   http://www.nature.com/scitable/topicpage/mtdna-and-mitochondrial-diseases-903
125   http://www.ncbi.nlm.nih.gov/books/NBK26904/
126   http://biology.stackexchange.com/questions/3186/given-atp-synthases-structure-how-can-3-33-

is created by 1/3 power of an electron pair. That is how ATP is made from . As noted earlier, four spent electrons are finally used to reduce oxygen to water. During this process of ATP production, superoxide, hydrogen peroxide, and hydroxyl free radicals are produced as reactive oxygen species when the reduction process uses only one electron. These free radicals cause cellular damage and inflammation.

Mitochondria are a bit alkaline and negatively charged. Electron transport from glucose to oxygen takes place in steps. Hydrogen and electron currents simply move protons for ATP production through a proton pumping molecular motor, the famous enzyme ATP synthase. **ATP Energy, about 200 milliVolt, is released in small increments. Actually, it is the sum of electrical potential and proton concentration through a spatially separated oxidation-reduction system.** The process is miraculously 90% efficient and the inner membrane of mitochondria is key substructure that helps pick up electrons on one side and transferring protons uphill to the other side in the intermediate space below the outer membrane. The hydraulics of downhill flow of protons helps make ATP.

1.10 Mitochondrial DNA Damage

Mitochondrial genome functions as a single dynamic cellular unit. They help us use exceedingly mobile water protons for our daily life functions of building, growth, and immunity. Unlike nuclear DNA, mitochondrial DNA is not coiled around any spool of histone protein [127]. It have its own loop very like old fashioned bacterial DNA. As such it is subject to easy damage by electrons that leak off the electron transport chain and become free radicals[128]. This situation is rather precarious for mitochondria in skeletal muscles, lungs, liver, neurons, and heart cells causing diseases[129],[130]. Other problems due to mitochondrial DNA mutation include inefficiency in ATP production, accelerated aging, cancer, cardiac hypertension, dementia, deafness, peripheral neuropathy, diabetes, migraines, epilepsy, optic neuropathy, and constipation. The fact is that good health is possible only with highly functional and healthy mitochondria.

---

protons-ultimately-synthesize-one-a
127   http://www.leica-microsystems.com/science-lab/mitochondrial-dna-molecules-are-packaged-individually/
128   http://nar.oxfordjournals.org/content/35/22/7505.full
129   http://www.nature.com/nrn/journal/v9/n7/fig_tab/nrn2417_F1.html
130   http://www.ncbi.nlm.nih.gov/books/NBK26894/

Considerations of Our Daily Food

1.11 A Day in the Life of Mitochondrial.

To repeat for emphasis let us start with a 2000 kilocalorie per day diet for a person weighing 70 Kg. If all energy nutrients were glucose, this person needs 2.98 moles of glucose per day plus all necessary vitamins, minerals, antioxidants, and precursors for cofactor nutrients. That is 536.8 grams or close to a pound and quarter of well sected food. Divide this gram number by molecular weight of glucose (180.155) to arrive at 2.98 moles. It is good to restate and summarise as to what our mitochondria does with 2.98 moles of glucose on each day.

a) Mitochondria produces 34 molecules of ATP from 1 molecule of glucose. Two others are produced in glycolysis making a total of 36. From 2.98 moles of glucose, total ATP per day is 107.28 moles of ATP.

b) Also, since one glucose processing by mitochondria produces 10 NADH, mitochondria extracts electrons in 29.8 moles or 19,771 grams (19.771 Kg) NADH.

c) By similar logic, $FADH_2$ requirement per day calculates to 2.98 X 2 X 786.55 MW = 4.687 Kg.

d) ATP and the electron carriers participate in myriads of reactions and evolution has mandated that they be recycles or else our life will be impossible. ATP recycle is almost 500 times a day.

e) Mitochondria manage 3 moles of proton per mole of ATP or a total of 321.84 moles of protons per day. This translates to 32.184 moles of electrons. Each mole of proton is 5.21 Kcal and 381 moles a day translate to 1,985 Kcalories.

f) Going back to 2.98 moles of glucose per day, each mole made with 48 moles of phontons during photosynthesis, our daily consumption of sun's energy by way of glucose alone is 143.04 moles of photons. We need 22 moles (1.5 lb) of oxygen per day to dispose of spent electrons from 2.98 moles of glucose [131].

---

131   http://advan.physiology.org/content/ajpadvan/271/6/S43.full.pdf

g) Let us keep in mind that only one mole of photon with 4.06 Kcal can raise the temperature of a liter of water by 40 degree C. Our daily life depends on a great deal of energy. Just think that only 150 mVolt across 4.5 billionth of a meter across inner mitochondrial membrane translates to 30 million volts across a meter. That is some power at nano-scale operation in biology.

h) Behind this power are electrons, protons, and free radicals. Let us never forget that we live by the spin of electrons and mitochondria manage the spins of electrons and free radicals. Current runs through electron transfer complexes like an electromagnetic compass and **Mitochondrial Inner Membrane Organizing System** (MINOS) continuously talks to mitochondria.

ATP, NADH, and $FADH_2$ are involved in numerous other signaling and communications' activitties and not just ATP production. Flavin mononucleotide or riboflavin 5-phosphate is another key vitamin derivative embedded in the structure of electron transport enzyme complex structures that accepts electrons from NADH. Underlying the key functions of these electron carriers is proper intake of vitamins niacin and riboflavin and mineral phosphate. Our cells have no more than 0.3 mole of NAD or 212 gram. Again what is critical is NAD^+/NADH ratio of 3:10 for mammals [132]. **It seems to be important in adding years to our life, preventing age associated diseases, and in securing values from calorie restricted diet** [133]. In simple terms NAD^+/NADH ratio is a shuttle for moving around hydrogen for storage or just simple transfer. We need 15-20 mg/day. Healthy mitochondria maintain critical proton gradient via NAD^+/NADH ratio.

NADH is a natural coenzyme and is best found in fresh foods, **rather exclusively from non plant foods like meat, chicken, and fish.** Human body can't make it. Brain cells have 50 micromoles/g body weight, heart cells 90, and red blood cells only 4 microMoles/g body weight. In general it is close to 0.3 millimoles in animal cell [134]. NADH is necessary for animals with locomotive power and high mitochondrial performance. Nucleotide core goes far beyond DNA as building block of the code of life, the DNA. Our entire electronic life revolves around nucleotides of one or the other kind -

---

132   http://en.wikipedia.org/wiki/Nicotinamide_adenine_dinucleotide
133   http://web.mit.edu/biology/guarente/references/15.pdf
134   http://en.wikipedia.org/wiki/Nicotinamide_adenine_dinucleotide

NADH, FADH$_2$, and FMN. Too bad that they are destroyed by modern food processing[135].

NAD when present at sufficient level prevents tumor growth and carcinogenesis [136], [137]. Enzyme PARP1 consumes NAD for DNA repair and its excessive activation is deleterious to pancreatic β-cells in Type I diabetes [138]. NAD+ depletion increases genomic instability, propensity to gastrointestinal cancer, and cellular energy crisis [139]. Another NAD+ dependent enzyme is Sirtuin which is actually a protein deacylase involved in regulating DNA decoding, cell division cycle, response to DNA damaging agents, and aging [140], [141]. NAD+ seems to affect the process of aging, the metabolism, and age related diseases [142]. This makes niacin (vitamin B$_3$) very important in day to day nutrition. SIRT3, SIRT4, and SIRT5 are found in mitochondrial matrix. This logic of molecular biology tells us to consume niacin or vitamin B$_3$ in sufficient amount from chicken, fish, and beef. The vegetarians can get enough of it from avocado, green peas, mushrooms, roasted peanuts, and sunflower seeds.

Human biology is a complex story of reduction-oxidation systems and just in time hydrogen storage and transfer. Key to our optimal biology is proper dose of nutrients such as vitamins B$_2$, B$_3$, folic acid, and vitamin K by way of our daily methylation diet. Vital signs and vital functions of our vital organs can be maintained only with good foods capable of delivering antioxidants, vitamins, and minerals such as iron, magnesium, calcium, copper, manganese, sulfer, and molybdenum. The electron transfer system in the mitochondria depends on them.

Immortal mitochondria control our life by controlling the present and future of our cells. We should hope to live long with a belief that each cell in our body is conscious and that the cell gets its power from mitochondria. Healthy mitochondria can help remake our life, behavior, and consciousness that goes with it. They must be fed well though not only with electrons but also with electron managing antioxidants and metabolic cofactors such that free radicals never exceed 1%. The key to good health is methylation diet.

135   http://web.mit.edu/athletics/sportsmedicine/wcrvitamins.html
136   http://www.ncbi.nlm.nih.gov/pubmed/10331640
137   http://link.springer.com/chapter/10.1007/978-1-4419-8740-2_10#page-1
138   http://diabetes.diabetesjournals.org/content/51/5/1470.abstract
139   http://www.hindawi.com/journals/jna/2010/157591/
140   http://www.ncbi.nlm.nih.gov/pmc/articles/PMC416462/
141   http://www.uniprot.org/uniprot/Q96EB6
142   http://jcs.biologists.org/content/124/6/833.full.pdf

1.12 Foods for Mitochondria

An emphasis on methylation diet in this book has the message of consuming controlled calorie diet containing all essential nutrients of fat and protein along with vitamins, minerals, and antioxidants. Calorie restriction diet simply implies less work and longer life of mitochondria for overall longevity [143]. Asian medicine and mineral micronutrients keep mitochondria active and efficient by their antioxidative and antiinflammatory effects [144]. Also, probiotic lactobacilli are known to effectively modulate mitochondrial function [145], [146]. Foods like yogurt, kimchee, and sour Kraut can combat mitochondrial dysfunction of chronic fatigue syndrome. Such fermented foods are known to prevent cancer and improve our immune system [147]. Even gut hormones affect cognition via mitochondrial function.

Naturally mitochondria *are major* pharmacological target for chronic disease control [148]. They can be trained to kill cancer cells, act as vectors for chemotherapy, and receive and promote drug functions and effects and the role of mitochondria in neurodegenerative diseases such as Parkinson's, Alzheimer's, and Huntington's is now more apparent than a decade ago. Use of antidiabetic sulfonyl ureas, immune suppression and anti-tumor drugs, antilipidemic medicines, antiviral agents, and drugs for potassium channel opening are good examples. *ATP per se regulates potassium channel functions, aging, and blood pressure.* Low blood glucose and low oxygen supply to brain cells is a problem for mitochondria [149], [150], [151].

Foods with antioxidants can prevent peroxidation and damage of mitochondrial DNA. For example, quircetin from apple and onion, a flavonoid antioxidant with anti-inflammatory and antihistamine power, seems to be a promoter of mitochondrial biogenesis [152]. This is why we must include berries, red grapes, purple fruits and vegetables, licorice, and onion in our daily antioxidant rich methylation diet [153].

---

143 https://www.fightaging.org/archives/2011/04/calorie-restriction-increases-mitochondrial-biogene-sis.php
144 http://www.nature.com/news/screen-uncovers-hidden-ingredients-of-chinese-medicine-1.10430
145 http://www.ncbi.nlm.nih.gov/pmc/articles/PMC2909492/
146 http://www.ncbi.nlm.nih.gov/pmc/articles/PMC3890654/
147 http://www.microbialcellfactories.com/content/12/1/71
148 http://pharmrev.aspetjournals.org/content/54/1/101.long
149 http://www.drmyhill.co.uk/wiki/brain_fog_-_poor_memory,_difficulty_thinking_clearly_etc
150 http://drmyhill.co.uk/wiki/CFS_-_The_Central_Cause:_Mitochondrial_Failure
151 http://www.cbn.com/health/naturalhealth/drsears_brainwellness.aspx
152 http://www.ncbi.nlm.nih.gov/pubmed/19516153
153 http://www.mitoresearch.org/treatmentdisease.html

We need to eat not only to get energy from electron bearing food molecules but also to quench reactive oxygen species and prevent routine damage to our DNA [154]. All 200 mutated DNA pass to the offspring from mother without any recombination [155], [156]. Methylation diet is the key to maintaining DNA stability, both nuclear and mitochondrial. Well designed methylation diet should provide all necessary nutrients (magnesium, manganese, zinc, iron, vitamin C, CoQ_{10}, vitamin K_2, vitamins C, E, and beta-carotene, pyrroquinoline quinone, alpha-lipoic acid, and even antioxidant carnosine from poultry, fish, and beef). N-acetyl cysteine and curcumine from turmeric are necessary for antioxidant glutathione, ubiquinone is necessary for Co Q_{10}, and pantothenic acid (B_5) is necessary for enzyme cofactor Co Enzyme A. Ubiquinol acts very much like vitamin C and beta-carotene. The value of isoprenoid antioxidants and vitamins will be considered in detail in chapter 5 on summation.

We now know that diet, exercise, and mindfulness promote mitochondrial health and enhance homeostatic controls [157]. This can be done by planned consumption of antioxidant rich methylation diet, exercise, yoga, and meditation. This book relies on last ten years of research in preparation of this primer on life supporting mitochondria, our vital signs, our vital organs, and mitochondrial diseases of brain, heart, lung, and kidney. Many references relevant to mitochondrial diseases and possible therapies for gene control are discussed in detail in chapter on summation.

Immortal mitochondria as John Kendew's thread of life runs the daily energetics of in terms of electrons, protons, ions, atoms, and molecules. It is about electrical current in every cell of our body, about birth and death of cells and mitochondria in them, about cross talk among cells and organelles within cells, and finally about making, repairing, editing mitochondrial and nuclear genes in our cells. Mitochondria are about repair of our organs and the proteome of proteins that regulates and sustains life. Much of today's research on these topics is possible because we now have the power of information theory. There are significant and authoritative book citations included in this chapter for readers who wish to gain fundamental understanding of DNA and their protein products. Also, included below is the list of major research institutions that our readers can consult for timely research on clinical and routine therapeutics.

---

154   http://www.ars.usda.gov/News/docs.htm?docid=17382
155   http://hihg.med.miami.edu/code/http/modules/education/Design/Print.asp?CourseNum=2&LessonNum=4
156   http://hihg.med.miami.edu/code/http/modules/education/Design/Print.asp?CourseNum=2&LessonNum=4
157   http://www.mindfulhealth.biz/store/#!/~/product/category=3151016&id=13557208

Major Research Institutions

Mitochondrial Protein Initiative: Italian Proteomics Association.

Mitochondrial Research Society

Society for Mitochondrial research and Medicine

Consortium for Mitochondrial research, University College, London

International Child Development Resource Center, Melbourne, FL 32934, USA

Biocenter, University of Basel, Switzerland

Medical Research Council, Mitochondrial Biology Unit, Welcome Trust John Hopkins Department of Cell biology

Harvard Medical School

2

We are designed to eat complex molecules of foods, produce electrons by breaking down their bonds, and live by electrons. This we accomplish by consuming water as the energy transformer of electron richfoods. An optimum daily water intake is necessary for optimum metabolic rate. Vitamins and minerals play a cruicial role. Mitochondria in our brain cells use vitamin A and D to produce electromotive force by using light. Water, light, and circadian rhythm, we now know, control our sustenance by electrons. Mitochondria of our salivary gland, stomach, pancreas, and small intestine get into action step by step the moment we think of eating. They expedite and facilitate breaking the bonds of food molecules to monomers like glucose, amino acids, and fatty acids and finally abstraction of electrons from them via a very complex process. Our body encounters varying energy cost for digestion and absorption of nutrients depending on the food type but this is one operating cost we should be glad to bear. It is amazing that the mitochondria at different places in our gastrointestinal tract control different specialized functions: enzyme amylase by salivary gland, hydrochloric acid by parietal cells in the stomach, bicarbonate and multiple enzymes by epithelial cells of pancreas, and hormone insulin. Nutrients are extremely important because they interact with genes, they help decode DNA and organize the protein sheath that covers the DNA, and routinely help manage the processes of gene expression and specific protein production. Vitamin and mineral rich methylation diet is a tool for DNA modification.

Electrons from our daily foods help produce life energy ATP but only with a appropriate diet of carbohydrate, fat, protein, vitamins, minerals, antioxidants, and other phytochemicals What matters is the right amount of nutrients at the right time. Calcium is critical to signaling by mitochondria and trace metals are necessary for electron transporting metallo-proteins of inner mitochondrial membrane. Even more critical are isoprene containing vitamins A, D, E, and K and omega -3 fatty acids. We are now learning that DHA (docosahexanoic acid) is a key molecule capable of converting sunlight into electronic signal. Light and water start mitochondria. Wholesome, and colorful fruits, vegetables, nuts, seeds and whole grains are good for our mitochondria. Such diets deliver vitamins, minerals, antioxidants, dietary fiber, and anticarcinogenic nutrients and help manage electrons, protons, and ions for producing life energy ATP. Such diets preserve stability of nuclear and mitochondrial DNA, expedite proper gene expression and production of proteins- enzymes, receptors, hormones, and neurotransmitters. Methylation foods run our metabolism optimally and yet precisely starting from gene expression to signaling for each and every reaction in our body. Daily nutrition preserves our biological state by serving stem cells for added longevity.

Chapter 2
Food for Mitochondrial Health

*Methylation diet times DNA modulation, produces energy as ATP,
and orchestrates the dance of electrons in enzyme complexes for
neuronal plasticity and stem cell preservation.*

Triveni P. Shukla

Our daily food is much more than source of calories. More critical are its functions in terms of perception and neurobiology of appetite, hunger, and satiety. Most important is the relationship of food nutrients and their level with DNA stability and gene expression. Cooking for taste, texture, and flavor matters just as much as the logical choice of foods for best delivery of nutrients depicted best by a Venn diagram. Flavorful calorie restricted methylation diet serves our body and its cells the best as long as we sleep well, get enough sun light, drink enough water, breath enough **paramagnetic oxygen**, and for sure include enough of **paramagnetic DHA** and other conjugated (alternate C=C double bond foods like conjugated linoleic acid) in our diet. The following paragraphs will show that good health is intrinsically tied to health of adult stem cell, neurotransmission and intelligence, and our conscious existence.

We learned in previous introductory chapter how energy in the bonds of carbohydrates, fats, and proteins are converted to chemical energy ATP, a process that involves electrons and protons. Beyond energy production, nutrients are also necessary for manufacturing and maintenance of DNA and DNA like basic structures of electron carriers, and of proteins that expedite and maintain the flow of electrons in mitochondria. They provide basic chemical groups for the manufacture of neurotransmitters and many other ion channel receptor and transporter proteins.

Nutrition in terms of essential amino acids, isoprenoid omega-3 and omega 6 fatty acids, isoprenoids vitamins, and metalloproteins is critical to our day to day health and life per se. Omega-3 fatty acid DHA is mitochondria's evolutionary companion in this regard. Actually, π-elections in alternating CH_2 bonds of isoprenoid nutrients and D-orbital electrons in trace transition metal in our daily diets are just as important in electronic movement and associated magnetism in our mitochondria as oxygen. We need an optimum combination of all **"paramagnetic"** nutrients including oxygen, DHA, and even free radicals in the aqueous ionic plasma in and around our cells. Gibb's free energy of ATP hydrolysis is the basis of our metabolism. No doubt nutritional biology is based on extraction of electrons from the bonds of glucose, fat, and amino acids for the formation of high energy ATP molecule by proton gradient. Nutrients function for metabolism both in and out side mitochondria in our cells, most critical being the nutrient for mitochondrial function [158].

Our cells need to make NADH, $FADH_2$, and $FMNH_2$ for electron shuttling, coenzyme A and lipoamide for acyl group, folate for one carbon units necessary for DNA methylation, S-adenosylmethionine for methyl group, and nucleoside triphosphate for nucleotides in DNA and RNA. Any deficiency causes poor health and disease.

Light and water start mitochondria and the electrons produced are connected, coupled, coordinated, and coherent. Foods we eat and hormones that our body produces are proxies to abstraction and addition of electrons in metabolic reactions. A key protein in this regard is MINOS (mitochondrial inner membrane organizing system) which interacts with water for energy conversion [159]. **The faster the electrons get through electron transport chain in mitochondria, the quicker is the set up of electric and magnetic fields in mitochondria.**

We should think of water as life's battery powered by sun and we should think that mitochondria tell our brain to have proper level of *paramagnetic* oxygen and DHA. The molecule of omega-3 fatty acid DHA is tied to our evolution as a conserved acyl component of signaling receptors. Its energies of π-electrons due to conjugation and with inductive effects of any substituents mean a lot to mitochondrial function and our existence

---

158   http://www.ncbi.nlm.nih.gov/pmc/articles/PMC1204426/
159   http://www.sciencedirect.com/science/article/pii/S0022283612003786

[160]. They are the basis of depolarization of retinal membranes and even overall constitution of our intelligence [161]. DHA can capture sunlight and electron current and send it to all places in the body by water and collagen network in our skin. Low DHA means a sick brain that doesn't know what to do with foods we eat because hormone leptin and the mechanism of cold thermogenesis have gone a bit amuck [162]. Melatonin release is during sleep hours in the night and, if uncontrolled, it uncouples the electron transport chain. If DHA is not replaced properly in our brain, leptin receptors are destroyed and hypothalamus is not set right for cold thermogenesis and energy allocation is out of order. Consequently the magnetic sense in the morning when light shows up is not up to the snuff. **Actually, not enough oxygen and not enough DHA means malfunctional mitochondria.** Low oxygen simply means less DHA no matter how much we eat. We get critical help from paramagnetic molecules such as oxygen, DHA, and the free radicals that mitochondria produces. Let us note that free radicals are used for cell signaling [163].

We need sun for a few hours a day to get appropriate dose of vitamin D_3. Also, we can and do suffer from poor neurotransmission and poor brain function when we have deficiency of essential amino acids. Essential fatty acids that we have come to know as omega-3 and omega-6 fatty acids are part of our brain structure and function [164]. Antioxidants that manage optimization and control electron transfer, electron shuttling, and free radical destruction on time and on demand are essential to our diet. Essential micro-minerals like iron, copper, magnesium, sulfur, and zinc are essential to structure and functioning of oxygen transporting hemoglobin and proteins of electron transport chain. Health values of isoprenoid antioxidant and vitamin molecules is well evidenced today by the produce section of a large retail store with many varieties fruits, vegetables, seeds, and nuts. This is a valuable trend in feeding mitochondria.

A good diet doesn't do it all. In order to stay healthy we must sleep well, manage our circadian rhythm well, and let sunlight during day time give proper direction to mitochondria in our cells. Circadian signals determine how we use electrons and thus the importance of minimum eight hour sleep. As a matter fact obesity is most likely because of altered circadian

---

160   http://www.terrapub.co.jp/onlineproceedings/fs/wfc2008/pdf/wfcbk_057.pdf
161   http://www.ncbi.nlm.nih.gov/pubmed/23206328
162   http://www.naturalnews.com/016353_omega-3_fatty_acids_mental_health.html
163   http://www.ncbi.nlm.nih.gov/pubmed/15051313
164   http://www.ncbi.nlm.nih.gov/pubmed/21279554

signaling and most of the signaling comes from mitochondria that have magnetic sense [165], [166].

Mitochondria as electromagnets in our cells have a lot to do with what happens to foods we eat and how is electronic energy allocated or appropriated. For example hormone leptin is connected to day light, water, and mitochondrial magnetism that organizes electron flow. Furthermore cold thermogenesis coordinated by environment engenders more magnetic mitochondria and higher rate of oxygen utilization [167], [168], [169].

Thermogenesis is a planned mitochondrial action. We need to think of thermogenesis as a physiological act of burning fat and reducing net calorie intake. Diet induced thermogenesis by foods like hot chili, black pepper, green tea, medium chain triglycerides of coconut oil, high fiber whole grains, ginger, and high protein foods including poultry, tofu, and lentils can help burn calories and help manage weight. **Exercise induces extra thermogenesis.** Even a calorie restricted methylation diet can be bad for mitochondria if not designed with only minimal level of refined sugar and high glycemic carbohydrates.

In context to all above, the best diet for our mitochondria is an antioxidant rich, low calories methylation or redox diet with complement of B vitamins, minerals, and vitamin A, C. D, E, and K , choline, and other antioxidants as phytonutrients. Vitamins and minerals through common foods have much better physiological value than supplements. **Methylation, addition of methyl group CH_3 to position 5 carbon of cytosine or guanine in our DNA, takes place billion times every second.** Obviously methyl donors like choline from lecithin or betaine, amino acid methionine, and folic acid are there to modify our DNA on demand and in time. Nutrients like B vitamins riboflavin, folate, B_6, B_{12}, choline, amino acids methionine, serine, cysteine, and glycine are necessary ingredients for methylation modification of our DNA. The reaction is tissue specific, non-random, and tightly regulated. Not all genes are active at all times and methylation is a tool for selective activation or even deactivation of genes. It can be caused by environment and stress for reprograming. Loss of control of DNA methylation causes ailments and diseases.

Methylation governs expression of specific genes via modification of specific sites on DNA. Methylation diets, it is easy to visualize, affect RNA

165   http://www.ncbi.nlm.nih.gov/pubmed/23869060
166   http://www.ncbi.nlm.nih.gov/pubmed/23159716
167   http://coconutrevival.com/?p=380
168   http://www.ncbi.nlm.nih.gov/pubmed/21558317
169   http://www.zafu.net/circadianrhythms.html

processing, affect our DNA, regulation of protein function particularly of histone of chromatin sheat which wraps our DNA in a bundle, and regulation of gene expression. As such it controls epigenetic effects of silencing a gene, inactivating X chromosome, and imprinting and reprograming. Methylation happens on 80-89% of CpG sites in human genome located as CpG islands in the DNA sequence. This is where most of promotors for ubiquitous genes are located. We now know that CpG methylation and transcription are inversely related. Methylation can even cause cancer which in a sense is represented by methylation state of DNA. A genome wide hypomethylation results in unstable chromosome vulnerable to mutation. We should recall our basic biochemistry of three hydrogen bond in GC base pair and two hydrogen bonds in AT base pair. Proton movements acroos these bonds have to do a lot with our daily life and health. The purine-pyrimidine base pairs are in a small space of 20 Angstrom such as to fit well in the DNA helix. Decoding and making of vital proteins happens in even a smaller space of 10-16 nanometers. Life is truly a nano-scale operation.

Our being in terms of embryonic development, genomic imprinting, X-chromosome inactivation, chromosome stability, and onset of a number of diseases depends on methylation. Methylation diet offers the best adult cell nutrition for long life including those of stem cells. Our health is the health of stem cells because some 79 diseases can be treated by stem cell therapy alone including arthritis, cancer, cardiovascular diseases, leukemia, autoimmune diseases, diabetes, lupus, and diseases of the cornea. Our daily diet must boost production of adult stem cells because we stay alive by our adult stem cells.

As key to homeostasis, stem cell mitochondria self regulate their function. Antiinflammatory nutrients including antioxidants (phycocyanins, cucurmin, silicate) and antiangiogenic nutrients B complex vitamins including folic acid, B_{12}, omega-3 fatty acids, minerals iron, selenium, and zinc are critical to adult stem cell nutrition. They can't tolerate high concentration of reactive oxygen species and oxidative stress. We need good blood circulation for timely delivery of stem cells, immune cells, and oxygen to all cells in our body.

Unfortunately we have run into a default diet over the last 60 some years that has caused deficiencies of vitamin D, mineral magnesium, and selenium along with possible deficiencies of iron, copper, sulfur, and manganese. Loaded with extra refined sugars, high glycemic carbohydrates, and saturated and trans fats the default diet makes mitochondria work over time. **Trans fats simply can't substitute for cis-DHA and too much glucose is a kind of physiological taxation on mitochondria.** Antioxidants like CoenzymQ$_{10}$, Pyrroloquiniline Quinone, selenium, various adaptogens, and probiotics can enhance mitochondrial health.

What we need to consume for the health of our mitochondria are antioxidants (Coenzyme Q10, melatonin, pyrooquinoline quinone, melatonin, glutathione), trace minerals , omega-3 fatty acids, and NADH (vitamin niacin). Poor intake of omega-3 is the reason for many of our brain disorders [170]. Common fruits and vegetable, plant and dairy proteins, grapes and wine, sprouts, and fermented foods can be incorporated in our weekly dishes for effective mitochondrial health and **not supplements.** In addition, such foods deliver critical nutrients of gamma amino butyric acid, melatonin, alpha-lipoic acid, coenzyme Q$_{10}$, glutathione, and N-Acetyl-carnitine.

Spice mixes like Dukha of Egypt, Curry powder of India, and Zetar of Palestine add not only the ethnically well tried flavors but also antioxidants, antibacterials, anticarcinogens, essential mineral and vitamin nutrients. We need to practice intelligent nutrition. No wonder why the top chefs on the globe are now perfecting the arts of flavoring our daily methylation dishes with herms, spices, and condiments.

Human body is built, sustained, and allowed to grow in good health by air we breathe for oxygen - the terminal electron acceptor, water we drink for abundant supply of protons, and food and beverage we eat for electronic energy stored in their bonds. In order to have a balanced metabolism, we must consume vitamins, minerals, and essential nutrients that our body can't make. **The latter are needed for inter-conversions of matter and energy by metabolic processes.**

Scientists are describing the quantum mechanics of smell that resides in the vibrations of small and big molecules of food as primary criteria of food selection by our brain [171], [172]. Quantum mechanics of smell is the main component of flavor and **flavor and smell are connected to** our brain in constant search for nutrition.

We must caution ourselves that carbohydrate foods make neurons swell and bring in glutamate excess causing hyper polarization and calcium efflux [173],[174]. Even worse are high fat diets that affect hydrogen peroxide production

170   http://www.terrapub.co.jp/onlineproceedings/fs/wfc2008/pdf/wfcbk_057.pdf
171   http://phys.org/news89542035.html
172   http://cup.columbia.edu/book/neurogastronomy/9780231159104
173   http://people.csail.mit.edu/seneff/EJIM_PUBLISHED.pdf
174   http://en.wikipedia.org/wiki/Glutamate_receptor

and create metabolic grounds for insulin resistance and oxidative stress [175]. To avoid such problems, we need to consume nuts and seeds, spices and herbs, grain and legume sprouts, and chocolate. Calorie restricted diets are good for cerebral biogenesis and redox state [176]. Methylation diets containing flavoproteins in particular repair free radicals and impact on magnetic sense of our cells [177]. Research shows that a flavorful calorie restricted methylation diet is ideal for mitochondria[178].

The very idea of war time FDA mandated fortification of wheat flour wirh iron, Thiamin (B_1), riboflavin (B_2), and niacin (B_3) during nineteen forties and 50 years later with folic acid (B_9) in 1998 is in effect meant for mitochondrial health. We now know of the critical importance of reduced iron and sulfur, NAD^+ from niacin, and FMN and FAD flavoproteins from riboflavin that maintain the functional efficiency of the ATP producing electron transport chain in mitochondria. There would not be any electron transfer without Iron-sulfur clusters in enzyme complexes of the electron transport chain. Too bad our daily default diet didn't contain enough vitamin and mineral fortified bread and we didn't consume enough fruits and vegetables in order to meet nutrient RDA_s during the 70_s, 80_s, and even 90_s. The consequence is an onslaught of chronic diseases and an epidemic of pain. Solution to many of these problems is properly designed methylation diet.

This chapter has footnotes on key considerations of diet based therapeutics of mitochondria in addition to reference citations for additional reading. There shall be a detailed coverage on antioxidants and omega three fatty acids in chapter 5.

Diet and Disease Connection

Good food and good life style aim at good health of mitochondria. Let us review, therefore, a list of all recently researched topics of food nutrients that affects oue health by their effects on mitochondria including

- acetyl carnitine involved in redox homeostasis

- alpha-lipoic acid in autonomic diabetic neuropathy

- amino acids and glutathione in Alzheimer's disease

---

175   http://www.ncbi.nlm.nih.gov/pubmed/23473496
176   http://www.pnas.org/content/103/6/1768.abstract
177   http://rsfs.royalsocietypublishing.org/content/3/5/20130037
178   http://link.springer.com/referenceworkentry/10.1007%2F978-1-4614-4788-7_78#page-1

- arginine in stroke and antioxodants in multiple sclerosis
- B vitamins in neurocognition and others related to dietary antidiabetic medications
- ATP production and neuromuscular disease
- Coenzyme Q and enhanced ATP production
- Creatinine and mitochondrial cytopathy
- Cucurmin from turmeric in metabolism of omega-3 fatty acids
- Diets as they relates to cardiovascular diseases
- Deficiency of B vitamin riboflavin in case of inefficiency of complex II of electron transport chain
- Diet connected to insulin resistance
- Diet in DNA repair and DNA demethylation
- Diets connected to alpha-actin gene
- Diet in autoimmune disease lupus,
- Diet connection to congestive heart failure
- Dietary polyphenolic antioxidants and aging of brain
- Dynamics of DNA methylation and demethylation
- Exercise for brain and muscular health by DNA shifting
- Flavolignans (silymarin) connected to stress reduction
- Folic acid as it relates to DNA repair and anti-carcinogenesis
- Gamma aminobutyric acid against depression
- Glutamate and production of reactive oxygen species
- High fat diet and obesity
- Low superoxide dismutase activity and stress
- Omega-3 fatty acid against multiple sclerosis
- Green tea theanine antioxidants
- Oxidative damage of DNA strand breakage
- Methylation diet against mental disorders

- Mitochondrial coupling and general functions

- Mitochondrial energy and basal metabolic rate

- NADH and diabetes

- Oxidative stress, diabetes and poor DNA repair

- Pesticides and Parkinson's disease

- Resveratrol against cancer

- Reactive oxygen species and cancer

- Taurine for health of mitochondria

- Trace minerals of copper, iron, and Selenium in osteoporosis

- Vitamin B_{12} and nervous system

- Vitamin D and problems of cancer, multiple sclerosis, and immune system.

We use about net 5% pure oxygen present in 11,000 liters of air we breathe daily [179]. Daily need of water for men is 3 liters and for women about 2.5 liters [180]. Essential amino acids such as arginine, cysteine, glutamate, proline, serine, and tyrosine, essential fatty acids such as omega-3 and omega-6 fatty acids, cofactors, minerals, and vitamins are required for efficient metabolic operations in general and those of mitochondrial function in particular.

Let us keep in mind that most of metabolism of Krebs cycle happens in the mitochondrial matrix and electron transfer happens in the mitochondrial inner membrane. There is convincing research indicating that the health of mitochondria is diet and lifestyle dependent. Naturally, nutrition plays a huge role for mitochondrial functions [181]. A diet for health maintenance and well being should eliminate excessive consumption of sugary foods and beverages because they reduce mitochondrial efficiency by simple overload [182],[183],[184], [185], [186]. Worst is the lack of exercise which reduces number

179   http://highered.mcgraw-hill.com/sites/dl/free/0073048763/232418/chapter01.pdf
180   http: http://biochemgen.ucsd.edu/mmdc/ep-15-16.pdf
33//www.mayoclinic.org/healthy-living/nutrition-and-healthy-eating/in-depth/water/art-20044256
181
182   http://www.ars.usda.gov/News/docs.htm?docid=17382
183   http://californiaagriculture.ucanr.edu/landingpage.cfm?article=ca.v065n03p141&fulltext=yes
184   http://www.naturalnews.com/031997_mitochondria_support.html
185   http://www.marksdailyapple.com/managing-your-mitochondria-nutrients-and-supplements/#ax-zz2wWx4nWJP
186   http://www.livestrong.com/article/336968-mitochondrial-repair-diet/

of mitochondria in active muscle cells and makes them inefficient and vulnerable to production of free radicals.

We can fine-tune mitochondrial functions by choosing a lifestyle that includes regular exercise, consuming colorful fresh fruits and vegetables, avoiding high glycemic refined sugar foods and beverages, controlling appetite and restricting daily calorie intake, and avoiding alcohol and smoking [187]. The tune up includes routine detoxification, balancing of hormones, and preventing inflammation.

The Health of Mitochondria

2.01 Maintaining healthy mitochondria

Poor function of mitochondria means poor energy production accompanied by more free radical production. Free radicals escape the electron transport chain and cause damage to both mitochondrial and nuclear DNA. Dysfunctions of mitochondria lead to cancer [188]. This can and does cause early cell death [189]. We can fight many diseases by feeding our mitochondria right kind of foods[190], foods that have been described as methylation diet in my book on "Our Genes Our Foods Our Lifestyle". The first step in mitochondrial tune up is to restrict daily intake of calories including those from refined sugar. Refined sugar consumption should be restricted to a maximum of no more than 20 grams per day [191]. Current consumption of more than 198 gram per day of carbohydrate of which 57 gram is refined table sugar is for sure a major cause of mitochondrial overload causing chronic diseases.

2.02 Calorie Restricted Diet for Mitochondrial Health

Longevity diet[192] and paleo diets[193] are simply subsets of methylation diet, a nomenclature we will stay by in this book. A sustained effort to consume at

---

187   http://www.lef.org/magazine/mag2010/feb2010_Reverse-Mitochondrial-Damage_01.htm
188   http://www.ncbi.nlm.nih.gov/pubmed/20732299
189   http://www.biologynews.net/archives/2005/12/04/getting_old_slowing_down_blame_inefficient_mi-tochondria.html
190   http://mda.org/disease/mitochondrial-myopathies/causes-inheritance
191   http://www.accessdata.fda.gov/scripts/cdrh/cfdocs/cfcfr/cfrsearch.cfm?fr=101.9
192   http://www.longevitydiet.info/
193   http://paleodiet.com/

least 30% less calories, say a total per day of only 1,500 Calories in case of a 150 lb weight person, simply spares mitochondria of excess work load by 25%. This is believed to add years to life span because a calorie restricted diet improves regeneration of mitochondria [194]. Proper protein intake under restricted calorie conditions has a significant multiplier effect [195], [196]. Furthermore, calorie restriction promotes mitochondrial gene expression [197]. Cardiac SIRTUINS (protein enzymes necessary for cellular activity) extend longevity when a restricted calories intake is maintained over long period of time [198]. We should commit to consuming 25-30% less calories high protein diet per day, say at 75% full stomach. This improves longevity by efficient and healthy mitochondria on one hand and desirable and timely gene expression on the other.

2.03 Methylation Diet Meets RDA of vitamins and Minerals

A diet based on six servings of fruits and vegetables as salads, fresh juices, canned V8, dips, salsa, mixed vegetable soup, and other side dish preparations of seeds, and nuts as daily snacks can easily deliver required RDA of vitamins and minerals along with many other phytonutrients. Amount and variety of fruits and vegetable consumption should exceed the per capita consumption of 2004 given in Table 2.04.01.

As described in Table 2.04.02 vitamins B$_1$ is great for managing Parkinson's and Alzheimer's disease and B$_2$ and B$_3$ are literally brain nutrients. A plateful of 500 g kale consumed is a valuable source of sulfur containing amino acids. Cruciferacea vegetables cabbage and cauliflower and deep green high chlorophyll spinach, kale, mustard green, chard, and collard green are excellent sources of B vitamins and coenzymes that serve as mitochondrial food.

194   http://www.ncbi.nlm.nih.gov/pubmed/22901095
195   http://www.ncbi.nlm.nih.gov/pubmed/22901095
196   http://www.sciencedirect.com/science/article/pii/S1097276512009057
197   http://www.hindawi.com/journals/ijcb/2012/759583/
198   http://www.hindawi.com/journals/omcl/2013/528935/

Table 2.04.01 Per Capita Consumption of Fruits and Vegetables

in lbs (2004, ER S report of 2006)

Commodity Fresh Frozen Canned

Foods	Fresh	Frozen	Canned
Asparagus	1.00	0.07	0.20
Beans, Snap	1.90	1.90	3.70
Carrots	8.90	1.60	1.20
Corn	9.60	9.1	8.2
Green peas		1.90	1.20
Mushroom	2.6-		1.60
Peaches and nectarines	5.10	0.55	3.60
Pine apple	4.4		4.80
Spinach	2.1	(Total for all) 0.93	
Tomatoes	19.30		70.40

2.04 Antioxidants for mitochondria

Antioxidants present in fruits and vegetables are well known to neutralize free radicals. Recent research suggests that they work differently in the body (*in vivo*) than in the laboratory. *It is now also known that some antioxidants, in particular the polyphenols, glutathione, and lipoic acid have a direct effect on mitochondria for higher efficiency in energy production and the effect is similar to that induced in mitochondria by exercise[199].*

Consumption of vegetables listed in Table 2.04.01 should almost double during our senior years because the nutrients in them (Table 2.02.02) prevent free radical production. **Beet greens, collard, kale and spinach are truly multivitamin and multi-trace mineral foods readily available in the produce section of today's retail food stores.** Furthermore, sea weed and algae to our daily dish helps secure trace mineral. **Two Brazil nuts, four almonds, and four walnuts for daily snack can supply daily requirement**

---

199   http://lpi.oregonstate.edu/infocenter/othernuts/la/

of antioxidant mineral selenium, mineral magnesium, omega-3 fatty acids. Common phenolic antioxidants (phenolic acid, high molecular weight tannins, flavones, and flavonols) can total up to 30-40 mg/g in commonly used herbs and spices including basil, mint, marjoram, oregano, rosemary, sage, and thyme [200].

Table 2.04.02 A Chart of Functions of Mitochondrial Nutrients

Nutrient	Function	Food Source	Daily Dose
Probiotics	Boost immune system. Probiotics build the second genome.	Pickles, sour kraut, yogurt; balance your daily bacterial intake.	1 cup Kefir or yogurt gives 500 billion bacteria. So will sour karat.
Omega-3 Fatty Acids	Myelin formation and key to signaling; LDL and HDL ratio mirrors omega-6 and omega-3 ratio. Brain is largely Omega-3 fatty acid.	Flax seed in soya sauce and vinegar, walnut, fish oil, salmon, and eggs.	3 grams per day
Antioxidants	Help mitochondria quench toxic free radicals gone amok off the ATP production chain.	Brazil nut and highly colored fruits and vegetables : peach, carrots, squash, and berries	300 grams can easily come from 500 gram fruits and vegetables.
Pyrroloquinoline Quinone (PQQ)	Growth of mitochondria, quitting down N-Methyl-D-Aspirate, and healing of brain	Fermented soybean (Natto), green tea, tofu, potato, carrot, edamami, and broad beans.	10-20 mg per day[201]

200   http://www.notulaebiologicae.ro/index.php/nsb/article/viewFile/5638/5520
201   http://www.benbest.com/nutrceut/MiscSupp.html

Nutrient	Function	Food Source	Daily Dose
Thiamine B_1	Needed for ATP production, needed along with B_{12} for making myelin. Good for mood control.	Sunflower seed, yeast, spinach, tomato, asparagus, black beans, kale, and mushrooms.	Up to 100 mg per day (not Stored)
Riboflavin B_2	Part of FADH for ATP production, helps eliminate toxins, good for mitochondrial health.	Almond, broccoli, asparagus, fish	Up to 200 mg per day
Niacin amide B_3	Boosts ATP production and fights autoimmune disorders.	Shrimp, mushrooms, potato with skin.	Less than 500 mg per day
Pyridoxin B_6	Builds neurons, helps make serotonin, GABA,	Garlic, cauliflower, mustard green, mushroom, kale, collard, chard	75 mg per day
Vitamin B_{12}	Makes myelin and hemoglobin and prevents anemia. Good for mood and impulse control.	Fermented foods, yeast, salmon, egg yolk, beef, and algae.	500 microgram per day
Folate B_9	Brain food; Prevents hyperhomocystenemia; helps generate neurotransmitters; helps detoxify.	Asparagus, dark green vegetables, and organ meats.	400 micrograms
Vitamin D	Helps manage MS, prevents depression and anxiety, and acts as antiinflammatory agent.	Sun shine, fortified milk, mushrooms	5000 IU

Nutrient	Function	Food Source	Daily Dose
CoEnzyme Q	Mitochondrial food, helps produce ATP for brain cells.	Wheat germ, green vegetables, kale, spinach, and organ meats.	Less than 200 mg per day
L-carnitine,	Helps burn fat; works with lipoic acid, quenches free radicals.	Beef is the best source, milk, cod, and poultry.	Less than 200 mg per day.
N-Acetylcysteine	Facilitates neurotransmission and impulse control.	Pepper, garlic, onion, broccoli, oat, wheat germ	2 gram per day
Glutathione	Help produce GABA; quenches free radicals; protects red blood cells, and empowers white blood cells,	Protein foods with glycine, glutamic acid, and cysteine: seeds, okra, green vegetables, dairy, eggs	No RDA but what you get from daily green vegetables is sufficient.
A- Lipoic Acid	Has anti-burning and anti-Itching function; serves as coenzyme in many reactions; acts as an antioxidant.	Spinach, broccoli, yeast	Daily vegetable provides enough, No RDA.
Resveratrol	Antioxidant and anti-aging nutrient	Grapes, red wine, peanut, and berries	Less than 200 mg per day
Creatine	Creatin phosphate helps produce ATP	Fish and meat	Less than 5 grams per day
Taurine	As a nutrient for neurotransmitters helps manage mood, anxiety, and pain.	Fish and Shellfish	Less than 1 gram/day

Nutrient	Function	Food Source	Daily Dose
Theanine	Reduces stress and anxiety; improves focus; induces calmness.	Green tea	Less than 500 mg per day
Trace Minerals	Zinc, boron, cobalt, copper, and molybdenum	Pumpkin seed, yeast, green vegetables, sea weed, fish	Needed in micrograms per day.
Magnesium	It is the muscle mineral. Controls mood, impulse, and pain.	Pumpkin and sesame seeds, and cabbage	Below 400 mg per day
Iodine	Brain Health, helps makes myelin and excrete toxins, bactericidal, and anti-carcinogen	Kelp, dried sea weed, sea foods, and red sea algae.	Traces. (Monitor thyroid hormone).
Selenium	Cofactor for glutathione peroxidase, antioxidant	Brazil nut, mushroom, tofu	100 microgram
Taurine, a non essential amino acid	As neurotransmitter ingredient reduces anxiety and pain.	Fish and shell fish	Less than 1 gram per day
Sulfur-vegetables	Production of GABA	Garlic, leak, onion, chive	3 Cups per day
Turmeric	Cures overdose of Tylenol, chronic fatigue syndrome, helps manufacture GABA via glutathione s-transferase	Polyphenol curcumin is found in turmeric, an ingredient of Indian curry powder.	Up to 3 gram per day of dry turmeric powder.

Consult Tables 2.04.02 for functions of nutrients, 2.04.03 for vitamin supplies, and 2.04.04 for mineral supplies for designing methylation diets of breakfast, lunch, snack, and dinner and boost health of mitochondria by fruits, vegetables, herbs, spices, and condiments. These are foods that have been part of our food chain for centutries.

Table 2.04.03 Vitamin Supplies from common Foods		
Food Source	**Vitamins**	**Health benefits**
Milk, Cheese, Eggs, Fatty fish Carrots, Pumpkin, Spinach, Broccoli Mango, Apricots	Vitamin A (Beta-carotene or retinal)	Vision, immune functions, healthy skin, teeth.
Pork , Legumes , Nuts Whole grains, Enriched cereal	Vitamin B-1(Thiamine)	Energy, nerve, heart, muscle
Meat, Eggs, Poultry, Fish Whole grains, Enriched breads, Cereals nuts , milk	Vitamin B-3 (Niacin)	Energy, nerves, digestion, skin.
Meat, Poultry, Fish Whole grains, Enriched breads , Cereals, Legumes, Green leafy vegetables	Vitamin B-6 (Pyridoxine)	Immune system, builds red blood cells, nerves
Meat, Poultry, Fish, Eggs Milk, Cheese	Vitamin B-12 (Cobalamine)	Normal nerve and blood function
Cereals , Legumes, Beans, Liver Dark-green leafy vegetables, Broccoli , Nuts , Oranges	Folic Acid (Folate, B Vitamin)	Tissues, heart, prevents neural tube defects in newborns.
Citrus fruits, Cantaloupe, Strawberries, Raspberries, Melons , Broccoli, Cabbage Dark-green leafy vegetables, Tomatoes , Sweet peppers, Potatoes	Vitamin C (Ascorbic acid)	Fights infection; helps skin, bones, helps absorb iron
Fortified milk , Eggs, Liver, , Salmon, Herring, Mackerel, Fortified margarine	Vitamin D (Calciferol)	Blood calcium levels, healthy bones, muscles, immune system, kidneys.

Sunflower seeds, Sunflower, Safflower, Peanut and Olive oils Almonds	Vitamin E (Tocopherol)	Antioxidant, healing, scarring, nerves, red blood cells.
Spinach, Salad greens, Cauliflower, Broccoli, Brussels sprouts, Cabbage Soybean ,Canola oil, Peanut butter, Margarine , Liver,	Vitamin K (Phylloquinone)	Helps blood clot, builds bones
Egg yolks, Organ meats , Brewer's yeast Legumes, Nuts	Biotin	Energy, skin, hair, fat and protein breakdown

In terms of the variety of nutrients, any flavorful dish is, in a sense, an antioxidant dish. A few antioxidants from common foods includes ellagitannins in raspberry and theoflavin-3-gallate in black tea, isoflavones in soya foods, flavone apigenin (4,5,7 trihydroxy isoflavone) in celery and parsley, flavonones hesperidins in citrus fruits, flavonols quircetin in onion, omega-3, omega-6, and omega-9 fatty acids in salmon and trout fish, steroid campesterol in buckwheat, vitamin E in most vegetable oils, monoterpine limonine in citrus fruits, capsaicin in chili, cucurminoids in turmeric, flavonoids in legume foods, and terpenes like lycopene in tomato, leutin in prune, astaxanthin, zeaxanthin, and well known beta-carotene in carrot. The point is to secure a balance by variety and appeal by alternate day use as breakfast, lunch, snack, or dinner. Including 3 cups of leafy greens (spinach, Swiss Chard), 3 cups of red beets, berries, and orange, and 3 cups of cruciferacea vegetables including broccoli, cabbage, and cauliflower should be the norm for preparing our weekly dishes of breakfast, lunch, snack, and dinner and beverages that go with them. The combination can serve very well as food for the mitochondria in forms of drinks, salads, dips, and cooked vegetables. Included in these preparations should be fruits such as beets, berries, apple, kiwi, and orange and vegetables of bright color such as broccoli, kale, spinach, cabbage, and cauliflower. Mineral antioxidants can come from a daily snack of Brazil nut, macadamia nut, and seeds of sesame, sunflower and pumpkin. Also, readily available dried fruits are good source of antioxidants as shown in Table 2.04.05 below..

Majority of antioxidants in our daily food come from plants that produce them for their own protection and defense [202]. As a matter of fact, all carotenoid pigments are antioxidants [203]. Antioxidants act by donating extra electron to make a pair of electrons from a lone electron in free radicals and thus quenching and rendering them harmless [204]. Common free radicals produced in mitochondria are hydrogen peroxide (H_2O_2, superoxide O^-, Singlet oxygen $^1O_2$, peroxinitrite, and nitric oxide. Antioxidants against them are vitamin E, Vitamin C, Vitamin A, glutathione, and minerals selenium, copper, Iron, manganese, and zinc. In addition, there are enzyme antioxidants superoxide dismutase, glutathione peroxidase, and catalase.

We need a combination of antioxidants for protection by different mechanisms In order to protect ourselves from DNA damage and oxidation of proteins and lipids . *For example lipid soluble vitamin E and ubiquinones scavenge peroxy radicals in mitochondria and water soluble glutathione and lipoic acid protect proteins from oxidative damage.* Flavonoids are powerful antioxidant and so is melatonin, the sleep hormone made from neurotransmitter serotonin. Even amino acids cysteine, methionine, and tryptophan have antioxidant power. Peptide glutathione is a very powerful antioxidant in human body.

202   http://rubisco.ugr.es/fisiofar/pagwebinmalcb/contenidos/Tema03/cloroplastos.pdf
203   http://elte.prompt.hu/sites/default/files/tananyagok/plants_fungi/ch03s04.html
204   http://news.psu.edu/story/141171/2008/08/18/research/probing-question-how-do-antioxi-
       dants-work

Table 2.04.04 Mineral Supplies from common Foods

Food Source	Minerals	Health benefits
Milk , Milk products , Dark-green leafy vegetables , Broccoli , Shrimp, Salmon, Clams , Orange juice ,Legumes , Tofu	Calcium	Healthy bones and teeth, Helps heart, muscles, and nerves
Yeast , Meat, Cheese, Eggs Whole grains, , Vegetable oil.	Chromium	Helps insulin work better
Cashew nut, legumes, kale, mushrooms, sesame seed, and sea foods	Copper	Health of bone and connective tissues
Salt water fish, Seafood Iodized salt	Iodine	Growth of nervous system, builds energy
Red meat, Organ meat, Egg yolk, Legumes, Green-leafy vegetables Enriched cereals, Bread , Dried fruits	Iron	Healthy bones and teeth, Helps heart, muscles, and nerves
Whole grains, Nuts Peas, Beans, Lentils, Legumes Dark-green leafy vegetables , Tea	Magnesium	Helps bones, metabolism, nerves and muscles
Almond, dairy foods, and edamami	Molybdenum	Mitochondrial function and other four enzymes functions..
Meat, Fish, Eggs , Dairy products, dried fruits,, Wheat Bran, Cereals, seeds, nuts	Phosphorus	Builds and maintains teeth and bones, needed for muscles and nerves
Root and Leafy green vegetables ,Tomatoes , Cucumbers, Zucchini, fruits, Eggplant, Pumpkin, and milk,	Potassium	Maintains normal blood pressure, heart beat and nerve impulses
Meat, Poultry, Fish , Whole grain cereals and Breads , Legumes , Nuts	Zinc	Needed for growth, immunity, digestion, and skin, improves sense of taste and wound healing

Table 2.15.05 Oxygen Radical Absorbance Capacity (ORAC) of Antioxidants Present in Our Daily Foods

Common Foods	Micromole in ORAC =Trolox Equivalent, TE per 100 grams	Common foods with antioxidants
Sumac bran	312,400	Allium: Garlic, leek, onion,
Spices, cloves, ground	314,446	
Cinnamon, ground	267,536	Anthocyanins: egg plant, grape, berries
Oregano, dried	200,129	
Turmeric, ground	159,277	Beta-carotene: pumpkin, mango, carrot,
Cocoa, dry powder, unsweetened	80,993	spinach, and parsley.
Unprocessed cocoa beans	28,000	
Black pepper	27,168	Catechins: Red wine and tea
Cinnamon, 1 tablespoonful	21,402	
Pecan, 100 g	17,940	Copper: sea foods, nuts, legumes, and milk
Raspberries, 1 cup	16,058	
Oregano, 1 tablespoonful	16,010	Cryptoxanthin: Red pepper, mango, pumpkin
Elderberries, 1 cup	14,697	
Lentils, 1 cup	13,981	Flavonoids: Tea, red wine, apples, onions
Red kidney beans	13,727	Citrus fruits
Turmeric, 1 tablespoonful	12,742	

Common Foods	Micromole in ORAC =Trolox Equivalent, TE per 100 grams	Common foods with antioxidants
Chocolate, 30 grams	12,060	Indols: Broccoli, cabbage, cauliflower
Pinto beans	11,864	
Blueberry, Cherry, Cranberry, raw, 1 cup	9,584	Lignans: sesame and flax seeds, whole grains
Artichoke, cooked, 1 cup; Pistachio 100 g	7,904	
Pomegranate juice 100%	5,923	Lutein: Spinach like leafy greens and corn
Prune, 1/2 cup	7,291	
Plum, dried	5,700	Lycopene: Tomato, pink grapefruit,
Black plum, 1	4,844	
Red wine	5,693	Manganese: nuts, sea foods, and milk
Blueberries, raw, and anthocyanins, 1 cup	9,019	
Sweet cherries, 1 cup	4,873	Polyphenols: Oregano and Thyme
Apples, red, quircetin, and other polyphenols	5,900	
Granny Smith, 1 apple	5,381	Selenium: Brazil nut, sea food, whole grains
Watermelon, a great source of lycopene	3,800	
Raisins	2,830	Vitamin C: Oranges, Kiwi, mango, berries
Blackberries, 1 cup	7,701	
Strawberries, 1 cup	5,938	Vitamin E: Avocado, vegetable oils, and nuts
Pears, 1 medium	5,255	

Common Foods	Micromole in ORAC =Trolox Equivalent, TE per 100 grams	Common foods with antioxidants
Pecans, 1 oz	5,095	Walnut: Omega-3 Fatty acid
Kale and spinach	1,700	
Broccoli and Brussels sprouts	980	Zinc: nuts, milk, lean meat

USDA and USDA define ORAC values as Trolox Equivalent (micromole TE per 100 gram). Trolox is a vitamin E analogue.

Freeze-dried fruits and vegetables have high ORAC values because of concentration of antioxidants.

Sources:
http://www.ars.usda.gov/is/AR/archive/feb99/aging0299.htm; http://www.ars.usda.gov/is/pr/1999/990208.htm
http://www.cancer.gov/newscenter/pressreleases/antioxidants ; http://brunswicklabs.com/artman/uploads/jf0116606.pdf

Note: Vitamin D function requires magnesium, magnesium and calcium control heartbeat. Magnesium relaxes and calcium helps contract muscles. Magnesium is critical to type 2 diabetes in relation to conversion of sugar to energy. It is critical to the energy process as a whole. Magnesium is next to potassium in concentration as a positively charged ion in our cells. Antioxidant enzymes glutathione peroxidase, superoxide dismutase, catalase, and coenzyme Q_{10} from sprouts can be routinely used to reduce oxidative stress.

There are many sources of free radicals including our metabolism and stress, processed foods, polluted air, drugs, pesticides, smoking , copying machines, cell phones, and electromagnetic radiation. A 70 Kg person consumes 504 grams or 352.8 liters liter of oxygen per day[205] . Up to 10% or 25 grams of this daily oxygen can become free radicals, a majority of 97% of which is superoxide. Extraneous exercise produces a lot of free radicals,

---

205   https://books.google.com/books?id=zFkJtWuBhGwC&pg=PA80&lpg=PA80&dq=daily+total+-free+radical+production+in+human+body&source=bl&ots=_cYDmHasSA&sig=VSnPEOjURN-WvKeJUMYCEorlyHhI&hl=en&sa=X&ei=UiOxVOvpCsmGyATknIDoAw&sqi=2&ved=0CB4Q6A-EwAA#v=onepage&q=daily%20total%20free%20radical%20production%20in%20human%20body&f=false

20 fold of normal daily production [206]. Obviously people committed to high intensity work out need to double their antioxidant consumption (Table 2.04.05). The ORAC data on common foods suggest that even a modest food budget can accommodate necessary antioxidant in our daily methylation diet by proper selection of fruits, vegetables, herbs and spices for cooking, and snacks of chocolate, and tree nuts. Senior citizens should raise their consumption of high ORAC foods at least by 25%.

We need to recognize that our body has an elaborate antioxidant delivery system in order to combat free radicals that are integral part of our evolution. The first line of defense are water soluble antioxidants such as vitamin C, glutathione peroxidase, superoxide dismutase, and catalase in the cell. Second line of defense is comprised of fat soluble vitamins A, E, D, K, and beta-carotene. The third line of defense comes from enzymes that break oxidized materials down into harmless compounds. The free radicals should not exceed 3% of total oxygen intake, 1% being the ideal objective. Fatigue, high blood pressure, and vulnerability to allergies is a good indication of high free radical concentration. An ordinary vegetable snack can fight away excess the free radicals.

Superoxide free radical that results from one electron reduction is the biggest problem. Hydrogen peroxide is the result of 2 electron reduction that is easily destroyed by enzyme catalase. Hydroxyl radical which results from 3 electron reduction is dangerous but produced only in small amounts. Nitric oxide, a beneficial free radical, is produced in very small amounts. We should recognize that all transition metals except copper can act as free radicals. Copper and iron lose electron rather readily and as such are capable of acting as free radicals. **Zinc is a very valuable mineral because it quenches free radicals.** Copper and zinc are part of enzyme superoxide dismutase. Reduction state wise O_2 becomes superoxide, superoxide becomes hydrogen peroxide, hydrogen peroxide becomes hydroxyl radical, and hydroxyl can be quenched into water. Although produced on purpose by our immune system for killing bacteria and viruses and by mitochondria for routine communication and signaling, an excess of free radicals containing highly reactive unpaired lone electrons must be destroyed by sufficient antioxidant intake via well designed methylation diet. Table 5.13.01 provides an extensive list of critical antioxidants.

---

206   http://www.scielo.br/pdf/rbme/v10n4/en_22047.pdf

Therapeutic Value of Our Daily Foods

Life began with oxygen but only with the help of a battery of antioxidants that are part of all life- bacteria, plants, animals, and humans. We now find that inflammation is caused by free radicals with unpaired electrons which habitually steel electrons from molecules of life and cause cancer, diabetes, cardiovascular disease, Alzheimer's disease, and autoimmune diseases.

Poor eating habits are responsible for too many free radicals in and around our mitochondria both in time and in amount. Their property of steeling electrons from stable molecules of DNA, proteins, enzymes, and lipids in our blood and brain makes us sick. We know that inflammation is the major cause of cellular stress, cellular dysfunction, and even chronic diseases [207].

A long-term preventive remedy is methylation diet that embodies all good attributes of various diets such as DASH, Mediterranean, Okinawa, Paleo, and Redox whose components deliver a combination of antioxidants that scavenge free radicals. Antiinflammatory foods included in these diets are

I.   Omega-3 fats from fish, flax seed, and walnut. Also egg for choline, olive oil , pecans, and peanut butter for monounsaturated fat. Walnut is a great source of omega-3 fatty acids. Also, dark Chocolate is a source of powerful antioxidants.

II.   Nuts (almonds, walnut, and Brazil nuts) for plant fats, proteins, and minerals for omega-3 fatty acids and monounsaturated fats.

III. A variety of fruits and vegetables: Fruits include apple, orange, banana, beet, blue berries, tart cherries, strawberries, black berries, and kiwi and common vegetables include avocado, broccoli, cabbage, carrots, kale, beans, beets, chard. Collectively they supply vitamins, minerals, and even omega-3 fatty acids. We should select as many cruciferacea vegetables as possible. Green vegetables such as cabbage are good source of sulfur for mitochondria.

---

207   https://www.lef.org/protocols/health_concerns/chronic_inflammation_01.htm

IV.   Fish, sea foods, and kelp for iodine in order to counteract effects of cruciferacea vegetables that compete for iodine receptors.

V.   Whole grains and legumes: beans, lentils, amaranth, quinova, and millet. Such foods are rich source of polyphenolic antioxidants. A good example is common tea that provides epigallocatechin gallate.

VI.   Flavors can come from herbs and spices such as garlic, onion, ginger, red wine, tea, tart cherries, nutritional yeast, and turmeric. Cinnamon, a great spice used in global food chain for centuries, should be incorporated in as many food formats as possible including crapes, muffins, coffee, smoothies, and beverages.

VII. Vitamin D_3 along with calcium is essential for bone health.

2.05 Anti-inflammatory Diet

Inflammation is a natural response to injury to our body. It is necessary for healing and it is part of our innate immunity, not the adaptive immunity though [208], [209], [210]. The variety depicted above delivers enough calcium but we must get our daily vitamin D_3 from fortified milk and cereals or even supplements as an anti-inflammatory food nutrient.

High sugar and high fat foods are inflammatory. They cause over activity of the immune system which in turn causes pains, fatigue, and damage to blood vessels. Evidence of inflammation is irritation, redness, burning sensation, swelling, pain, and in severe cases even loss of function. Infection may cause inflammation also but inflammation is not infection. Good foods are necessary to keep inflammation under control before it damages our cells and organs and molecules life such as DNA, proteins, and lipids.

---

208   http://www.siumed.edu/~dking2/intro/inflam.htm
209   http://www.ncbi.nlm.nih.gov/pubmedhealth/PMH0009852/
210   htt http://www.ncbi.nlm.nih.gov/pubmed/10528314p://trinitychiro.com/media/Diet_and_Inflammation.pdf

2.06 Food Supplements

Fat burning and blocking, appetite suppressing, and metabolism boosting supplements are of only questionable value[211], [212]. Hoodia, and hydroxycitrate are being questioned as to their health value. Even values of beta-glucan, guar gum, and leptin are over rated. Instead we need to consume appropriate amount of antioxidants by natural methylation diet, follow a lifestyle that is punctuated with exercise, meditation, and social interaction. We will examine this topic in section 5.13 under summation in much more in detail. Polyphenols and pyrroquinilin quinone shall receive extensive coverage in view of their nutritional value.

2.06.01 Coenzyme Q: The Mitochondrial Nutrient

Use of ubiquinone for for cellular energy metabolism has been under serious study for a long time[213]. NADH-Ubiquinone oxidoreductase (complex I of the electron transport chain in mitochondria) is a respiratory chain enzyme that helps transfer two electrons from NADH to Ubiquinone[214]. It is the key reaction for proton translocation across the inner mitochondrial membrane. *Also, complex I and II are major source of free radicals that originate via electron transfer from FMNH (Flavin Mononucleotide).*

CoEnzyme $Q_{10,}$ the scientific name of ubiquinone, is a major food supplement in the retail food stores. Highly recommended supplements of up to 3 gram per day are indicated for treating congestive heart failure. However, a good and practical alternative is to get this key nutrient from our daily foods such as peanut (not overly cooked), spinach, salmon, tuna, and wheat germ [215],[216]. A smaller RDA of 100 mg per day is well accepted and this can easily come from our well designed calorie restricted methylation diet.

211   http://breakingmuscle.com/health-medicine/science-says-weight-loss-supplements-do-not-work
212   http://www.ucdmc.ucdavis.edu/welcome/features/20090513_dietpills/index.html
213   http://www.ncbi.nlm.nih.gov/pubmed/10528314
214   http://www.ebi.ac.uk/interpro/entry/IPR000260
215   http://umm.edu/health/medical/altmed/supplement/coenzyme-q10
216   http://www.healthsupplementsnutritionalguide.com/Coenzyme-Q10.html

2.06.02 Antioxidant Pyrroloquinoline Quinone (PQQ)

PQQ, an antioxidant, found in our daily foods such as broad beans, carrot, potato, papaya, and parsley helps maintain mitochondrial health. Fermented soybean as natto, green tea, and edamami deliver high amounts sufficient to help grow new mitochondria, make nerve growth factors, prevent oxidation of beta-amyloid proteins, prevent development of alpha-synuclein protein responsible for Parkinson's disease, reverse cognitive impairments, and quite down N-methyl-D-aspartic acid receptor effects of synaptic plasticity and memory [217]. A summary of antioxidants often talked about in the popular press is included in Table 2.06.02 below. This should help in selection of foods for a good methylation diet. Section 5.13 in summation has a detailed coverage on this powerful antioxidant.

2.06.03 D-Ribose

D-Ribose can boost energy production and D-ribose food supplements are available [218]. It is used with creatine for energy release[219], for treatment of chronic fatigue syndrome [220], and for improved mitochondrial function in general [221]. However, our daily foods of milk, cheddar cheese, cream cheese, mushroom, eggs, and yogurt can supply enough D-ribose for a healthy mitochondria. To heart patients in particular, a Coenzyme Q_{10} supplement is more advisable than D-ribose.

217   http://www.altmedrev.com/publications/14/3/268.pdf
218   http://www.swansonvitamins.com/d-ribose
219   http://warddeanmd.com/mitochondrial-restoration-part-iii-d-ribose-and-creatine-increase-mito-chondrial-energy-production/
220   https://www.seekinghealth.com/media/Use%20of%20Ribose%20in%20CFS%20and%20Fibromyal-gia.pdf
221   http://lifewave.com/pdf/ThetaNutrition/(3)Enhancing-Mitochondrial-Function-With-D-Ribose.pdf

Table 2.06.02 A list of Antioxidants from common Foods

Terpenoid		Food Sources
	Carotenoid	
		Alpha-Carotenes (carrots). Beta-carotene from green vegetables, gamma-carotene, delta-carotene, lycopene from tomato, neurosporine, and phytoene and phytofluene from sweet potato, ,
	Xanthophylls	Canthaxanthine from paprika, cryptoxanthin from mango and papaya, zeaxanthin from eggs and spinach, Astaxanthin from yeast and krill, and leutin from spinach and turnip.
	Triterpenoids	Saponins from soy beans, Oleanolic acid from garlic and clove, and Ursolic acid from apples and basil.
	Monoterpenes	Limonene from citrus and cherry and perillyl alcohol from caraway seeds and citrus
	Sterols	Phytosterols from almond and cashews, campestrol and Stigmasterol from buckwheat, tocopherol and vitamin E from plant fats, gamma linoleic acid from black currant, and omega -3 fatty acids from flax seed
Phenolics		
	Natural Mono-phenols	Apiole from celery and parsley, carnasol from rosemary and sage, carvacrol from orange and thyme, and rosemarinol from rosemary.
	Polyphenols	Flavonols: Flavonols from red, blue, and purple pigments, quircetin from onion and beans, gingerol from ginger, kaempferol from tea, myristein from wine and berries, fisestin from cucumber and strawberries, rutin from citrus and orange, isorhametin from red turnip

Terpenoid		Food Sources
		Flavonones: hisperedin from citrus, naranginin from citrus, catechins from tea, eggalocatechins from tea, and Theaflavin from black tea.
		Flavononols: apigenins celery and parsley, tangertin from tangerine, and luteolin from beet sugar and artichoke.
		Flavone-3-ols: catechin from tea, Theaflavin from black tea, thearubigins, and proanthocyanindins
		Anthocyanindins: delphinidins from egg plant, pelargonidin, cyanidin, and malvadin from berries
		Isoflavones from peas, beans, soy, and peanut
		Flavolignans: Silymarin from artichoke,
		Lignans: Matairesinol from flax seed, and seciisolariciresinol from zucchini and flax seed
		Stilbenoids: Resveratrol from grapes and wine, pterostilbenes from grapes and blue berries and Piceatanol from grapes.
		Cucurbinoids; piceatanol from grapes,
		Cucurbinois: cucurmin from turmeric and mustard
		Hydrolysable Tannins; Ellagitannins
	Aromatic Acids	
		Salicylic Acid from peppermint
		Vanillin from vanilla beans
		Tannic acid
		Phenolic acids
		Hydroxycinnamic acid
	Capsaicin	Capsaicin from chili pepper and red pepper

Terpenoid		Food Sources
	Phenyletha-noids	Tyrisol and hydroxytyrisol from olive oil, and oleocanthal from olive oil
	Alkylresorci-nols	Alkylresorcinols from rye and wheat.
Glucosino-lates		
	Isocyanates	Isocyanates, sulphoraphane, and Thioiso-cyanates from cruciferacea vegetables, indols, and organosulfides
	Allium from garlic Diallylsulfides from garlic.	
Indols		Indol-3-carbinol from cabbage, kale, and mustard.
Betaines		Betaine from sugar beats
Betaxanthin		Betaxanthin from red and yellow beet-roots.
Chlorophylls	Chlorophyllin	Chlorophyllin from asparagus, brussels sprout and deep green vegetables.

The following list names antioxidants which have been reported to exhibit antiaging properties.

Apigenin, baicalein, chrysin, 3 hydroxyflavone, 6 hydroxyflavone cyanidin, 3 glucoside, delphinidin, diosmin, eriodictyol, fisetin, gossypetin, hesperetin, hesperidin, isokaempferide, isorhamnetin, kaempferol, luteolin, morin, myricetin, naringenin, pelargonidin, quercetin, resveratrol, rhamnetin, scutellarein, and wogonin. Some of them function as cholinesterase Inhibitors and neuroprotective agents.

2.06.04 Resveratrol

Resveratrol, a polyphenolic antioxidant found in red wine inhibits apoptosis (programmed cell death) by acting as a SIRT-1 enzyme agonist. Resveratrol has been studied for its potential role in the treatment of diabetes, cardiovascular disease, neurodegenerative disease, cancer, obesity, and aging [222], [223]. However, not enough clinical trials have been completed to establish its use and determine possible side effects and risks. However, it is being marketed as an anti-aging food supplement [224] rather vigorously. Supplies are made from Japanese knotweed. Red grapes and wines can supply up to 2 mg per serving . The huge hype continues [225] based largely on research works at the Harvard University. We have a long way to go before resveratrol treatment of heart disease and diabetes becomes approved by Food and Drug Administration clearing concerns about safety in routine use. The big hope for the near future is that resveratrol based drugs can act on sirtuin (silent information regulator) genes that may promote longevity. In the mean time it is wise to stay natural and consume red grapes, blue berries, and pistachios for daily intake of resveratrol.

2.06.05 Alpha Lipoic Acid

Alpha-lipoic Acid or thioctic acid is naturally present in our body [226]. It is a powerful antioxidant. Furthermore, lipoic acid is involved in insulin signaling and glutathione synthesis. Also, it is bound to enzymes that function as cofactors in mitochondrial electron transfer chain. Carnitine and alpha lipoic acid supplements may normalize levels of Krebs cycle enzymes in aging populations [227]. **Alpha-lipoic acid, when administered with vitamin E, coenzyme Q_{10}, and melatonin, has been found to enhance cerebral mitochondrial electron transport in case of mice [228], [229].** Actually, new research shows that It may slow down the progression of multiple sclerosis

222   http://onlinelibrary.wiley.com/doi/10.1002/mnfr.201100143/abstract
223   http://www.ncbi.nlm.nih.gov/pmc/articles/PMC2083123/
224   http://www.longecity.org/forum/topic/49947-review-article-of-resveratrol-based-human-clinical-tri-als/
225   http://www.health.harvard.edu/blog/resveratrol-the-hype-continues-201202034189
226   http://lpi.oregonstate.edu/infocenter/othernuts/la/
227   http://www.ncbi.nlm.nih.gov/pubmed/15919137
228   http://www.ncbi.nlm.nih.gov/pubmed/11445263
229   http://www.plosone.org/article/info%3Adoi%2F10.1371%2Fjournal.pone.0060722

also [230], [231]. *Good sources of alpha-lipoic acid are brewer's yeast, broccoli, Brussels sprout, peas, spinach, and tomato-* all common to a well designed methylation diet. Over-the-counter supplements are not necessary.

2.06.06 N-Acetyl-Cysteine

Carnitine carries fatty acids to mitochondria for energy production and it is believed to be involved in cardiac and cerebral functions. Our kidneys regulate carnitine level and preserve it in case of deficiency. Good sources of N-Acetyl-carnitine are milk, cheese, chicken, beef, other animal foods.

N-Acetyl-carnitine, a kind of antioxidant, is marketed as a drug and also as food supplement for maintaining health, reducing weight, and enhanced longevity [232]. However, carnitine or N-acetyl carnitine should be taken under a physician's advice only because of possible adverse side effects of bleeding, chest tightness, and brochoconstriction [233].

2.06.07 Adaptogenic Foods

Although not approved by FDA in US for treatment of any disease, use of adaptogenic herbs and vegetables is gaining popularity simply because they have a long history of use in human food chain. It appears that evolution has integrated active ingredients in such foods as food molecules of control and balance at the cellular level. They are known to quench free radicals, prevent DNA damage, maintain homeostasis, improve perception, modulate efficient use of oxygen, improve antibody titer for better immune system, support adrenal function, reduce stress, and detoxify.

It is a matter of general belief now that adaptogenic foods stabilize homeostasis and physiological processes, affect sympathetic nervous system, reduce sensitivity to stress, induce longevity, increase libido, fight fatigue, and even act as anticarcinogens against cancer. Indications are that

---

230   http://www.overcomingmultiplesclerosis.org/Community/Forum/viewtopic.php?f=3&t=4370
231   http://www.ncbi.nlm.nih.gov/pubmed/18537699
232   http://www.mskcc.org/cancer-care/integrative-medicine/disclaimer?msk_disclaimer_herb=1&destination=%2Fcancer-care%2Fherb%2Fn-acetylcysteine
233   http: http://www.yourliferegained.com/articles/adaptogens///www.sfrbm.org/frs/ErcalNAC.pdf

they normalize the hypothalamus-pituitary axis for cellular control and help reduce stress by endocrine control [234], [235].

Oxidative stress is well known to introduce inefficiency in mitochondrial function. *Major adaptogenic foods that reduce stress are Korean ginseng, Siberian ginseng, Chinese penyin, mushrooms, Okinawa's bitter guard, true aloe, and India's Aswagandha.* Other common foods that may also have adaptogenic role are blueberry, tulsi or holy basal of India, ginger, garlic, truffles, and even tomato and potato. Most reports on such effects are from Chinese, Korean, Indian Ayurveda, and Russian publications. Most of these foods contain antioxidants like coenzyme Q_{10}, vitamin C, and N-dimethylglycine believed to fight stress, trauma, and anxiety [236], [237]. The literature is replete with health value of phytosterol, tocotrienol, beta-sistosterol, cucurbitans, various saponins, flavonoids and flavone glycosides, sesamin, and syringaresinol. Reports to the effects of (1) antioxidant and antiinflammatory sesamin from sesame oil for reducing blood pressure, (2) cucurbitans found in cucumber and winter squash for preventing breast, colon, and prostate cancer, and (3) syringaresinol, another lignan for inhibiting Helicobacter pylori and relieve problems of stomach ulcer support the idea that adaptogenic foods do provide health values.

Cucumber, sesame seed, and winter squash are very common foods and they have been part of our common recipes for centuries. **Found in beans and liver, N-dimethylglycine is under serious studies for its effects on enhanced performance of immune system [238].** Also, ginseng is known to increase level of superoxide dismutase and quench reactive oxygen free radicals [239]. **An important aspect of adaptogenic foods is that in most cases their active ingredients are isoprenoid or terpenoids structures suited for electron mobility.**

US Food and Drug Administration and European Medicines Agency are coming close to accepting the concept in theory that adaptogens work via cell receptors and the stress protective action of adaptogens is believed to be due to their effects on gene transcriptions involved in cellular signaling via G-Protein Coupled Receptors [240], [241]. Furthermore, adaptogens have

---

234   http://www.uptodate.com/contents/hypothalamic-pituitary-axis
235   http://www.ncbi.nlm.nih.gov/pmc/articles/PMC3181830/
236   http://www.yourliferegained.com/articles/adaptogens/
237   73http://www.sciencedirect.com/science/article/pii/S1756464613000133http://www.naturalnews.com/adaptogens.html
http://www.ncbi.nlm.nih.gov/pubmed/19531970
238   http://dmgdoctor.com/information/about/
239   http://www.ncbi.nlm.nih.gov/pubmed/19531970
240   http://www.ncbi.nlm.nih.gov/pubmed/23430930
241   http://journal.frontiersin.org/Journal/10.3389/fnins.2013.00016/full

beneficial interactive effects via Heat Shock Protein (HSP) chaperonin, cortisol, and vasodilator nitric oxide. HSP_{60}, a particular heat shock protein, is a mitochondrial chaperonin that transports and refolds proteins from cytoplasm [242]. How wonderful! Evolution has endowed us with protein molecules that help shape other protein molecules for better and fuller function at the cellular level. As a matter of fact FDA allowed functional claims on such items in 1998.

Bitter gourd common to Okinawa diet leads the list of natural adaptogenic foods in Japan[243], [244]. As a person born and raised up to my 20th birth day in India, I can attest many a common uses of bitter guard in Indian cousin. In my home here in the United States, my wife presents bitter gourd in a variety of culinary formats of stuffed, relish, and curried versions. *There is serious research on nuclear receptor protein PPARs (peroxisome proliferator activator receptor) from bitter gourd , a vegetable present in almost all major retail food stores in the US today [245], [246].* Active ingredients are conjugated linoleic acid and triterpines. Another adaptogen under study is Tulsi or Holy Basil that contains apigenin ,eugenol, and luteolin [247]. I was given tulsi extract as a cure all against stress, fever and cold, cough, sore throat, and sore throat during my childhood years in India.

Even mushrooms are gaining importance in terms of their tonic and adaptogenic activities due to terpenoids and specific polysaccharides present in them [248], [249]. We do need, however, much more clinical and pre-clinical confirmatory testing on adaptogenic herbs and vegetables to be used as human food. No doubt that we should incorporate common adaptogens of long history in human food chain in our daily methylation breakfast, lunch, and dinner recipes.

2.06.08 Nutritional Yeast

Deactivated yeast as flakes or yellow powder is sold as commercial food product and food ingredient . It is a very good source of protein and water

242   http://www.phosphosite.org/proteinAction.do?id=4118
243   http://www.sciencedirect.com/science/article/pii/S1756464613000133
244   http://onlinelibrary.wiley.com/doi/10.1002/ptr.2650070405/abstract
245   http://www.ncbi.nlm.nih.gov/pubmed/21128828
246   http://link.springer.com/article/10.1007%2FBF02256331#page-1
247   http://www.sacredearth.co.za/sacred-tulsi/
248   http://www.lindazurich.com/medicinal-mushrooms-remarkably-effective-myco-adaptogens/
249   http://www.ncbi.nlm.nih.gov/pmc/articles/PMC1203343/

soluble vitamin B complex [250]. Very common in Australia and New Zealand, nutritional yeast is nutty and cheesy in flavor and creamy in texture. On average, two tablespoons provides 60 calories with 5 g of carbohydrates (of which 4 g is fiber). One serving also provides 9 g of high quality complete protein, providing all nine essential amino acids the human body cannot produce. It is also a source of <u>selenium</u>, chromium, and <u>potassium</u> [251]. In Australia Vegemite, dark brown food paste from brewer's yeast, is a matter of stylish cousine.

2.06.09 B Vitamins necessary for Mitochondria

Our water based evolution incorporated mitochondria as basis of our life that depends largely on water based B vitamins such as B_3 (niacin) , the backbone of NADH/NAD$^+$ electron carrier system, B2 (riboflavin) as part of FAD and FMN electron transfer systems, B_6 (Pyridoxin) which participates in close to 100 enzyme functions, B_9 (folic acid) is central to DNA methylation, and the brain vitamin vitamin $B_{12,}$. Thus members of Vitamin b complex are central to mitochondrial function and our methylation diet should be complete with respect to RDAs of these vitamins.

2.06.10 Gamma Amino Butyric Acid

Gamma amino butyric acid (GABA) is an important inhibitory neurotransmitter in that it regulates neuronal excitability throughout the nervous system. Although it doesn't penetrate blood-brain barrier its excitatory or inhibitory role is a function of brain development. **High GABA has the effect of relaxation and reduced anxiety.**

GABA binds ligand gated and G protein coupled receptors at the inhibitory synapses in the brain and opens ion channels for chloride ions into the cell and potassium ions out of the cell. **This induces negative transmembrane potential and hyper-polarization.** *GABA effects are an active area of research in pain management* [252], [253], [254].
Foods that can deliver good amounts of GABA are tea, fermented foods,

250   http://nutritiondata.self.com/facts/custom/1323565/2
251   http://umm.edu/health/medical/altmed/supplement/brewers-yeast
252   http://www.med.nyu.edu/content?ChunkIID=222543
253   http://www.denvernaturopathic.com/news/GABA.html
254   htt http://www.ncbi.nlm.nih.gov/pmc/articles/PMC3402070/p://www.gammaaminobutyricacid.org/

and germinated brown rice. Lifestyle choices of meditation and yoga enhance GABA levels in our brain cells [255].

2.06.11 Melatonin and a Good Night Sleep

Melatonin, patented by MIT some 20 years ago, is a hormone produced by pineal gland for regulating sleep, circadian rhythm, and even other reproductive hormones in case of women [256]. Therefore, **use of high melatonin foods such as banana, barley, oats, oranges, pineapple, sweet corn, tart cherries, and tomatoes in our weekly diet is a good dietary practice.** *Strawberries, tomatoes, and walnut are fairly good source for melatonin capable of delivering 1 to 11, 3 to 114, and 3 to 4 nanogram per gram respectively [257].* It is noteworthy that varieties and particular supplies do make a difference. *High tryptophan foods are good for the production of melatonin in our body.* Severe fasting below 300 calories per day and excessive alcohol consumption can restrict melatonin production and, therefore, calories restriction for weight control should be in a range of 1,200 to 1,400 calories per day for an average 150 lb person. For adequate melatonin production we need to consume diets that supply appropriate RDA_s of folate, magnesium, zinc, and other vitamins and minerals [258]. **It is an ampiphilic hormone (N-acetyl-5-methoxytryptamine) with positive and negative charges and readily quenches free radicals as a potent antioxidant** [259]. **It is two times more potent antioxidant compared to vitamin E** [260]. Montmorency variety of tart cherries grown in US have 13.5 ng of metatonin per gram (more than what is found in blood) with an ORAC value of 5000.

2.06.12 Omega-3 Fatty Acids

Excessive use of soy bean and cotton seed oils has increased the ratio of omega-6 to omega-3 essential fatty acids to 10:1 in our default diets. The ideal ratio is 3:1. DHA omega-3 fatty acid, our evolutionary companion, is a necessary dietary need in case of neurological disorders. *Flax seed, walnut,*

255   http://www.psychologytoday.com/blog/evolutionary-psychiatry/201303/yoga-ba-gaba
256   http://www.ncbi.nlm.nih.gov/pmc/articles/PMC3402070/
257   http://www.ncbi.nlm.nih.gov/pmc/articles/PMC3402070/
258   http://adcaps.wsu.edu/campaigns/sleep-foods/
259   ww.nutritionandmetabolism.com/content/2/1/22
260   http://www.ncbi.nlm.nih.gov/pubmed/7934611

egg, salmon, trout, cloves, broccoli, cauliflower, chia seed, soy bean, basal, oregano, and Brussels' sprout are good sources of omega-3 fatty acids. Alpha-Linolenic acid from flax seed and walnut are the best readily available common sources.

Alpha-Linolenic acid of flax seed and walnut is converted in the body into EPA (eicosapentanoic acid) and DHA (docosahexanoic acid). These brain foods enhance memory and strengthen brain cell structure above and beyond functions of controlling clotting and building cell membranes [261]. Both EPA and DHA are antiinflammatory. Even omega-6 is necessary for lowering low density lipoprotein (LDL cholesterol) and improving cardiovascular health (reduced blood pressure, prevention of coronary heart disease and atrial fibrillation). These polyunsaturated fatty acids are classified as essential for daily metabolism [262].

2.06.13 Key Minerals

Iron, copper, zinc, manganese, and magnesium are essential for the health of mitochondria. Magnesium aspartate is a muscle mineral salt as a muscle relaxant in its own right. Magnesium sulfate is the chemical in many supplements. Since aspartic acid is a neurotransmitter, magnesium in this form should be consumed carefully and under a physician's advice. A review of vital minerals is summarized in Table 2.04.04.

2.06.14 NADH

NADH is also known as coenzyme 1. It is generated during glucose breakdown in glycolysis and Krebs cycle as a source of high energy electrons carrier as input to operation of mitochondria [263]. NADH supplements are there in the market but the best practice is our daily vitamin B_3 or niacin intake of about 14 mg. By law wheat flour is fortified with niacin in USA and most Western countries. Most cold cereals are also fortified. Other good and common sources are peanuts, mushroom, green beans, sunflower seeds, wheat bran,

261   http://www.hsph.harvard.edu/nutritionsource/omega-3/
262   http://umm.edu/health/medical/altmed/supplement/omega3-fatty-acids
263   htt http://www.nadh-apotheke.eu/NADH-Studien/NADH%20stimulates%20endogenous%20dopa-
      mine%20biosynthesis%20by%20enhancing%20the.pdf
45 p://www.nadh-apotheke.eu/NADH-Studien/NADH-Coenzym-1-EBook-en.pdf

fish, chicken, beef, and liver. Given this variety, it is not difficult to design our daily methylation dish for sufficient delivery of NADH.

Coenzyme NADH is present in our cells both in free and bound forms in a range of about 0.3 to 0.4 millimoles or 0.20 to 0.25 gram [264]. It is a key coenzyme in ATP energy production by mitochondria [265] and is used daily [266], [267]. NADH is the main source of high energy electrons for the human body[268] . **It is recycled 500-750 times per day [269] just as ATP is recycled [270].** Average ATP in human body is no more than 0.2 mole or 250 gram but the daily turnover is in a range of 50-75 Kg or 100-150 Moles per day representing a 500-750 times recycling rate per day .

It is a memory retention coenzyme. NADH stimulates dopamine synthesis [271]. The life and death of cells in our body depends on NADH dependent mitochondrial function. Heart and central nervous system are most vulnerable when mitochondrial efficiency goes down.

2.06.15 Thermogenic Foods

In theory all foods are thermogenic but we can certainnly increase the thermogenic effect by consuming foods requiring extra expenditure of energy and thus reducing net calorie gain. Examples of such foods are whole grains and high protein foods like legumes, lentils, white egg, chicken, turkey, and lean meat. Also, there is sufficient research which shows that spices and chili [272], black pepper containing peperine, green tea containing polyphenolic and epigallaocatechin gallate, coconut oil with medium chain triglycerides [273], [274], ginger[275], and foods with high calcium and vitamin D, [276] are thermogenic. **Two gram ginger at breakfast provides enough gingerone**

264   htt http://www.nadh-apotheke.eu/NADH-Stud
41 http://www.nadh-apotheke.eu/NADH-Studien/Extracellular%20metabolisation%20of%20NADH%20 by%20blood%20cells%20correlates%20with.pdf
265
266   http://www.nottingham.ac.uk/ncmh/BGER/pdf/Volume%206/BGER6-6.pdf
http://aem.asm.org/content/75/3/687.full
267   ht http://www.nadh.com/site7/FAQact10.htmtp://www.biomedcentral.com/1472-6750/11/101
268   http://www.ncbi.nlm.nih.gov/books/NBK26904/
269   http://en.wikipedia.org/wiki/Adenosine_triphosphate
270   http://www.bmb.leeds.ac.uk/teaching/icu3/lecture/19/
271
272   http://ajpregu.physiology.org/content/ajpregu/292/1/R77.full.pdf
273   http://www.meltorganic.com/wp-content/uploads/2011/06/Medium-chain-fatty-acids-Functional-lip-ids-for-the-prevention-and-treatment-of-the-metabolic-syndrome.pdf
274   http://www.examiner.com/article/best-thermogenic-foods-diet-balancing-tech-niques-for-weight-management
275   http://www.ncbi.nlm.nih.gov/pubmed/22538118
276   http://www.health.com/health/gallery/0,,20553780,00.html

for thermogenic effects. Diet induced thermogenesis coupled with exercise is the best way to increase metabolic rate, burn fat, and manage weight.

2.06.16 Glutathione

Glutathione is as an antioxidant, an evolutionary friend of ours. There is a case study that reveals protective effects of glutathione and its ability to help us evolve and survive. Professors Timothy Mousseau of University of South Carolina, Anders Moller of CNRS in France, and Iamael Galvan of Donna Research station in Spain have found something very revealing. They found that birds near Chernobyl in Ukraine after nuclear explosion had better survival rate than the ones in Fukushima , Japan. The birds in Ukraine had time to evolve but not the ones in Fukushima as evidenced by genetic damage undone by higher glutathione production that neutralizes radiation chemicals. Birds from low exposure areas in Ukraine had glutathione level of only 450 microgram per gram of body mass compared to a high 735 microgram per gram of body mass in birds from high exposure areas. The higher the exposure the higher the glutathione level just as Darwin would have predicted. What does this finding say about human exposure to herbicides, pesticides, and food process born carcinogens? There is no definitive study but the case of glutathione supplement is no doubt made. It should be emphasized that vitamins A and C should be part of routine diet for natural antioxidant glutathione to function effectively.

2.07 Methylation diet for Mitochondrial Health

I prepared a master table for my book on Our Genes Our Foods Our Lifestyle". It is incorporated in this book as Table No. 2.07.02 below. This table can serve as a guide to creating methylation diets and preparing daily dishes. Methylation diet, it is clear from this master table helps prevent major chronic diseases and ailments and mitigates deficiencies of Vitamins B complex including B_{12}, Vitamin D, vitamins A and C, and minerals magnesium, manganese, selenium, copper, and zinc. The idea is to secure a nutrient balance.

Almost 40% Americans have vitamin B_{12} deficiency, 54% suffer from pain, and 64% suffer from constipation. As pointed out earlier methylation diet eliminates problems of nutrient deficiency, promotes proper gene expression, maintains a stable DNA and genome, and fights epigenomic problems. Simply stated methylation diet keeps us healthy by supplying enough of vitamins A, B Complex, C, D, E, folate, and minerals calcium, iron, magnesium, and zinc..

Carrots, bitter gourd, and cucumber have great health values as methylation foods. They are abundantly available as providers of fiber, beta carotene, Vitamins A, D, C, B_1, B_6, folate, minerals calcium, magnesium, and zinc, and phytochemicals cucurbitans, lariciresinol, and pinoresinol. Cucumber and carrots are readily available in our retail stores and and bitter gourd is now noticeable too. Twice a week consumption of side dishes of cucumber, carrot, and bitter gourd are big promotors of mitochondrial health. Coenzyme Q_{10}, as a mobile electron carrier, is best known for therapeutic use in case of mitochondrial diseases. It strengthens muscles and decreases fatigue. Table 2.07.01 lists many other mitochondrial foods including vitamins of B complex, folic acid, vitamin E, Lipoic acid, and mineral selenium and their suggested daily intake.

Table 2.07.01 Foods and Food Supplements in Mitigating Mitochondrial Diseases

Supplements	Daily Dose	Remarks
Coenzyme Q_{10} mg	750	350 mg dose twice a day.
L-carnitine, g	3.75	1.25 g 3 times a day; Improves fatty acid metabolism.
Thiamine, B_1, mg	300	Increase vegetable intake.
Riboflavin, B_6, mg	400	
Niacin amide, B_3, mg	350	Avoid Niacin. May cause flushing.
Folate, mcg	2,000	
Vitamin E, IU	750	May interfere with Coenzyme Q_{10}. Antioxidants prevent DNA damage.
Selenium, mcg	50	Two brazil nuts every day
Lipoic Acid, mg	400	
Source: Cleveland Clinic and averages from a variety of sources.		

Table 2.07.02 Food Nutrients and the Mechanism of Their Curative Action

Food	Key Nutrient	Mechanism	Cure
Adaptogenic foods			**Promote epigenome stability and homeostasis.**
Asafoetida	**Ferulic acid, asaresinotanol**	Antioxidants	Ant flatulent, antibacterial, anticonstipative
Artichoke	Sylimarin, dietary fiber	antioxidants	Prevents skin cancer
Asparagus[277],[278]	Vitamin C, E, Folic acid, B_{12}, Rutin, (Swedish Study)	Antiinflammatory Effective against Pancreatic cancer Histamine production	Telomerase activator Enhances immune system Improved complexion.
Asparagus roots	Cytoastrogenol	Folic acid	Boosts telomerase activity.
Asvagandha	alkaloids, steroidal lactones, saponins, and withanolides	Adaptogenic	Prevents DNA damage Found in Indian steroid adaptogen ashvagandga.
Astragalus	Cycloastrogenol, fiber, telomerase activator,	Antioxidants	DNA damage control, anti-aging food, Anti HIV, antiinflammatory, and liver protective food.
Chinese berries	Achisandra berries	Antioxidants	Liver protective medicine in China

---

277   http://www.nutrition-and-you.com/asparagus.html
278   http://www.livestrong.com/article/17504-nutritional-value-asparagus/

Food	Key Nutrient	Mechanism	Cure
Garlic		antiinflamma-tory	Promotes heart health
Ginger		antiinflamma-tory	Prevent pain and promotes heart health
Licorice		Antioxidants	Prevents DNA damage
Tomato	Lycopene, lutein	Antioxidants	Eye health
Shitake, Mistake Mushroom	Vitamin D and B vitamins	Free radical quenching	Prevent DNA damage
Antiangiogenic Foods			
Almond Oil [279]	Vitamin E, A, B_1, B_2, B_6, Omega-3 and Omega-9	Antioxidants and essential vitamins	Very good for hair care. http://pubs.acs.org/doi/abs/10.1021/ie50382a014?-journal-Code=iechad
Dark Chocolate	Polyphenols	Antioxidants	Cures cough, prevents DNA damage
Kale		antioxidants	
Red grapes	Resveratrol	antioxidants	Heart health value
Tomato	Lycopene, lutein		
Turmeric	Curcumin	Antiinflamma-tory and anti-carcinogenic	Prevents cancer Cures joint pain
Anticarcinogen-ic and Antioxi-dant Foods			
Fruits	Vitamins, min-erals	Essential nutri-ents	Heart disease and cancer

279 http://pubs.acs.org/doi/abs/10.1021/jf051692j

Food	Key Nutrient	Mechanism	Cure
Vegetables	Vitamins, minerals, phytonutrients	Essential phytonutrients	Heart disease and cancer
Antiinflamatory Foods			
Black and blue berries [280]	Tuft University[281]	Communications Between neurons	Brain Health
Antioxidants	Carotenoids, vitamins A C E K and minerals selenium and zinc, Eugenol, limonine, orientin, vicerin	Free radical scavenging	Control DNA damage Manage telomerase length.
Dahi (India), Cheese, Kimchi, mother's milk, sour Kraut, Yogurt	Probiotic food	Builds immune system	Digestive health and enhanced immunity
Oyster	Zinc and Iron	Enzyme function	Prevents DNA damage
Ash, poplar, and weed goldenrod extract	Salicin (aspirin like) chemical	Antiinflammatory	Reduces arthritic and joint pains.
Almond and peanut butter	Magnesium	Muscle relaxant	Prevents colon cancer
Almond	Copper, magnesium, manganese, vitamin E, protein, dietary fiber	Antiinflammatory	Muscle health due to magnesium, lowers cholesterol for heart health.

280   http://nutritiondata.self.com/facts/fruits-and-fruit-juices/1848/2
281   http://www.cookinglight.com/eating-smart/nutrition-101/brain-foods/blackberries-polyphenols

Food	Key Nutrient	Mechanism	Cure
Apple (berries, red grapes, tomato, pea pods)[282]	Quircetin, pectin soluble fiber, Cornell University	Regulates blood flow	Promotes weight loss, Fights dementia, Alzheimer's, Prevents H. Pylori stomach ulcer
Asafoetida	Ferulic acid, ubelliferone, and asaresino-tannols	Antioxidant Antispsmodic antiinflammatory	Lowers blood pressure and removes blood clots, helps builds bone density [283].
Avocado	olive oil, fat soluble beta-carotene and lycopene, fiber, folic acid, vitamins K and C, B_5, and B_6.	Excellent methylation food http://www.avocadosoy.net/clinical-trials.html, Multiple Studies	Heart healthy food
Avocado[284, 285]	Vitamin B_3	Various mechanisms	Heart healthy food Reduces inflammation
Banana	Potassium, vitamins B_6, C, dietary fiber, lutein, carotenoids, zeaxanthin,, magnesium, manganese, molybdenum	Good source of trace minerals and monounsaturated fat.	Reduces risk of breast cancer
Basal	Vitamin K, Eugenol, limonene, flavonoid, Orientin, and vicerin	**Antioxidants and adaptogens**	Prevent DNA damage

282   http://www.nutritionj.com/content/3/1/5
283   http://examine.com/supplements/Ferula+asafoetida/
284   http://www.whfoods.com/genpage.php?tname=foodspice&dbid=5
285   http://www.californiaavocado.com/nutrition/

Food	Key Nutrient	Mechanism	Cure
Baker's yeast	Folic Acid	Methionine synthesis	Fights allergy
Barley	Beta-glucan soluble dietary fiber, Selenium	Antioxidants	Reduces cholesterol
Beans	Antioxidants, dietary fiber, Copper, magnesium, manganese, molybdenum folic acid	Dopamine, serotonin, melatonin synthesis	Blood sugar control, Nerve function
Beet roots[286], [287]	Betaine, folic acid, manganese, potassium, dietary fiber, multiple studies	Antioxidants Increased blood flow	Prevents DNA damage Prevents lung and stomach cancer, increased blood flow, promotes brain and cardiac health
Bell Pepper	**High Vitamin C and Carotenoids**	**Antioxidants** **Antiinflammatory**	Build immune system, prevents cardiovascular diseases
Black currant, borage oil	**Gama linoleic acid and Omega-6**	antiinflammatory	Builds bone, eye, skin, and hair health, improves bone health
Black Pepper, peppercorn	**Peperine, bioperine, chromium**	**Antioxidants**	Interferes with shelf-renewal of cancer stem cells, antidiabetic, induces weight loss, promotes energy metabolism, reduces pain.
Bosswella serrata	**Oil and terpenoids**	**Antiinflammatory**	Cures osteoarthritis.

286   http://www.whfoods.com/genpage.php?tname=foodspice&dbid=49
287   http://www.sciencedirect.com/science/article/pii/S1756464611000673

Food	Key Nutrient	Mechanism	Cure
Brans (Rice, cereals)	**Phytosterols**	**Lowers cholesterol**	Promotes heart health
Blueberries	Pterosilbene, Ellagic acid antioxidants	Reveratrol like action.	Improves cognition and memory, Reduce stress Boosts immune system Protects capillaries from oxidative damage
Brazil Nut	Protein, dietary fiber, Selenium, folic acid, vitamin E, magnesium, manganese	antioxidant	Prevent DNA damage Cognitive function, cell signaling, turns on gene Nrf2 that regulates hundreds of other genes.
Broccoli, broccoli sprouts, cauliflower, kale[288, 289]	Sulphoraphane, indol-3-carbinol Multiple studies	Histone acylation Fights free radicals, Produces cancer killing enzymes, antioxidants	Cancer prevention Genomic stability Indol-3-carbinol inhibits growth of estrogen responsive cancer.
Brown rice	Polyphenols, phytosterols	antioxidants	Low glycemic food
Buck Choy	Bracissin, anthocyanins	Anticarcinogens	Reduced risk of cancer Reduced estrogen.

---

288   http://www.cancer.gov/cancertopics/factsheet/diet/cruciferous-vegetables
289   http://www.diagnosticpathology.org/content/9/1/7

Food	Key Nutrient	Mechanism	Cure
Buckwheat	Polyphenol anti-oxidants	Quenches free radicals.	Reduces stress, Prevents DNA damage, prevents muscular degeneration, prevents cancer, improves cognition.
Butter	Conjugated linoleic Acid	Body fat reduction, improves insulin control.	Reduces obesity, improves weight loss
Buttermilk	Probiotic Lactic bacteria	Our second genome	Digestive health
Cabbage[290] **(Swedish Study)**[291]	**Isocyanate, vitamin K**	**anticarcino-genic**	Protects against prostate and pancreatic cancer
Cacao	**Theobromine**		Boosts mental capacity.
Canola Oil	**Monounsaturated fat and oil**	**Antiinflamma-tory**	Promotes heart health
Card mum, very common in Indian diet.	**Pine, linatol**	**Antioxidant** **Antibacterial** **Lowers cholesterol**	Promotes heart health. Improves weight loss.
Carrots, red and yellow	**Provitamin A, Beta-carotene, Vitamins A, K, and C**	**Antioxidant, reduce risk of cancer, and heart disease.**	Reduces risk of cancer, reduces risk of heart disease, DNA repair.

290   http://www.whfoods.com/genpage.php?tname=foodspice&dbid=19
291   http://www.bugwood.org/arthropod2005/vol1/6d.pdf

Food	Key Nutrient	Mechanism	Cure
Cashew Nut	Monounsaturated good fat, Copper, B_5, B_6, riboflavin, and thiamine, manganese, zinc, selenium, tryptophan	Antioxidants and precursors for neurotransmitters	Control DNA damage Improves neuronal activity
Celery-onion-bell pepper trinity	Apiol, flavonoid	Antioxidants prevent blood lipid damage	Promotes weight loss, reduces blood pressure
Cereals	Dietary fiber, Copper, manganese, magnesium, selenium, vitamin B_1	Improve digestion and immune system	Good vitamin supplement
Cheese, egg, beef,	Conjugated Linoleic Acid	anticarcinogenic	Prevents atherosclerosis, Builds immune system.
Cheese, Yogurt	Vitamin B_{12}	Methionine synthesis, anti-stress vitamin	Fights allergy, mental health, memory
Chick pea and red pepper hummus	Protein, iron, vitamin C	Antiinflammatory	Builds red blood cells
Chicken Soup, beef, trout	Amino Acid Cysteine Coenzyme Q_{10}	Antiinflammatory	Promotes muscle health
Chia Seed	Omega-3 Fatty Acid	Protein and fiber for appetite control	Helps burn fat, improves metabolism

Food	Key Nutrient	Mechanism	Cure
Chili Pepper, cayenne pepper	Capsaicin, carotenoids, Vitamin A, C, B vitamins, magnesium, potassium, and iron	Mediates and boosts metabolism, multiple effects in cardiovascular health	Blood sugar control, improves insulin function, reduces cholesterol, helps maintain blood sugar, improves cognition, protects from cancer, and acts as anticlotting agent, fights pain, induces weight loss, increases metabolism.
Chocolate	Polyphenols	Antioxidants	Prevents DNA damage
Cinnamon[292],[293]	Proanthocyanins, Eugenol, Cinnamaldehyde, UC Santa Barbara	Analgesic Antidiabetic Hypocholesteremic	Prevents stress, reduces adipose tissue (Lund University)
Citrus peel	Flavonoid mobiletin , limonene, and tangeretin; vitamin C	Antioxidant, Inhibits key proteins that promote cancer of skin,	Reduces cholesterol, LDL associated apoloprotein B, and triglyceride.
Cloves	Eugenol, Omega 3 fatty acids, Manganese	Antibacterial, anti-diabetic	Promotes digestive health

292   http://www.ia.ucsb.edu/pa/display.aspx?pkey=3022
293   http://www.whfoods.com/genpage.php?tname=foodspice&dbid=68

Food	Key Nutrient	Mechanism	Cure
Coconut, green Freeze-dried [294]	**Cococin, vitamins, minerals, High lauric acid**	**Emulsion stability** **Creaminess**	Promotes Skin Health **http://www.nsf. ac.lk/newsletter/ VOL3NO3/conut. pdf**
Cocoa powder	Antioxidants, arginine, fiber,	Antioxidants: Prevent DNA damage and promote heart health.	Reduces stress and promotes heart health.
Coconut Oil	Low calorie medium chain fatty acids	Helps burn calories, doesn't go in adipose fat	
Compfrey Ointment	Allantoin	antiinflammatory	Promotes growth of healthy tissue.
Cottage cheese	Selenium, protein, vitamins and minerals	Antioxidants and protein nutrition	
Cranberry	Anthocyanins	Antibacterial, anticarcinogenic	Cures urinary infection, prevents cancer
Curry Powder[295, 296]	Curcumin Multiple studies	Anticarcinogens Antioxidant antiinflammatory	Prevents Alzheimer's
Coffee, tea[297298]	Antioxidants Finish Study	Central nervous system stimulation and cognition	Promote memory Reduce dementia

294   ww.nsf.ac.lk/newsletter/VOL3NO3/conut.pdf
295   http://www.bioportfolio.com/resources/pmarticle/697359/A-systematic-review-and-meta-analysis-of-randomized-controlled-trials-investigating-the.html

296   http://nutritiondata.self.com/facts/spices-and-herbs/185/2
297   http://www.womenshealthnetwork.com/fatigueandinsomnia/effectsofcaffeine-references.aspx
298   http://www.amazon.com/Tea-Therapy-Remedies-Traditional-Medicine/dp/1602201471

Food	Key Nutrient	Mechanism	Cure
Collard Green	Calcium, fiber, antioxidants	Fiber and anti-oxidant effects	Promotes cardio-vascular health
coriander	Phthalides, coumarins, terpenol	Antibacterial anticholesteremic	Promotes digestive health Prevents cancer
Cucumbers	Lignans laricires-inol, pinorecinol, cucurbitacins, Vitamins A, B_1, B_6, C, folate, Calcium and Magnesium	Anticarcinogenic Antiinflammatory Antidiabetic hypochlesteremin	Prevents cancer, lowers cholestrol and joint pain. Consume cucumber and carrot in combination.
Cumin	Luteolin, peperine, pipene, terpine, Iron	antioxidants	Prevents prostate cancer Improves digestive health
Dark Chocolate	Polyphenols	Antioxidants, A natural opiate anandamide	Prevent DNA damage Promotes heart health, Reduces stress, reduces pain.
Dietary fiber	Butyric Acid in colon	Histone deacylation	Longevity
Dill seed	Quircetin, Kaempferol	antioxidants	Prevents DNA damage
Edamami	Antioxidants, isoflavones	Antioxidant and protein nutrition	Promotes weight loss Enhances cardio-vascular health.

Food	Key Nutrient	Mechanism	Cure
Egg yolk	Choline Well established	Neurotransmission, Methyl group donor	DNA Methylation
Egg White	Almost pure protein	Satiation	Low food intake and weight control.
Egg, peanut, green vegetables	B_5	Energy production	Anti-stress vitamin
Fruits and vegetables	B_6, Cox 2 Inhibitors, prebiotics	Antiinflammatory foods, Methionine synthesis Homocysteine in blood	Fights allergy
Crimin Mushroom	B_2 or Riboflavin	Homocysteine in blood	
Garbanzo beans	Molybdenum, protein, dietary fiber, choline, vitamin A and C	Maintains oxidation state and oxygen transfer	Supplies protein and amino acids for endogenous endomorphins
Garlic	Allinase	Anticarcinogens	Boosts immunity, Protects blood cell membranes, fights cancer.
Ginseng	An adaptogen	Antiinflammatory and reduces stress	Prevents DNA damage
Ginger	Gingerol, Gingerone	Antioxidant antiinflammatory	Digestive aid Fights arthritic pain, protects DNA
Gouda, Jalsberg Cheese	B_{12}, vitamin K	antiangiogenic	Protective of lung cancer

Food	Key Nutrient	Mechanism	Cure
Grapes	Resveratrol	Antiinflamma-tory Helps produce nitric oxide vasodilator	Promotes heart health Anti aging anticarcinogenis
Green Peppers	Vitamin C, beta-carotene, lycopene	Antioxidants	Very high vitamin C, fights allergy
Green Tea	Epigallocate-chin-3-gallate, Vitamin A and C	Antioxidants	Promotes heart health and prevents cancer, DNA repair and gene stability, kills cancer cells.
Gouda, emen-thaler, and Adam Cheese	Menaquinone and Menatertre-none	Anticarcinogen Antiangiogenic	Prevents cancer Promotes heart health Fights diabetes.
Flax Seed	Lignan, Omega-3 Fatty acid, B_6, copper, manga-nese, Lignan,	Antiinflamma-tory Antioxidants, reduces choles-terol.	Promotes Cardiac and brain health, reduces cardiac arrest, lowers blood pressure, prevents pros-tate cancer, and promotes kidney health. Builds immune system.
Fenugreek	Dietary Fiber and antioxidants	Slows glucose absorption	Satiety and hun-ger control
Fermented Soy Products[299], [300]	Nattokinase, enzyme from Natto., (Univer-sity of Chicago Work)		Breaks fibrin down, the blood clotting enzyme.

299   http://www.chicagoreader.com/Bleader/archives/2010/12/23/one-bite-natto
300   http://undergroundhealthreporter.com/natto-benefits-live-longer-like-japanese/#axzz3759Qrhhg

Food	Key Nutrient	Mechanism	Cure
Fruits and Vegetables: broccoli, yellow squash, red bell pepper, leafy greens, tomato, potato peals, and citrus fruits	Prebiotic Fiber, sulphoraphane, isothiocyanates, Probiotic bacteria Vitamins A, C, Coenzyme Q$_{10}$, Selenium	Antioxidants Anticarcinogenic, antiangiogenic, improved glucose and fat metabolism, homocysteine reduction	Prevent cancer, boosting of immune system, improved cellular communication, good gene expression, cellular mobility by binding tubulin protein for digestive health, arterial elasticity,
Garlic	Diallyl sulfide, allicin, vitamin c, chromium	Histone acylation Antiplatelet enzyme, antidiabetic.	Cancer prevention, reduction of blood pressure, protects arteries and veins, prevents clotting
Ginger	Gingerol	Blocks postaglandins	Antiarthritic and antihypertensive
Grape juice[301, 302]	Polyphenols U of Cincinnati	antioxidants	
Honey	Low glycemic sugar	Satiation	Antidiabetic
Hop extract from brewery	Perluxan	Inhibits proinflammatory chemicals.	Fast pain relief.
Horse Radish	Ally isocyanate, glucosinolates, Vitamin C, calcium, magnesium, and phosphorus	Anticarcinogenic glucosinolates prevent cancer.	10X better than broccoli Helps liver do detoxification.
Inulin (Jerusalem Artichoke)	Oligosaccharides	Lowers cholesterol and regulates blood sugar.	Promote colon health

301   http://www.phytochemicals.info/plants/grape.php
302   http://www.psychiatry.uc.edu/FacultyStaff/FacultyProfile.aspx?epersonID=MTQ1OA%3D%3D

Food	Key Nutrient	Mechanism	Cure
Isomaltulose	Low glycemic sugar		Wight and obesity control
Kohlrabi	High vitamin C, fiber, folic acid, minerals, sulphoraphane, Indol-3-carbinol, vitamins, isothiocyanates, B and B vitamins.	Antioxidant vitamin C, and other phytochemicals	Healthy connective tissue, teeth and gum, prevents asthma and bronchitis.
Kokum	Luteolin, flavones, apigenin, antioxidants, hydroxycitric acid	Balm formulations \n\n Promotes cell oxygenation	Soft skin
Leafy Green Vegetables	Zeaxanthin	Powerful antioxidant	Prevents skin cancer.
Legume, peas, soy, beans	Folic acid and fiber, \n\n Indol-3-carbinol	Homocysteine control	Reduced cholesterol and reduced risk of heart attack. \n\n Protects breast, ovarian, and colon cancer.
Lentils	B vitamins and folic acid	DNA methylation	Weight and obesity control
Licorice	Anethol, Glycirrhizin, isoflavone	Nutrient dense antiinflammatory food	Protects liver and reduces cholesterol
Lipowheat Ceramide	A fat like molecule	Inhibits enzyme elastase, rehydrates	Smooth and soft skin
Meat, mushroom, green vegetables	Coenz Q10, B_2,	Critical to electron transport chain function.	Energy metabolism, ATP production, great for skin, hair, and eye health
Maple syrup		Antioxidants	

Food	Key Nutrient	Mechanism	Cure
Mango powder	Citric acid, malic acid, oxalic acid	Natural acidulant	Digestive aid
Millet	Fiber	Bile acid secretion	Removes cholesterol
Mint[303]	Menthone and menthol. Mint chutney is great marinating agent.	Regulates gut bacteria. Quenches free radicals.	Antibacterial against sinusitis, bronchitis, and pneumonia. Digestive aid.
Mushroom	Vitamins A, B, and C, Protein, dietary fiber, copper, potassium,. iron, selenium, and zinc.	Anticarcinogenic	Prevents cancer
Mustard, garden green, kale	Selenium, protein, oil, good emulsifier, B_2, B_5, B_3, Vitamin C and K	Antioxidants Anticarcinogens and antiinflammatory	Open tumor cell receptors to chemotherapy drugs for effect and efficiency.
Natural Food Colors	Carotenoids used for ages	Antioxidants Antiinflammatory	Prevent DNA damage
Nonfat dry milk	Calcium, B_{12}, protein		Satiety and weight loss
Nutmeg	Atropine like bioactivity	Antifungal	Digestive aid
Nuts and seeds	Minerals and vitamins Widely approved	Antioxidants, good fat, and trace minerals	Mental health and improved HDL
Oats	Beta Glucan Soluble fiber	Satiety enhancer	Reduces blood pressure, reduces cholesterol , digestive health, boosts immunity

303　http://www.ajol.info/index.php/tjpr/article/viewFile/93279/82692

Food	Key Nutrient	Mechanism	Cure
Olive Oil [304]	Oleocanthal and Squaline (Monell Chemical Senses Center, Philadelphia PA)	Anticarcinogenic antiinflammatory	Relieves pain, Heart health Mental health
Onion	Quircetin	Antioxidant	Antidiabetic
Oranges	Vitamin C, hesperidins	Antioxidants	Prevents DNA damage, prevents cancer, prevents vericose veins, improves digestion.
Oregano	Vitamin K, carnasol, quircetin, thymol	Antioxidants antifungal	Digestive aid
Oysters	Zinc, protein, Vitamin A	Prevents zinc deficiency	Heals wounds and cures infant diarrhea
Papaya			
Parsley	Apigenin, apiin, cresoviol, luteolin, flavonoids, vitamins A, C, and K	Antioxidants	Prevents DNA damage Builds immune system, enhances white blood cell
Peanut Butter, peanut	Unsaturated plant fat, protein, fiber	Nutrient dense, good fat	Promotes heart health Induces weight loss.
Pine bark extract	Pycnogenol	Antioxidant Nitric oxide vasodilator	Lowers blood pressure, Reduces osteoarthritic pain.

304   http://www.monell.org/news/news_releases/trpa1_receptor

Food	Key Nutrient	Mechanism	Cure
Pistachio [305]	Protein, fiber, oleic acid, vitamin E, K, B_6, and thiamine, and minerals	Antioxidants (Stanford University)	Reduces stomach fat Increases HDL
Pomegranate	Antioxidants Elagic Acid to Urolithin A & b conversion by gut bacteria		Prevents DNA damage, prevents prostate cancer, improves heart health, speeds up skin cell synthesis
Potato	Potassium, copper, B vitamins, starch	Vitamin c and Potassium	Cures acne, promotes digestive health.
Protein, high	Methionine, tyrosine, tryptophan, phenylalanine, arginine	Dopamine synthesis Satiation, produces vasodilator nitric oxide	S-Adenosyl Methionine for stable epigenome Antidiabetic, satiation, antihypertensive
Prune/dried plum	Boron, vitamin K, antioxidants	A natural laxative with antioxidant power	Bone density improvement.
Pumpkin Seed	Zinc, protein, Vitamins A, C, E, K, and Folic Acid	Works with anabolic receptors	Protects bladder health, Reduces pain
Red Yeast	Statin like monacolin K, trade name cholestin	Lovastatin like mechanism of action	Reduces cholesterol
Red grape skin	Resveratrol	Antiinflammatory COX II inhibitor.	Reduces pain.
Red Wine	Resveratrol	Histone deacylation	Longevity

---

305   http://www.musclemagfitness.com/nutrition/healthy-eating/lower-ldl-cholesterol-naturally-on-the-pistachio-diet.html

Food	Key Nutrient	Mechanism	Cure
Rice Bran [306], [307],[308]	A good source of phytosterol oryzanol, tocotrienol, ferulate, vitamins and minerals	0.8 gram per day FDA and (Pennington Biomedical Research Center)	Heart Health promoter Reduces cholesterol
Rosemary	20 antioxidants	Antiinflammatory, antibacterial,	Improves cognition and memory
Salmon, sardines [309],[310],[311]	Omega-3 Fatty acids U of Los Angeles	Antiinflammatory	Brain structure and function Improves memory and cognition.
Sage oil extract	Rosemaric acid, cornosol, thymol, carvacol	Inhibits enzyme that destroys neurotransmitter acetylcholine	Improves cognition, neuroprotective, cures Alzheimer's
Salt, Black		Carminative Anti-flatulent	
Sanguisorba			Cures diarrhea
Sea food, milk, egg, meat, fish	L-Taurine	Brain and blood cell function	Crosses blood brain barrier, reduces cholesterol, prevents congestive heart failure, reduces blood pressure.

306   http://nutritiondata.self.com/facts/cereal-grains-and-pasta/5725/2
307   http://www.californiariceoil.com/nutrition.htm
308   http://www.disabled-world.com/fitness/rice-bran.php
309   http://www.whfoods.com/genpage.php?tname=foodspice&dbid=104
310   http://www.mayoclinic.org/diseases-conditions/heart-disease/in-depth/omega-3/art-20045614
311

Food	Key Nutrient	Mechanism	Cure
Sesame Seed	Molybdenum, copper, calcium, iron, zinc, manganese, vitamin B_6, and C, protein, dietary fiber, choline	DNA methylation	Skin health, bone health, Oral and digestive health Heart health by blood pressure reduction, Prevention of DNA damage.
Shitake mushroom	Lentinan Vitamin D	Anti-carcinogenic, slows down tumor growth.	Boosts immune system Improves cognition
Soy, barley, wheat, rye,[312]	Lunacil, isoflavones (Dr. Benito, UC Berkeley)[313]	Anticarcinogenic	Kills cancer cells
Sprouted Grains	B_{12}, Folic acid, Other B vitamins, vitamin A and K, manganese	DNA methylation	Stable DNA
Soy products and fiber	Genistein Proteins, Saponins, isoflavones to uquol conversion by gut bacteria, iron, molybdenum, manganese, potassium, zinc, niacin, folic acid,	Methylation, regulates ell death, cell cycle control, and DNA repair.	Cancer prevention Estrogen like effect, prevents breast and prostate cancer, Regulates tumor suppressor gene, anti-protozoal (Girardia) agent.

312   http://celiacdisease.about.com/od/Gluten-Free-Grains/f/Is-Soy-Gluten-Free.htm
313   ww.sunstar.com.ph/bacolod/lifestyle/2014/01/30/filipino-scientist-who-found-switch-325792

Food	Key Nutrient	Mechanism	Cure
Spinach, green pepper, soy foods	Pyrroloquinoline quinone	A very powerful antioxidant	Prevents DNA damage
Spinach, Swiss chord, kale	Folic acid, vitamin k, luteolin, magnesium	Blood clotting	Promotes weight loss, Prevents calcification of arteries, promotes bone health, fights Hodgkin's lymphoma, Prevents dementia, Enhances immune system.
Squash, yellow veg	carotenoids		Prevents cancer
Stevia sweetener	Steviol base sweet glycoside	Antioxidant and antiinflammatory	Antidiabetic
Strawberries	Antioxidants, ellagic acid		Antidiabetic Boosts immune system Protects capillaries from oxidative damage.
Sugar beet	Betaine	Breakdown of toxic products from SAM synthesis	Protects from osmolytic stress.
Sunflower seeds	Folic acid, selenium, copper, B_{12},	Methionine synthesis Homocysteine in blood	Fights allergy

Food	Key Nutrient	Mechanism	Cure
Sweet Potato	Copper, Iron, magnesium, manganese, protein, good fat, dietary fiber, vitamin A, and carotenoids.		Promotes eye health Promotes heart health
Tarragon	Charvicol, poly-phenol	Antioxidants	A great heart healthy spice
Tea, black & Green	Catechins, theanine, flavo-noids		Prevents DNA damage Improves cogni-tion
Thyme	Geraniol, borneol, thymol, carvacol, and vitamin K	Antimicrobial, antioxidant,	Carminative and antispasmodic
Tomato [314], [315]	Lycopene, chro-mium	Antioxidant (Harvard Med School)	Promotes heart health, prevents breast, and lung cancer.
Turmeric	Curcumin, folic acid, Vitamins C, K, and B_6	Antioxidant, antibacterial, Antiinflamma-tory, anticar-cinogenic	Prevents cancer Fights osteo-arthritic pain, prevents enlarge-ment of heart, protects liver, digestive health promoter, reduc-es osteoarthritic pain.
Vinegar	Acetic Acid, ap-ple cider, pickled cucumber	Antidiabetic and anti-ath-erosclerotic	Prevents lung and prostate cancer, promotes weight loss.

Food	Key Nutrient	Mechanism	Cure
Walnuts	Vitamin E, Omega-3 fatty acids Manganese, copper, tryptophan	Antiinflammatory antioxidants	Cardiovascular health, Brain structure and function Cognition, memory, immune system enhancement
Watermelon	Lycopene	Antioxidant lycopene	Promotes eye health
Watercress	Isothiocyanates	Anti-carcinogen	Triggers enzyme that stop cancer cell growth.
Whey Protein (hydrolyzed)	Ace inhibitor like polypeptide	Immunoproteins enhance immune system	Blood pressure control
White kidney beans		Prevents DNA damage.	Helps weight loss
Whole grain	Antioxidants Omega-3 fatty acids Polyphenol antioxidants minerals	Antioxidants, minerals, and fiber	Digestive, cardiac, and mental health
Yogurt	Vitamin B_{12},	Our second genome	Digestive aid
Yumberry and honeyberry		**Antioxidants**	
	Citicholine mononucleotide		Neuroprotective effect, improved cognition.

Food	Key Nutrient	Mechanism	Cure
Fruits, vegetables, and whole grain	Dietary Fiber	Gene expression and help produce telomerase	Enhanced immune system, enhanced humoral immunity, increased immunoglobulin concentration, short chain fatty acid supply.
Spinach and collard	Alpha-Lipoic Acid	Boosts ATP production	Promotes skin health, promotes weight loss
Fruits & Vegetables	Isocyanates	Affect genes that produce telomerase	Effective in preventing cancer cell growth.
Fruits and Vegetables	Bioflavonids	Block the receptor sites	Prevent infection
Coconut and palm kernel oil with 8-12 carbon long fatty acids	Medium chain Triglycerides	Eases fat metabolism	Anti aging cream formulations for healthy skin
Bacterial Exopolysaccharide	Abyssine	Polysaccharides postpone cellular aging	Anti aging ingredient in BB cream

The diet we design and select for daily consumption should stabilize our genome, help populate and establish our microbiome, and fix our epigenome[316], [317]. To live with our nuclear and mitochondrial genes well, we need to avoid smoking, toxins, and unnecessary medications (acid blockers, water pill HCTZ (hydrochlorithiazide for blood pressure, and Delantin for seizures). As long as we eat leafy dark green vegetables, deemphasize animal protein and highly processed foods, use caffeine and alcohol in moderation, improve stomach acid by herbal digestive bitters, and if necessary, take anti-homocysteine supplements (folic acid, B_6 and B_{12}) our DNA should

---

316   http://learn.genetics.utah.edu/content/epigenetics/nutrition/
317   http://advances.nutrition.org/content/1/1/8.full

remain stable and undamaged [318], [319]. The best practice is to get it all from methylation diet comprised of commonly available foods and not the expensive supplements.

Just to safeguard further we should ask our physicians to watch Mean Corpuscular Volume (MCV below 95) and urinary methylmelonic acid carefully. **High numbers indicate folate and B$_{12}$ deficiency**. In cases of Alzheimer's disease, a physician may choose to prescribe SAM-e or S-Adenosyl Methionine.

All foods must be washed in warm water or blanched as delivered by the hot water heater in our houses before use. The practice is absolutely necessary for more contaminated foods like berries, celery, and lettuce. It is true that healthy mitochondria can transform and detoxify xenobiotic foods but light blanching in the kitchen is an added safeguard.

We should keep in mind that we also get valuable Omega-3 fatty acids from dark green vegetables, cloves, and cinnamon. Spice mixes like Dukha of Egypt, Curry powder of India, and Zetar of Palestine add not only flavor but also essential mineral and vitamin nutrients. A good spice mix is a kind of vitamin and mineral supplement. Examples of complementary side dishes based on Table 2.15.02 are

- A cup of fresh red grapes and 1/2 a cup of roated almond for antioxidants and hunger control.

- Lemon and rosemary added to hummus to be used in snack dips for good fat, fiber, and protein.

- A combinations of fruit pastes, dried pineaple, cranberries, date paste, lentil and legume flours in the form of fruit loopes and bars.

- One hard boiled egg with guacamole spread and strips of red pepper.

We need to alternate these items interspersed throughout the week for sustaining the health of our mitochondria.

318   http://www.ncbi.nlm.nih.gov/pubmed/22359306
319   http://jn.nutrition.org/content/132/8/2333S.long

2.08 Probiotic Foods

Probiotics are foods that carry healthful bacteria, the Lactobacilli present in our foods used routinely for centuries as our evolutionary friends. Actually, the bacteria in our nose, stomach, and the colon have been integral part of our physiology thoughout our evolution. All combined they weigh 3-4 pounds, same as our brain, and build more than 50% of our immune system via additional 1 million co-inhabiting functional genes. We can't ignore them because we can't live without them.

Our gut bacteria remodel our intestines and make them better atabsorbing nutrients Our thermoregulation is controlled by these companion so called symbiotic bacteria. They control our thermostat says Dr. Mirko Trajkovsky of Geneva University 320. Actually, we know that obese people have different microbiome (set of bacteria) compared to non-obese people.

Our over dependence on antibiotics is making these good bacteria go extinct [321], [322]. Even the helix shaped stomach ulcer bacteria (Helicobacter pylori) that is known to control immunity, weight, and height is systematically killed by antibiotics [323]. The unpleasant result is chronic diseases of asthma, allergy, diabetes, obesity, and even cancer .

We now have credible research that shows that human microbiome, the right combination of bacteria, and mitochondria are critically connected [324] and, therefore, a daily dose of probiotics (cheese, yogurt, kefir, kimchi, South East Asian miso, South American curtido, and sour kraut) and dietary fiber prebiotics should be considered critical components of methylation diet for mitochondria [325]. We need to regularly repopulate our digestive system with probiotics because they help digest, absorb, produce vitamins K2, B_1, B_3, B_6, B_{12}, and vitamin B_9 or folic acid, and finally help transport minerals and vitamins [326]. Prebiotics should be consumed more often after any antibiotic treatment. Such foods become extra source of valuable antioxidants and minerals when combined with herbs and spices.

---

320   http://www.cell.com/cell/pdfExtended/S0092-8674(15)01484-1
321   http://commonfund.nih.gov/hmp/index
322   http://www.examiner.com/article/new-study-elucidates-evolution-of-human-gut-microbes
323   http://www.the-scientist.com/?articles.list/categoryNo/2625/category/The-Scientist/tagNo/227,10/tags/extinction,microbiology/
324   http://www.ncbi.nlm.nih.gov/pubmed/24416709
325   http://www.sciencedaily.com/releases/2011/05/110503132658.htm
326   http://forums.phoenixrising.me/index.php?threads/the-human-microbiome-acquired-mitochondrial-disease.28498/

Lifestyle as a Therapeutic Factor

2.09 Insulin and Leptin Resistance

A good methylation diet can remedy the condition of insulin resistance defined as production of insulin by beta cells of pancreas in amount that doesn't compensate for insulin that is not detected at the surface our cells [327]. In case of type II diabetes, secretion of insulin and resistance to its recognition at the cellular level and glucose production by liver are closely related phenomena.

Leptin resistance in addition to insulin resistance make matters worse for diabetics. Leptin is an appetite and weight control hormone produced by white adipose (fat) tissue whose levels vary exponentially with fat mass. Leptin resistant diabetics loose the homone's effect on appetite control even high levels.

Diabetics who consume high fat diets can create a situation of elevated free fatty acid in their blood stream and thus a high level of fat metabolites which interfere with leptin signaling. New research shows that triglycerides induce leptin resistance at the blood-brain barrier [328]. A good methylation diet for diabetics and non-diabetics alike should deliver no more than 25 to 30 % fat calories in a methylation diet.

2.10 Low Cortisol and Stress free Life Style

Corticoprotein releasing and adrenocorticotropic hormones control the adrenal gland and the super command of the hypothalmus in brain. Glucocorticoid cortisol production under stress is regulated by these hormones for increasing glucose in the blood stream and eventual utilization by the brain [329], [330]. This hormone affects digestion, immunity, and even reproductive performance.

---

327   http://www.jci.org/articles/view/10761
328   http://diabetes.diabetesjournals.org/content/53/5/1253.full.html
329   https://www.nlm.nih.gov/medlineplus/ency/article/003695.htm
330   http://www.todaysdietitian.com/newarchives/111609p38.shtml

Methylation foods comprised of asparagus, avocado, berries, beef, cashews, chocolate, garlic, green tea, oatmeal, oranges, oysters, strawberries, and walnut reduce cortisol and help fight stress. Diet induced benefits increase by regular exercise and mindfulness. A regular commitment to 30 minute aerobic exercise and yoga and 30 minute regime of programmed meditative mental activities are necessary complements to methylation diet for its maximum effect and health value. Exercise, meditation, and mindfulness keep stress hormone cortisol in balance [331]. The morning cortisol level should not get higher than 20-23 mcg/dL.

2.11 Foods for Nerve Growth Factors

There are stem cells in our brain that have the power to accelerate production of nerve growth factors (NGF) that help sprout axons and dendrites. High NGF leads to better repair of axons, dendrites, and nerve cells for cognition, coordination, and memory [332]. Nerve growth factor and Brain derived Neurotrophic Factors (BDNF) are the key to growth of our neurons [333], [334], [335]. **We know that that Lion's Mana mushroom is great for NGF production other than Vitamins B complex, E, and antioxidant polyphenol supplies from daily methylation foods [336].** Mushrooms deliver vitamin D, B vitamins including folic acid, choline, and minerals magnesium, copper, and zinc. Just imagine the importance of maintaining the health of 4 square yard nerve fibers in an area of one square inch of our skin that contains 600 pain sensors, 1300 nerve cells, 900 nerve endings, 36 heat sensors, and 75 pressure sensors [337]. No wonder why skin health is the best barometer of good health. A good methylation diet can potentially take care of all 120 billion neurons in our brain.

---

331   http://www.health.harvard.edu/staying-healthy/exercising-to-relax
332   http://www.scientificamerican.com/article/the-nerve-growth-factor/
333   http://enchantedmind.com/html/science/brain_food.html
334   http://nervehealthsupport.com/nerve-growth-factor/
335   http://www.ncbi.nlm.nih.gov/pubmed/23466052
336   http://www.ncbi.nlm.nih.gov/pubmed/23510212
337   http://www.foursigmafoods.com/lions-mane-nutrients-for-your-nerves

2.12 A good Night Sleep

Axons and dendrites are pruned during sleep and this pruning improves memory building and cognition [338], [339]. We must sleep well and long to stay healthy, say at least 7-8 hours a day. A high protein methylation diet induces sleep and a good night sleep per se is antiinflammatory.

2.13 Foods for Sodium Channel Blockers

Mitochondria run Krebs cycle, electron transfer chain, the proton pump for making ATP, lipid metabolism, urea cycle, and metal group biosynthesis . Only mitochondria can help us fight degenerative diseases of cognition. Our daily foods must strengthen our ever functioning mitochondria. Polyphenols in methylation foods have the effect of blocking sodium channel and serve as an antiarrhythmic medicine [340]. Red wine is a good source of polyphenolics [341].

Sodium channel blocker drugs in case of epilepsy and arrhythmia should always be used with great caution. Methylation diet can help greatly in this regard by maintaining the health of mitochondria for our vital signs. Mitochondrial health is fundamental to healthy living and health of our brain and muscle cells.

2.14 Quinones and Isoprenoid molecules in Mitochondrial health

Isoprenoid quinones are fat soluble molecules present in membrane structures in general [342], [343]. These molecules are involved in electron and proton transfer and translocation. Ubiquinone of mitochondrial electron transport chain is a benzoquinone and vitamin K_s are phytyl naphthaquinones. They are the key to running our daily metabolism.
In case of coenzyme Q_{10}, Q refers to quinone and 10 indicates the number of isoprenoid repeats. Other examples are pyrroquinoline quinone, and

---

338   http://www.scientificamerican.com/article/new-hypothesis-explains-why-we-sleep/
339   http://www.economist.com/node/7138780
340   htt http://www.ncbi.nlm.nih.gov/pmc/articles/PMC2014645/p://www.ncbi.nlm.nih.gov/pmc/articles/PMC2014645/
341
342   http://www.ncbi.nlm.nih.gov/pubmed/20599680
343   http://www.sciencedirect.com/science/article/pii/S0005272810006365

retinoids (vitamin A) [344]. Coenzyme Q_{10} is needed for proper energy production by mitochondria.

While the isoprenoid tail embeds the quinones in fat layer of inner mitochondrial membrane, the non-protein quinone groups help carry electrons and transport over the chain where it picks up electrons from complex I and II and transfers them to complex III [345], [346]. Of the three major quinone, vitamin E, vitamin K, and coenzyme Q_{10}, the latter has the maximum number of 10 isoprenoid or terpene repeats.

Methylation of DNA (or demethylation), mitochondrial biogenesis, function of electron transport chain in the inner membrane of mitochondria, and oxidative stress govern our day to day health. Methylation diet and exercise, it is well established now, can cure much of our common ailments. This chapter has ample references on the values of mitochondrial foods like L-arginine, L-carnitine, creatine, theanine, coenzyme Q_{10}, taurine, gamma amino butyric acid, resveratrol, polyphenols, flavolignan sylimarin, folate, B vitamins including vitamin B_{12}, glutathione, omega-3 fatty acids, vitamin D, alternative medicine nutrients including cucurmin, and trace minerals. Our daily methylation diet, exercise, and mindfulness are the solutions to our chronic health problems including diabetes II and cognitive impairment during our senior years. Routine foods can be made more therapeutic by proper selection of methylation nutrients and culinary practice. Section 2.15 below is devoted to make this point.

2.15 Recipe Design for Mitochondrial Health

A fitting preamble to this section is FDA's recommendation of a daily intake of "six servings of fruits and vegetables" While the recommendation per se is fine its daily execution by a majority of consumers in the US like industrial society has been unattainable where at least 4.5% of all 75 million or more blue and white collar workers labor hard under the neon light in the night from 11 PM to 7 AM the next morning. How should they manage six servings of fruits and vegetables? The answer in my view is extensive variety of easy to make dips, salad, sauce, soup, and stew from vegetables and cocktails and compote from fruits. Fruits can become our daily syrup in many dishes. Such dishes can be either full lunch, dinner, or just side dish of one or two

---

344   http://lipidlibrary.aocs.org/Lipids/isoprene/index.htm
345   http://www.benbest.com/nutrceut/CoEnzymeQ.html
346   https://www.tamu.edu/faculty/bmiles/lectures/electrontrans.pdf

vegetables. Dark chocolate, green tea, nuts, seeds, and blue berries can be used as daily snack items. Nuts and seeds snacks deliver fiber, trace mineral and vitamins. A variety of fruits and vegetables ensure a wide spectrum of antioxidants of selective solubility in water and lipid structures of our cells and planned weekly recipes for breakfast, lunch, snacks, and dinner including any desserts can thus constitute a methylation diet for antioxidant delivery.

The language of food is bound to culture, religion, and tradition. A chef knows this the best. he or she practices and chronicles creative complexities often tied to human expression that bespeak of our evolutionary continuum of food selection and consumption. Time tested therapeutic value of a dish that has been in food chain for centuries doesn't need validation by randomized block clinical trials. A good dish loses least of nutrients, produces appetizing flavors, and concentrates all major nutrients necessary for DNA methylation. Internet gives us the advage to examine recipes by chefs of repute listed in the block below and to design recipes of our own using readily available local fruits and vegetables.

To make this point, values of dishes included in this section shall be highlighted with respect to nutrient density and presence of key vitamins, mineras, and phytonutrients. Modifications are suggested in order to optimize serving size and inclusion of alternate ingredients particularly in regard to daily protein and dietary fiber delivery by a low fat, low cholesterol, and low sodium methylation diet.

World famous chefs: Florian Trento and Christof Syre, Hong Kong; Christof Syre, Exec Chef, Reagent, Hong Kong; Sanjeeva Kapoor and Neeraj Katyal, India; Antonio (Tom) Carloccio, Italy; Jean Geoges Vongerichten; Fruits and Vegetables man; Gary Farrell and Nigel Keen, Australia; Grant Achatz; David Chang; Fergus Henderson; John Besh; Rene Redzepi; Alain Ducasse, Paris; Daniel Boulud, La Cirqui; Ferran Adria of El Bulli, Spain; Heston Blumenthal, Fat Duck, London, UK; Thomas Keller, Yountville, California USA
US Chefs: Fabio Viviani, Suzanne Gorin, Michael Garnero, Nancy Clark, davin Alexander (pumpkin cake), Cat Cora (white bean chicken blanca), Rocco Dispirito (Vietnamese), Richard Blais (vege burger), Jacque Torres (chocolate Bar, cardmom date bar), Elizabeth Falkner (Moracan date bobbons), Gordon Ramsey and Rachael Ray (antiinflammatory Diet).

Old chicken soup is much better than an expensive supplement of chondritine sulfate. Campbell Soup Company, the king of tomatoes, wants us to go after Latin inspired varieties, carrots that taste like ranch, high protein fruity yogurt in a tube, green juice from kale, and pouches of flavored skillet sauce and soup. Marketing hype notwithstanding there is some value in the effort but I would rather follow Chef Rene Redzepi of Noma Restaurant in Copenhagen and cook foods ad hoc in variety and in cost effective style for maximum nutrition of vitamin B complex. I will choose to eat fruits and vegetables in variety and drizzle chopped seeds and nuts on side and main dishes wherever I can because fruits and vegetables are the major source of methylation nutrients, antioxidants, minerals, vitamins, and other phytonutrients. They offer variety of flavor, juiciness, and succulence. Look at the power of V8. A juice concentrate is a pure and simple concentrate of nutrients. The ingredient list for such soups may include mushroom, various roots, vegetables, fruits, and herbs and spices. I have compiled a few complementary and critical recipes for this section from public domain with a sincere belief of soothing our soul and fighting chronic problems of diseases and pain. There are authoritative pamphlets and monographs on the topic of food selection including American Dietetic Association on vegetarian diets, nutritional updates for physicians on plant based diets, nutritional profile of Indian vegetarian diet, and many a meta-analyses on status of zinc and mineral nutrition of vegetarians. These works give us solid reasons for maximizing nutrient values from the produce section of the local retail store. The variety is unlimited and we can eat well and stay within our norms of culture and religious beliefs in Hinduism, Confucianism, Buddhism, post-Christian Taoism, Judaism, or Islam.

Select a chef's recipe and modify it for your personal nutrition. For instance pregnant women must have probiotics, iron, Vitamin B_{12} (yogurt, cereals), 400 mcg per day of folate, 1000 mg calcium (milk, yogurt, leafy vegetables), 75 mg of vitamin C (fruits and vegetables), 25 g of fiber (whole grains, fruits), 310-320 mg magnesium (nuts, seeds, and green vegetables), and 4.7 g of potassium (banana, oranges, leafy greens). We have to stay imaginative and make our fritters or coated and fried snacks, gnochi, pizza like gratin, and quiche for maximum nutrient density for methylation ingredients.

Let us review a few fancy features of non-conventional quick dishes for our daily nutrition.

- Vegetables including broccoli, spinach and kale, pine apple in order to deliver minerals like manganese.

- Vegetables soups and vegetable broths can be routinely used for cooking rice and preparing pizza dough.

- Variety of low fat cheeses by way of tofu, Indian panir, or finely diced chicken for enhanced proteins for satiety and essential amino acid delivery.

- Flavor can come from garlic and herbs added over cheese topping.

- Beverages and smothies can be made with chilled broth, fruits, nuts, and seeds.

- Nutritious dumplings can be made for for added color.

- Dips can be prepared from soaked/marinated nuts and seeds and vegetables. Hummus is a great example.

- Tofu and grilled tuna bits can be used as as topings over many a savory snacks items.

- Both canola and olive oils have high smoke point of 468-470 Deg F. As such they degrade slowly when used for frying at 360 to 380 degree F and are less prone to rancidity, loss of vitamin E, and production of carcinogens like acrylamide. Heat induced rancidity simply means free radicals. We should avoid stale and rancid foods [347], [348]. Rancidy is known to deplete vitamin E. There are case studies on the effects of rancid foods on serious health problems like cancer in India, Morocco, Spain, Taiwan, and Tunisia. We should never consume foods like cakes, cookies, and even high fat bars past the expiration of their shelf-life. Store fats and oils properly and always confirm fortification with natural antioxidants.

- Virgin olive oil contains natural polyphenols and offers protection against rancidity [349],[350]. Hydroxytyrosol is the major phenolic [351].

---

347   http://peterborten.com/all/oxidation-educate-your-nose/
348   http://nutritionnutsandbolts.com/2012/08/01/rancid-fat/
349   http://www.whfoods.com/genpage.php?tname=foodspice&dbid=132
350   http://www.sciencedirect.com/science/article/pii/S0955286312002975
351   http://www.ncbi.nlm.nih.gov/pubmed/15749387

We need to be mindful of daily protein intake for efficient methylation diet. There are many ways to compliment and supplement for protein via dips, sauces, and whole grain bread but we need to know how much and wherefrom:

- 1/2 cup buckwheat gives 3 g protein, 1 cup amaranth gives 9.7 g protein, 1 cup quinova gives 8 gram, 1 cup edamame gives 8 g.

- one egg gives 6 g protin, 2 TBL hemp seed gives 7 g, , and two slices of Ezakiel bread based on sprouted grains gives 8 g.

- 2 TBL hummus gives 2.2 g protein.

2.15.01 RDA$_s$ of Methylation Nutrients

We live by enzyme proteins made under instruction of our DNA which uses methylation reaction as a tool to program its doing in time, both long term chronological events like onset of puberty, development of mammary glands, and menopause and short term cicadiam rhythm of going to bed and getting up. The suprachiasmatic nucleus of the hypothalamus in our brain controls our cell specific clocks. **Hundreds of rhythmically expressed genes follow their cycles of sleeping and waking up, cellular proliferation, detoxification, and metabolism in general.** A chronic purturbation of this organization has consequences to our health. This can be reduced by our daily nutrients.

Scientists are busy calculating that 10^{80} atoms in our body are not enough to account for 100 terabytes of memory by thousands of synaptic connections of 8.6×10^{10} neurons. Each synaptic activity involves a gene expression and DNA and its histone sheath must respond each time. Obviously our mind with a volume of 1.2 million cubic millimeters works in amazing ways when it comes to daily expressions of our genes underly each synaptic activity. **Let us keep in mind that thousands of genes work at any given time in rather rigorous control and some 1 million enzyme proteins are tied to this activity. Close to 43% of these genes follow a daily schedule detrmined largely by nutrients like vitamins A, C, D, B complex, iron, selenium, hydroxytyrosol of virgin olive oil, cholesterol, betaine,** choline, folic acid, S-adenosyl methionine, and antioxidants like quercetin, naringenin, hesperatin, and tea catechins. It is these nutrients that comprise methylation nutrients. It is these nutrient that modify DNA by methylation reaction in order to make epigenetic tags for putting or not putting a gene in action. A methylation diet thus controls our daily life, health, and well being [352], [353], [354], [355]. Let us turn our body into as good a temple as possible and prevent it from degrading to a shed.

Foods we use in our methylation diet must deliver mitochondria protecting nutrients. A well designed breakfast, lunch, snack, dinner, dessert, and occasional beverage can for sure meet our daily needs as listed in Table 2.15.01A.

Table 2.15.01A RDA$_s$ of Methylation Nutrients [For vitamin A 1 IU X 0.3 = mcg , for vitamin E 1 IU X 0.9 = mcg, and for vitamin D, 1 IU X 0.025 = mcg]		
Nutrients	**RDA**	**Nutrient rich Foods**
Minerals		
Copper	900 mcg	Tree nuts (850 mcg/oz), raw mushrooms (344 mcg/cup), chocolate (198 mcg/Oz)
Chromium	35 mcg	Broccoli (22 mcg/cup), whole wheat English muffin (3.6 mcg/muffin).
Iodine	150 mcg	Beef (2.32/3 oz), oyster (5 mg/6 oyster), raisins
Magnesium	400 mg	Brown rice (86 mg/cup), Oat Bran (96 mg/cup), almond (78 mg/Oz
Manganese	2.3 mg	
Molybdenum	11 mcg	Black beans (30 mcg/cup), Split peas (48 mg/cup), tree nuts (42 mg/cup
Potassium	2000 mg	Potato (926 mg/medium potato), Artichoke (343 mg/medium), Plums (637 mg/1/2 cup), raisins (598 mg/1/2 cup), banana (422 mg/medium).

352   http://www.intechopen.com/books/olive-oil-constituents-quality-health-properties-and-bioconversions/biological-properties-of-hydroxytyrosol-and-its-derivatives
353   http://nutrigenomics.ucdavis.edu/?page=information/Concepts_in_Nutrigenomics/Diet_and_Gene_Expression
354   http://www.ncbi.nlm.nih.gov/pubmed/10089110
355   http://onlinelibrary.wiley.com/doi/10.1111/prd.12001/abstract

Selenium	50-75 mcg	Brazil nut 544/6 kernels, salmon 40 mcg/3 oz, eggs
Zinc	11 mcg	Oysters, beef, turkey, cashews
Vitamins		
Vitamin A	900 mcg	Butter squash (572/1/2 cup), sweet potato (961 mcg/1/2 cup), carrots (538 mcg/1/2 cup), Kale (143 mcg/cup), and Eggs (91 mcg/i large egg).
Vitamin C	90 mg	Citrus (100 mg/cup), grape fruit76 mg/cup), strawberry (85 mg/cup), red pepper (96 mg/cup).
Vitamin D	15 mcg	Salmon (13.3 mcg/3 oz), cereals and milk aRE FORTIFIED
Vitamin E	15 mcg	Olive oil (1.9 mg/TBL), Canola oil (2.4 mg/TBL), Almond (4.3 mg/oz).
Vitamin K	120 mcg	Broccoli or chord (220 mcg/cup), Kale (547 mcg/cup), Parsley (246 mcg/cup)
Choline	425 mg	Eggs (126 mg/egg), milk (135 mg/cup).
B1 (Thiamine)	1.2 mg	Lentils (0.67 mg/1/2 cup), rice (0.26 mg/cup
B2 (riboflavin)	13 mg	Milk (0.34/cup), Cereals (0.9/cup), almond (0.23/oz, eggs (0.27/large0
B3 (Niacin)	16 mg	Peanuts (3.8 mg/oz), salmon (8.5 mg/3 oz), cereal (20 mg/cup)
B5 (Pantothenate)	5 mg	Chicken 90.98/ 3 oz), milk (0.52/cup), sweet potato (0.88 mg/med)
B6 (Pyridoxin)	1.3 mg	Salmon (0.48 mg/3 oz), banana (0.43 mg/medium), potato (0.7 mg/med), cooked spinach (0.44 mg/cup).
B7 (biotin)	8 mcg	Consume high protein foods
B9 (folic Acid)	400 mcg	Cereals (300 mcg/cup), asparagus (134/six), spinach (132 mcg/1/2 cup), Shrimp (34 mcg/10 shrimp).
B12 (Cyanoco-balamine)	2.4 mcg	Salmon (2.1 mcg/3 oz), clams (84 mcg/3 oz), eggs 0.6 mcg/large egg).

RDA for key nutrients is listed in Table 2.15. 01B. Recipes included in this subsection are selected for these nutrients and, whereever possible, the nutrient amount of nutrient is included. We need to always decide on a combination of recipe ingredients that delivers enough methylation nutrients.

Table 2.15. 01B Key Nutrients for Mitochondria		
#	Nutrients and Foods	Recommended RDA
	Alpha-Lipoic Acid	100 mg
	DMAE	100 mg
	Coenzyme Q10	30 mg
	N Acetyl Cysteine	600 mg
	Vitamin C	1000 mg
	Vitamin E	200 IU
	Selenium	200 mcg
	Folic Acid	100 mcg
	Vitamin B6	55 mg
	Vitamin B12	1000 mcg
	Probiotics	1010 Live Bacteria

Methylation foods containing copper, sulfur, magnesium, selenium, amino acid methionine, coenzyme Q_{10}, vitamin B_2, folic acid, choline, and riboflavin cure and prevent cognitive disorders, malgrain headache, and multiple sclerosis. Research shows that methylation diet is necessary for brain plasticity by creating a functional epigenome necessary for desirable gene expression which in turn controls adaptation and neuroplasticity. The function of epigenome depends on acelation and deacelation of histone sheath of DNA, methylation of DNA and component genes, and production of Bdnf (Brain Derived Neurotrophic factors) that activate molecular changes in circuits of nerve cells. Table 2.15.02 summarizes the methylation nutrients in simple foods of broccoli and papaya. Almond, apple, asparagus, barley, blackberry, brazil nut, and sweet potato are other common food packed with methylation nutrients (see extensive list in Tables 2.15.03 and 2.15.04).

Table 2.15.02 Example of - Broccoli and Papaya, A Nature's Package of Nutrients

Table 2.15.02 Broccoli and Papaya by Nutrient Density				
Nutrients	**Papaya by reduction**		**Broccoli by roasting**	
	As Is	To Half Volume	As is	40% moisture
Carbohydrate	10	20	6.6	13.2
Fiber	2.15	4.3	2.6	5.2
Protein	0.71	1.52	3.3	6.6
Vitamin A, mcg	198	396	560	1120
Vitamin c, mg	62	124	90	180
Folate, mcg	38	76	60	120
Vitamin K			100	200
Choline, mg	6	12	18.3	36.6
Omega-3	31	62		
Iron			0.77	1.54
Magnesium	10	20	21	42
Calcium	24	48		
Zinc			0.44	0.88

Diet based epigenetics plays a huge role in mitochondrial function and mitochondrondrial biogenesis itself depends on methylation of promotor gene PGC1α [356], [357]. DNA methylation in particular controls adaptive energy production, type II diabetes, immunity, and hormone balance. It balances body functions in general. Obesity in particular is a metabolic disease. Mitochondria derived fatty acids are involved in its epigenetic regulation. Insulin resistance in type II diabetes and dysfuction of skeletal muscle mitochondria can be corrected by our daily diet [358]. No doubt balanced foods are our medicine. Short chain fatty acids in particular prevent obesity by acting as histone deacytilase inhibitor [359]. Recipes that deliver nutrients in Table 2.15.02 help methylate human DNA and prevent many other diseases.

356   http://www.ncbi.nlm.nih.gov/pmc/articles/PMC3057551/
357   http://jcs.biologists.org/content/125/21/4963.full.pdf
358   http://www.symbiosisonlinepublishing.com/nutritionalhealth-foodscience/nutritionalhealth-food-science27.php
359   http://www.ncbi.nlm.nih.gov/pubmed/12769690

A very common Ingredient like vinegar goes beyond shelf-life, taste, and flavor accentuation when used properly in cooking as to the amount and the step. Wherever possible raw food should be brought to room temperature for proper heat transfer (low temperature differential) and sufficient time to allow extraction of nutrients during cooking. Time tested cooking techniques enhance not only the flavor and texture of finished food but also the total deliverable nutrient density by concentration and reduction for a conventional serving size.

2.15.03: Snacks of Nuts and Seeds deliver Trace Minerals

Nutrition information on nuts and seeds in Table 2.15.03 points out that just one oz of mixed nuts and seeds per day can meet RDA requirements, eliminate deficiencies, make mitochondria efficient.

2.15.03 Natures Package of Mineral and vitamin Nutrition (all entries or on one Oz or 28 g Basis)

Food Item	Source of Nutrient	Amount	Food Item	Source of Nutrient	Amount
Almond	Vitamin E, mg	7.32	Caraway Seeds	Calcium, mg	208
	Folate, µg	14		Magne-sium, mg	1.86
	Choline, mg	14.5		Zinc, mg	1.86
	Magnesium, mg	75			
	Iron, mg	1	Peanuts	Vitamin E, mg	1.9
	Zinc, mg	0.85		Niacin (B3), mg	3.8
	Copper, mg	0.26		Choline, mg	15.0
	Manganese, mg	0.64			

Brazil Nut	Selenium, µg	538	Poppy seed	Calcium, mg	391 mg
	Calcium, mg	45		Magnesium, mg	95
	Zinc, mg	1.13			
	Copper, mg	0.48			
	Iron, mg	0.67	Pumpkin seeds	Magnesium, mg	72
				Iron, mg	0.9
				Zinc, mg	2.83
Chia seed	Dietary fiber, g	11	Sunflower seeds	Vitamin E, mg	32
	Calcium, mg	177		Folic acid, µg	62
	Zinc, mg	1		Choline, mg	15
				Betaine, mg	10
				Fiber, g	2.4
Date	Carotenoids, µg	31			
	Magnesium, mg	15			
	Zinc, mg	0.12	Walnuts	Omega-3, g	2.5
	Fiber, g	1.87		Omega-6, g	10.7
				Choline, mg	11
Dried Prunes	Vitamin K, µg	16		Zinc, mg	0.86
	Choline, mg	2.83		Copper, mg	0.45
	Fiber, g	1.93			
Flax seed	Omega-3 , g	6			
	Omega-6, g	1.6			
	Lignan fiber, g	7.3			
	Folate, µg	23			

	Zinc, mg	1.1			
	Selenium, µg	6.8			

We need to have ready access to major methylation nutrients in food items that we can afford and then watch the nutrient density of our recipes week by week with respect to vitamins, cofactors, trace minerals, prebiotic fibers, and probiotic fermented foods.

2.15.04 Use of Nature's Packages for Rejuvenation of Mitochondria

Tables 2.15.03 and 2.15.04 can be used routinely in designing and modifying recipes of great chef's week by week for our personal taste and nutrient requirements. Let us force ourselves to remember that an enhanced daily nutrient delivery can easily come from simple imagination and modification in cooking, serving, and serving size selection methods. The great chefs do it all the time. A few examples are that can be further modified with alternate available foods.

- **A high protein breakfast of eggs or sprouted grain and legume patties. Mixed cold cereals with fruity Greek yogurt and serve yourself a breakfast. Top it with shreaded nuts and seeds. Another example is hot oatmeal with brown sugar and berries.**

- **Servings of herbed and spiced main and side dishes of breakfast for as many common nutrients and phytonutrients as possible.**

- **A snack of mixed nuts or fruit smoothies each day.**

- **An appetizer of mixed vegetables every alternate day. The key is variety.**

- **A bowl of rice cooked in vegetable broth rich in mineral and vitamin nutrients. We can call it rissoto for methylations by adding beans, peas, nuts, and seeds.**

- **A dessert of dark chocolate each evening.**

- A serving of probiotic from the list of yogurt, sour kraut, and kimchi.

- Servings of drinks of spiced broths and soups can meet our daily mineral and vitamin requirements.

Table 2.15.04 Methylation Food Nutrients That Rejuvenate Mitochondria

[For vitamin A i IU X 0.3 = mcg , for vitamin E 1 IU X 0.9 = mcg, and for vitamin D, 1 IU X 0.025 = mcg]															
	Vitamins					Minerals									
Nutrients	Vit A (mcg)	Vit C (mg)	Vit E (mg)	Folate (mcg)	Vit K (mcg)	Iron (mg)	Pot (mg)	Cal (mg)_	Phosph (mg)	Selen (mcg)	Zin c (mg)	Chro m (mcg)	Mg (mg)	Cop (mcg)	Mol (mcg)	Man (mg)
RDA	1000	90	15	400	50	8	2000	600	460	65	10	30	100	340	17	2.3
Food Nutrients for Mitochondrial Health per 100 gram Basis															
Almonds			7.43	14			200	75	137		0.87		76			
Amaranth				22		2.1	135	47	148	5.5	0.8		65			

Table 2.15.04 Methylation Food Nutrients That Rejuvenate Mitochondria

[For vitamin A i IU X 0.3 = mcg , for vitamin E 1 IU X 0.9 = mcg, and for vitamin D, 1 IU X 0.025 = mcg]

Nutrients	Vitamins					Minerals										
	Vit A (mcg)	Vit C (mg)	Vit E (mg)	Fol ate	Vit K (mcg)	Iron (mg)	Pot (mg)	Cal (mg)	Phos ph (mg)	Sele n (mcg)	Zin c (mg)	Chro m (mcg)	Mg (mg)	Cop (mcg)	Mol (mcg)	Man (mg)
RDA	1000	90	15	400	50	8	2000	600	460	65	10	30	100	340	17	2.3
											6					
Apple	98	8.4				0.22	195	11	20				9			
Asparagus	905	8	1.35	134	45.5	0.82	202	21	49	5.5	0.54			0.15		
Avocado, 1 oz	293		4.16	163	42	1.1	975	24	105		1.29		58	0.38		
Bamboo shoots						0.29	640		24	0.50	0.56					
Banana			0.2	45		0.31	422		26		1.2		60			
Barley				16		1.33	93		54	8.60		13	121	46	0.4	1.78
	Also 1/2 cup barley supplies 16 g fiber, 31 g protein, 2.82 mg vitamin B$_2$, and 0.4 mg B$_1$															
Beans				128		2		50						196		
	Less than 0.5 % fat, 19-22% protein, 8-9% dietary fiber. A 200 gram serving of beans including garbanzo beans doubles these major nutrients and supplies more than twice the RDA of iron and folate.															
Beef																
Black eye pea														180		
Blackberries	308	30.2	1.68	36	29	0.89	233	42	32		0.76		29	0.24		
Black currants	238	202.7	1.12			1.27	361		66		0.30		27			
Boysenberries	88	202.7	1.15		10.3	1.12	183		36		0.29		21			
Breadfruit		63.8		31	1.1	1.19	1,078	37	66		0.26		55	0.18		
Beetroot				68		0.67	229		32	0.60	0.3		20			
Bok choy	7,223		0.15	70	58		631	158	49				19			
Broccoli	1,207		1.13	84	110		229		52	1.2	0.35		16			
Brussels sprouts	1,209		0.67		219	1.87	495	56	87		0.51		31			
Butternut squash	22,868	31	2.64	39	2	1.23	582	84	55	1	0.27		59			
Bell																

Table 2.15.04 Methylation Food Nutrients That Rejuvenate Mitochondria

[For vitamin A i IU X 0.3 = mcg , for vitamin E 1 IU X 0.9 = mcg, and for vitamin D, 1 IU X 0.025 = mcg]

Nutrients	Vit A (mcg)	Vit C (mg)	Vit E (mg)	Folate (mcg)	Vit K (mcg)	Iron (mg)	Pot (mg)	Cal (mg)	Phos ph (mg)	Sele n (mcg)	Zin c (mg)	Chro m (mcg)	Mg (mg)	Cop (mcg)	Mol (mcg)	Man (mg)
			Vitamins							Minerals						
RDA	1000	90	15	400	50	8	2000	600	460	65	10	30	100	340	17	2.3
Peppers																
2 tsp Black Pepper																0.74
Brazil nuts			1.62	6			187	45	206	543	1.15		107	0.50		
Broccoli																
Brazil nut																
Brown rice																1.76
Brussels sprout																
Buckwheat				30		2.20	460		347	8.80	2.40		231	1.10		
Cashews			0.26	7	9.70	1.89	187		168	5.6	1.64		83	0.62		
Chestnuts	22		0.42	59	0.66	0.76	497		90		0.48		28			
Cantaloupe	2,334	25.7			1.7	0.14	184		10		0.12					
Cherries	88	9.7			2.9	0.50	306	18	29				15			
Cloves/2 tsp																2.53
Chinese pear		10.4	0.33		12.4		333	11	30				22	0.14		
Coconut				21		1.94	285		90	8.10	0.88		26	0.34		
Cranberries	60	13.3	1.2		5.1	0.25	85		13							
Cabbage		28.1	0.1	22	81.5	0.13	147	36	25				11			
Carrots	13,286		0.8	11	10.7		183		23							
Cauliflower				27	8.6											
Celery	782		0.53	33	56.7		426		38	1.5						
Chinese broccoli	1,441		0.42	87	74.6		230	88	36	1.1			16			
Chinese cabbage	1,151			63		0.36	268	38	46				12			
Corn	310					0.53	257		91			0.73	31			
Cucumber	55				8.5		76	8	12							
Chicken																
Cocoa																
Coffee																
Collard green																0.97
Daikon radish				25			419	25	35				13			
Edamami			0.5		20						1		50	0.25		0.75

Also 1/2 cup edamami supplies 4 g fiber, 8.25 g protein, 43 mg choline, 3.5 mg choline like betaine

Table 2.15.04 Methylation Food Nutrients That Rejuvenate Mitochondria

[For vitamin A i IU X 0.3 = mcg , for vitamin E 1 IU X 0.9 = mcg, and for vitamin D, 1 IU X 0.025 = mcg]

Nutrients	Vitamins					Minerals										
	Vit A (mcg)	Vit C (mg)	Vit E (mg)	Folate (mcg)	Vit K (mcg)	Iron (mg)	Pot (mg)	Cal (mg)	Phosph (mg)	Selen (mcg)	Zinc (mg)	Chrom (mcg)	Mg (mg)	Cop (mcg)	Mol (mcg)	Man (mg)
RDA	1000	90	15	400	50	8	2000	60	460	65	10	30	100	340	17	2.3
Dates				28	4		964		91	4.4			63	0.30		
Figs	91				3	0.24	148	22	9	1			11			
Gooseberries	435	41.5	0.56	9			297	38	40	0.9	0.18		15			
Grapefruit	2,132	79.1	0.30	23		0.21	320	28	18		0.16		18			
Grapes		16.3	0.29		22	0.54	288		30		0.11		11	0.19		
...	...	...	...	...		...	...	...	...	...		...	56			
Eggs																
Eggplant			0.41	14	2.9	0.25	122									
Fennel	177			23		0.64	360		44				15			
Flaxseed						0.59	84		66							
French beans				133			655	112	181	2.1			99			
Grapes																
Green pepper	274	...		...	...		...	...								
Hazelnuts			4.26	32	4		193		82				46	0.49		
Kale	17,707	53	1.1	17	1,062	1.17	296		36	1.2			23			
Egg																
Grapes																
Grape Tomato	130	32		52	250											

Also 1 cup grape tomato supplies 2.58 g fiber, 2.58 g protein, **45 mcg vitamin D**, 0.25 mg B$_6$, and 0.2 mg pyridoxin.

Also 1/2 cup kiwi supplies 7.8 g fiber, 31 g protein, 3.5 g fat, 0.3 mg thiamin, 0.4 mg B$_6$, and 32.5 mg choline

Nutrients	Vit A	Vit C	Vit E	Folate	Vit K	Iron	Pot	Cal	Phosph	Selen	Zinc	Chrom	Mg	Cop	Mol	Man
Kiwi	60	64	1.01	17	27.8	0.21	215	23	23		1.25		36	0.25		0.5
Kohlrabi																
Leek	1,007		0.62		31.5	1.36	108	37	21				17			
Lentil				90		1.6			6			0.65	18	0.12	18	0.25

Also 1.4 cup lentil supplies 3.9 g fiber, 15.5 g protein, only 1.6 g fat, 0.2 mg B$_6$, and 16 mg choline.

Nutrients	Vit A	Vit C	Vit E	Folate	Vit K	Iron	Pot	Cal	Phosph	Selen	Zinc	Chrom	Mg	Cop	Mol	Man
Lima bean			0.36	156	3.8	4.49	955	209			1.79		81	0.45	142	
gLemon	18		0.13			0.50	116		13	0.3			7			
Lime	34	19.5					68		12	0.3						
Lichee		136	0.13			0.59	325		59	1.1		0.13	19	0.13		
Macadamia nuts			0.15				104		53				37	0.21		

Table 2.15.04 Methylation Food Nutrients That Rejuvenate Mitochondria

[For vitamin A i IU X 0.3 = mcg , for vitamin E 1 IU X 0.9 = mcg, and for vitamin D, 1 IU X 0.025 = mcg]

Nutrients	Vit A (mcg)	Vit C (mg)	Vit E (mg)	Folate (mcg)	Vit K (mcg)	Iron (mg)	Pot (mg)	Cal (mg)	Phosph (mg)	Selen (mcg)	Zinc (mg)	Chrom (mcg)	Mg (mg)	Cop (mcg)	Mol (mcg)	Man (mg)
RDA	1000	90	15	400	50	8	2000	600	460	65	10	30	100	340	17	2.3
Millet				19		0.63	62		100				44			
Mango	1,584	57.3		29		0.27	323		23				19			
Mulberries			51	1.22		10	2.59	272		53		0.17	25			
Mushroom				6			11		30	3.3						
Mustard green																
Nectarine	475					0.4	287		37					0.12		
Oats				56		4.27	429	54	523		3.97		177	0.62		
Okra	453		0.43	74	64			216		51			58			
Olive						0.28										
Onion				9												
Orange		69.7	0.24	39			237		18				13			
Papaya	1532	86.5	1.02	53	3.6		360		7	0.8			14			

Also 1/2 cup papaya supplies 1.16 g fiber, and 0.17 mg Pantothenate,

Peanuts						0.64	187		101		0.94		50			
Pecans							116		79				34	0.34		
Parsnip			1.56	90	1.6		573	58	108		0.41					
Passion fruit	3,002	70.8				3.78	821		160		0.24			0.20		
Pear				8	0.3	212		20			0.18		12	0.14		
Peas	1,282		0.22		41.4	2.46	434	43	187	3000	1.9		62			
Peach	489		1.09		3.9	0.38	285		30		0.26		14	0.10		
Pepper	140	115	1.45										10		4.6	0.1

1 cup bell pepper also supplies 0.25 mg Pyridoxin, 0.08 mg riboflavin, 0.28 mg pantothenate, 0.8 mg niacin, and 0.05 mg thiamin.

Pineapple		78.9		30	1.2	0.48	180		13		0.2			0.18		
Pine nuts				10	15.30		169		163				71	0.37		
Pistachios	74		0.55	14	3.70		295		137							
Plum	569		0.43	8	11	0.28	259		26		0.17		12			
Pomegranate		28.8	1.69	107	46	0.85	666		102		0.99		34	0.45		
Pumpkin	12,		1.9	22	2.0	1.4	564		76		0.5		22			

Table 2.15.04 Methylation Food Nutrients That Rejuvenate Mitochondria

[For vitamin A i IU X 0.3 = mcg , for vitamin E 1 IU X 0.9 = mcg, and for vitamin D, 1 IU X 0.025 = mcg]

Nutrients	Vitamins					Minerals										
	Vit A (mcg)	Vit C (mg)	Vit E (mg)	Folate (mcg)	Vit K (mcg)	Iron (mg)	Pot (mg)	Cal (mg)	Phosph (mg)	Sele n (mcg)	Zinc (mg)	Chrom (mcg)	Mg (mg)	Cop (mcg)	Mol (mcg)	Man (mg)
RDA	1000	90	15	400	50	8	2000	600	460	65	10	30	100	340	17	2.3
seeds	230		6			0					6					
Potato																
Quinova				77									118	0.36		1.79
Rice, brown																
Rice, wild																
Raisins					1.5	0.81	332		43				14	0.14		
Raspberries			1.07	26	10	0.85	186		36		0.52		27	0.11		
Red Wine																
Salmon										43						
	Also 4 oz (113.4 g) salmon supplies 26 g protein, 0.64 mg Pyridoxin, 0.92 mg Pantothenate, 4.54 mcg biotin, **5.67 mcg vitamin B$_{12}$, 12.8 mcg or 513 IU of vitamin D, and 1.25 g omega-3 fatty acids.**															
Sesame seed				9		1.31	42	88	57					0.36		
Spelt			0.26				143		150		1.25		49	0.21		
Sunflower seeds			7.40	67	0.80		241	20	327				37			
Spaghetti squash	170		0.19		1.2	0.53	181	33			0.31					
Split peas															148	
Spinach	2,183	8.40	0.61	58	145		167						24			1.68
Starfruit	81	45	0.2	16			176		16					0.18		
Strawberry		84.7	0.42	35	3	0.59	220	23	35	0.6	0.2					
Sunflower seed			12							18			110	0.60		0.65
	Also 1/c or 35 g sunflower seed supplies 5 g fiber, 8 g protein, 25 g fat , 0.52 mg thiamin, 2.92 mg niacin, and 0.45 mg pyridoxin.															
Summer squash	2,011		0.22	41	7.9		319	40	52	0.40				0.11		
Sweet potato	21,909		0.81		2.6		542	43	62	0.36			31	0.18		
Swiss Chard																
Taro	79		2.4	23	1.0		615		87	0.2			34			

Table 2.15.04 Methylation Food Nutrients That Rejuvenate Mitochondria

[For vitamin A i IU X 0.3 = mcg , for vitamin E 1 IU X 0.9 = mcg, and for vitamin D, 1 IU X 0.025 = mcg]

Nutrients	Vitamins					Minerals										
	Vit A (mcg)	Vit C (mg)	Vit E (mg)	Folate (mcg)	Vit K (mcg)	Iron (mg)	Pot (mg)	Cal (mg)	Phos ph (mg)	Sele n (mcg)	Zin c (mg)	Chro m (mcg)	Mg (mg)	Cop (mcg)	Mol (mcg)	M an (mg)
RDA	1000	90	15	400	50	8	2000	600	460	65	10	30	100	340	17	2.3
			8								4					
Tea																
Tomato			0.66	18	10	0.33	292	12	30		0.21		14			
Turnip		18.10		14	1.0		276	51	41				14			
Walnut	Walnuts			0.20	28	0.20	0.82	125	28	98				45	0.45	
	Also 1 oz walnut supplies 2 g fiber, 4.5 g protein, 18 g fat containing 2.72 g omega-3 fatty acid, and 5.7 mcg biotin.															
Watermelon	1,627	23.2				0.69	320		31		0.29		29	0.12		
Whole Wheat													11.2	0.02		0.21
	One pita bread or 35 gram whole wheat flour solids supplies 5 g protein, 5 gram fiber, 0.3 g fat, polyphenolic antioxidants.															
Winter squash	10,707		0.25	41	9.0		494	45	39		0.45					
Wheat durum						3.5	431	34	508	89	4		144	0.55		1.11
Wheat, red						3.6	340	25	332	70	3		124	0.41		
Yellow squash	190	24.50	2.48		4.1		282	27	41				25			
Yogurt				25		0.2	500									
	I Cup yogurt (245 g) supplies 12 g protein, 2.5 g fat, 0.12 mg thiamin, 0.5 mg riboflavin, 0.3 mg niacin, 1.5 mcg B_{12}, and 3.17 mcg vitamin D															

Notes

1. Salmon, trout, sardines, and mackerel are good sources of omega-3 fatty acids along woth protein and vitamin B_{12}.
2. Molybdenum is essential for electron transport, sulfite detoxification, nitrite reduction, and molybdenum-iron binding in general. It accepts or donates two electrons at a time.
3. Regular use of whole grain flours of barley and wheat, oat cereal, and garbanzo beans (hummus) supplies sufficient level of manganese. It is necessary to quench free radicals by superoxide dismutase. Helps prevent osteoporosis and rheumatoid arthritis.
4. Thirty percent of enzymes in human body require transition metals.

Now that we have a way to select ingredients for a methylation diet let us look at selected diets for a day and then for a week. Finally examine a few recipes. There is no strict protocol here except that of variety and portion control. We can change selections for any day of the week from the list of recipes in sections 2.15.07 and 2.15.08.

2.15.05 Model Methylation Diet for a Day

Almost every recipe of a day's breakfast, lunch, snack, dinner, dessert , and beverages can be pinned down as to its power of nutrient delivery. We can select recipes for variety of nutrition, texture, and flavor season by season in view of our personal needs.

Table 2.15.05 Model Methylation Diet for a Day

	Vitamins					Minerals										
Nutri-ents	Vit A (mcg)	Vit C (mg)	Vit E (mg)	Fo-late (mcg)	Vit K (mcg)	Iron (mg)	Pot (mg)	Cal (mg)_	Phosph (mg)	Selen (mcg)	Zinc (mg)	Chrom (mcg)	Mg (mg)	Cop (mcg)	Mol (mcg)	Man (mg)
RDA	1000	90	15	400	50	8	2000	600	460	65	10	30	100	340	17	2.3
A Selection of Breakfast, Lunch, and Dinner That Satisfy Rejuvenate Mitochondria (Most vitamins and Mineral RDAs)																
Breakfast		Lunch			Dinner				Remarks							
Yogurt, 8 Oz Papaya, 1/2 Cup Kiwi, 1/2 Cup Walnut 1 oz, Skim milk, 4 oz		Whole grain Pita, 1 Lettuce, 1 Cup Orange/red Pepper, 1 Grape tomato, 1 Cup Edamami, 1/2 Cup 1 TBL unsalted Sun-flower seed Salad dressing with vinegral, olive oil, salt and pepper			Salmon, 4 oz broiled in yogurt sauce Cooked Barley, 1/2 Cup Lentils, 1/4 Cup Baby Buck Choy, 1 cup steamed				A great methylation diet. Breakfast, lunch, and dinner combined supply balanced nutrition in terms of fiber, protein, omega-3 fatty acids, vitamins and trace minerals. Vitamin D and B$_{12}$ supplies from salmon are very impressive. Please check table on methylation food nutrients above.							

2.15.06 Model Methylation Diets for a Week

A day by day weekly choice of dishes for breakfast, lunch, snack, dinner, and desserts is listed in table 2.15.06. The target is the day's total intake of methylation ingredients for meeting RDA$_s$ of nutrients of fat, carbohydrate, sugar, dietary fiber, probiotics, vitamins, and minerals. Let us review a week's list for common foods in terms of their nutrient power given in Table 2.15.04. The list acounts for variety, flavor, and nutrient delivery. Like in a hotel room, a mini serving of dark chocolate after dinner can be our daily dessert. Alternatives in case of missing items in the pantry can always selected on the basis of information in Tables 2.15.03 and 2.15.04.

	Breakfast	Lunch	Snack	Dinner	Dessert
Sunday	Eggs	Hummus	Mixed nuts	Salmon	Greek yogurt
Monday	Cheese & pineapple	Pasta, egg plant relish	An orange	Vegie burger	Dark chocolate
Tuesday	Oatmeal	Lentil soup	Fruits & vegetables	Fish dish, Salmon	Dark chocolate
Wednesday	Buckwheat pancake	Turkey sandwich	Fruits, nuts	Vegetable Dish	Dark chocolate
Thursday	Berries and yogurt	Cheese & cracker	Stuffed artichoke	Vegetable dish	Dark chocolate
Friday	Boiled eggs & juice	Bean salad, bread	Mixed nuts	Baked potato and broccoli	Dark chocolate
Saturday	Banana, oatmeal	Lentil soup	Stuffed artichoke	Salad and Vegetable Stew	Dark chocolate

Mixed nuts must include Brazil nuts for selenium, items in bold can be switched around in a given week, and a serving of plain and live yogurt should should be used twice a week. Savory dishes can be spiced with kimchi or any other fermented and pickled relish.

Table 2.15.06 Weekly Model Methylation Dishes

SUNDAY

Nutrients	Vitamins					Minerals										
	Vit A (mcg)	Vit C (mg)	Vit E (mg)	Folate (mcg)	Vit K (mcg)	Iron (mg)	Pot (mg)	Cal (mg)	Phosph (mg)	Selen (mcg)	Zinc (mg)	Chrom (mcg)	Mg (mg)	Cop (mcg)	Mol (mcg)	Man (mg)
RDA	1000	90	15	400	50	8	2000	600	460	65	10	30	100	340	17	2.3

Weekly Selection of Breakfast, Lunch, and Dinner That Satisfy Rejuvenate Mitochondria (Most vitamins and Mineral RDAs)			
Breakfast	**Lunch**	**Dinner**	**Remarks**
Breakfast: Egg white veggie scramble.	Lunch: Hummus veggie pita sandwich of one half whole-grain pita spread with one teaspoon mustard, stuffed with vegetables bell pepper, sprouts, lettuce, two slices of avocado; two tangerines; unsweetened herbal tea. Snack: One sheet of graham cracker with a nut and seed dip.	Dinner: A three-ounce grilled salmon fillet with citrus glaze (orange juice and honey); one half cup cooked brown rice; one cup cooked winter squash or toasted artichoke (topped with lemon, olive oil, onion, salt, or balsamic vinegar). Dessert: One half cup fat-free plain Greek yogurt with two teaspoons fruit spread.	A high-protein breakfast, high-protein vegetable-based lunch, snack for mineral nutrition, and high-omega dinner. The Greek yogurt and fruit dessert two hours before retiring is a great complementary addition.

As an alternative, we can use a breakfast of four ounces of orange juice, multigrain pancake, green tea; a lunch of salad with vinaigrette dressing, grilled chicken, fresh fruits, strawberries; and a dinner of roasted vegetables, mushrooms, meatloaf, mixed salad, and two cups of spiced pear. What a simple dinner!

MONDAY

Nutrients	Vitamins					Minerals										
	Vit A (mcg)	Vit C (mg)	Vit E (mg)	Folate (mcg)	Vit K (mcg)	Iron (mg)	Pot (mg)	Cal (mg)	Phosph (mg)	Selen (mcg)	Zinc (mg)	Chrom (mcg)	Mg (mg)	Cop (mcg)	Mol (mcg)	Man (mg)
RDA	1000	90	15	400	50	8	2000	600	460	65	10	30	100	340	17	2.3

Weekly Selection of Breakfast, Lunch, and Dinner That Satisfy Rejuvenate Mitochondria (Most vitamins and Mineral RDAs)			
Breakfast	**Lunch**	**Dinner**	**Remarks**
Breakfast: Low-fat cottage cheese with pineapple chunks.	Lunch: Pasta with eggplant-tomato relish with four ounces of tofu; one tablespoon low-fat Greek yogurt; water with mint and lemongrass. Snack: One piece of fresh fruit or one cup mixed vegetables with two teaspoons of vinaigrette.	Dinner: Three ounces of grilled chicken or three ounces of tofu; one medium baked potato; two cups toasted greens topped with one tablespoon of vinaigrette, followed by unsweetened herbal tea.	Begin day two with a high-protein breakfast, high-protein lunch via Greek yogurt, and a snack of vegetables. A dinner of a small portion of chicken or equivalent tofu with herbal tea completes the day.

A alternative is a breakfast of bran flakes, soy milk, one cup banana, whole-wheat toast, apricot fruit spread; a lunch of corn spaghetti, olive roll, and fresh orange; a snack of a peach-pineapple-apricot crisp; and a dinner of grilled salmon, green snap beans, whole-wheat couscous, and a pumpernickel roll. The dessert can be skipped.

Tuesday

Nutrients	Vitamins					Minerals										
	Vit A (mcg)	Vit C (mg)	Vit E (mg)	Folate (mcg)	Vit K (mcg)	Iron (mg)	Pot (mg)	Cal (mg)	Phosph (mg)	Selen (mcg)	Zinc (mg)	Chrom (mcg)	Mg (mg)	Cop (mcg)	Mol (mcg)	Man (mg)
RDA	1000	90	15	400	50	8	2000	600	460	65	10	30	100	340	17	2.3

Weekly Selection of Breakfast, Lunch, and Dinner That Satisfy Rejuvenate Mitochondria (Most vitamins and Mineral RDAs)			
Breakfast	**Lunch**	**Dinner**	**Remarks**
Breakfast: One cup oatmeal with low-fat Greek yogurt, coffee or green tea or clove toddy.	Lunch: One cup lentil soup, two cups mixed salad greens, herbal tea. Snack: One medium orange.	Dinner: Veggie burger on whole-wheat bun, spinach salad with onion and orange, dressed with one teaspoon olive oil.	Tuesday: Breakfast provides both protein from Greek yogurt and soluble dietary fiber from oats, lunch delivers vegetable proteins from lentils and vegetables, lunch provides protein and antioxidants, and the dinner of vegetable burger and vegetable salad is a combination of light food for the day.

An alternative is a breakfast of nut bread, two slices of fruit bits; lunch of grilled chicken, mixed green salad, vinaigrette dressing, large apple; a snack of whole-grain crackers with one half tablespoonful peanut butter; and dinner of pork tenderloin, chicken, or tofu with wild rice pilaf, steamed asparagus, and cinnamon applesauce. Use fruits for dessert or skip it.

Wednesday

Nutrients	Vitamins					Minerals										
	Vit A (mcg)	Vit C (mg)	Vit E (mg)	Folate (mcg)	Vit K (mcg)	Iron (mg)	Pot (mg)	Cal (mg)	Phosph (mg)	Selen (mcg)	Zinc (mg)	Chrom (mcg)	Mg (mg)	Cop (mcg)	Mol (mcg)	Man (mg)
RDA	1000	90	15	400	50	8	2000	600	460	65	10	30	100	340	17	2.3

Weekly Selection of Breakfast, Lunch, and Dinner That Satisfy Rejuvenate Mitochondria
(Most vitamins and Mineral RDA$_s$)

Breakfast	Lunch	Dinner	Remarks
Breakfast: Buckwheat pancake, sliced kiwi.	Lunch: Turkey sandwich (1 slice of bun, 2 oz turkey) with tomato and mustard. Snack: One piece fresh fruit: banana or apple. May include Brazil nuts.	Dinner: Baked fish, Mediterranean mashed potato with broccoli.	Wednesday: A high-antioxidant breakfast, high-protein lunch, fruit-based snack, and fish protein and powerful broccoli dinner is just right for multiple nutrients. The snack may include Brazil nuts for selenium and other minerals from pumpkin and sunflower seeds.

An alternative is a breakfast of fried egg sandwich, grilled whole-wheat muffin, grapefruit, blackberry banana smoothie; a lunch of tofu steak sandwich, seven-vegetable slaw, one cup sliced kiwi/blueberries; a snack of fruit and spicy nut trail mix, with one half cup orange juice; and a dinner of curried winter squash soup, cracked wheat bread, and spinach and mushroom salad with vinaigrette. No dessert.

Thursday

Nutrients	Vitamins					Minerals										
	Vit A (mcg)	Vit C (mg)	Vit E (mg)	Folate (mcg)	Vit K (mcg)	Iron (mg)	Pot (mg)	Cal (mg)	Phosph (mg)	Selen (mcg)	Zinc (mg)	Chrom (mcg)	Mg (mg)	Cop (mcg)	Mol (mcg)	Man (mg)
RDA	1000	90	15	400	50	8	2000	600	460	65	10	30	100	340	17	2.3

Weekly Selection of Breakfast, Lunch, and Dinner That Satisfy Rejuvenate Mitochondria
(Most vitamins and Mineral RDA$_s$)

Breakfast	Lunch	Dinner	Remarks
Breakfast: Fresh berries and nonfat yogurt.	Lunch: One ounce low-fat cheese with five whole grain crackers. Snack: Stuffed artichoke (bread crumbs, diced provolone or Gouda cheese, beans, parsley, olive oil, garlic).	Dinner: Sweet and sour vegetables with tofu tossed green salad and orange.	Thursday: Berries with antioxidants and yogurt with probiotics begin the day, lunch adds protein and fiber value of beans by midday, an artichoke and cheese snack adds protein and phytochemicals, and a light dinner is a great combination for the midweek.

An alternative is a breakfast of two slices of whole-wheat toast with peanut butter and strawberry fruit spread, apple-cranberry juice; a lunch of chipotle chicken chili, baked tortilla chips, fruit juice, oatmeal raisin cookie; a snack of toasted nuts and seeds; and a dinner of restaurant crostini (Italian ciabatta bread), sea bass wild rice pilaf, steamed broccoli, fruit sorbet, and expresso. Go for yogurt with fruits for dessert if you feel like.

Friday

Nutrients	Vitamins					Minerals										
	Vit A (mcg)	Vit C (mg)	Vit E (mg)	Folate (mcg)	Vit K (mcg)	Iron (mg)	Pot (mg)	Cal (mg)	Phosph (mg)	Selen (mcg)	Zinc (mg)	Chrom (mcg)	Mg (mg)	Cop (mcg)	Mol (mcg)	Man (mg)
RDA	1000	90	15	400	50	8	2000	600	460	65	10	30	100	340	17	2.3

Weekly Selection of Breakfast, Lunch, and Dinner That Satisfy Rejuvenate Mitochondria
(Most vitamins and Mineral RDAₛ)

Breakfast	Lunch	Dinner	Remarks
Breakfast: Boiled eggs, berries, and orange juice.	Lunch: Mediterranean bean salad, two slices whole-grain bread, and one pear. Skip snack	Dinner: Baked potato and broccoli salad with two tablespoons low fat dressing of your choice.	Friday: The day begins with a high-protein breakfast, the lunch adds fiber and protein, and a light dinner completes the day.

An alternative is a breakfast of apple-crunch oatmeal, pineapple juice, six ounces green tea, carrot wheat germ muffin, hard-boiled egg, black grapes; a lunch of tortilla wrap, large banana, spicy shrimp, celery sticks, lime water; a snack of multi-fruit crumble and coffee; and a dinner of lemon grouper, vegetables, romaine lettuce salad, orange juice, blueberry-banana smoothie, and roasted cashews.

Saturday

Nutrients	Vitamins					Minerals										
	Vit A (mcg)	Vit C (mg)	Vit E (mg)	Folate (mcg)	Vit K (mcg)	Iron (mg)	Pot (mg)	Cal (mg)	Phosph (mg)	Selen (mcg)	Zinc (mg)	Chrom (mcg)	Mg (mg)	Cop (mcg)	Mol (mcg)	Man (mg)
RDA	1000	90	15	400	50	8	2000	600	460	65	10	30	100	340	17	2.3

Weekly Selection of Breakfast, Lunch, and Dinner That Satisfy Rejuvenate Mitochondria
(Most vitamins and Mineral RDAₛ)

Breakfast	Lunch	Dinner	Remarks
Breakfast: Sliced banana oatmeal.	Lunch: One cup lentil soup, two cups mixed salad greens, herbal tea. Snack: Stuffed artichoke (bread crumbs, diced provolone cheese).	Dinner: Sweet and sour vegetables with tofu tossed green salad, orange.	Saturday: High-soluble fiber breakfast complements a vegetable protein lunch with added vegetables, followed by a high-protein artichoke snack. A light dinner completes the day.

An alternative is a breakfast of grapefruit juice, marbled eggs, whole-grain toast, fruit spread, green tea; a lunch of chicken salad, oat groat bread, iced green tea/lemon; a snack of popcorn, two cups fruit and spicy nut trail mix; and a dinner of avocado shrimp salsa, tomato dip/corn chips, chicken chili, pineapple. Go for a light dessert only if you have had a physically active day.

The recipes above for each day of the week represent a nutrient-wise, complete and yet restricted-calorie methylation diet for appropriate gene expressions and mitochondrial health. Also, included in this weekly list are food ingredients for building desirable variety of antioxidants, dietary fiber, probiotics, good fat, protein, essential amino acids and fatty acids, essential minerals, and vitamins that the American population is generally deficient in. Each recipe gives a breakdown of per serving nutritional information, with notations of proven health effects and values in terms of nutrient deliveries. The recipes can be used as alternates in the weekly list of breakfast, lunch, snack, or dinner wherever possible without increasing total calories for the day. The main criteria of diet design are to deliver high amounts of fiber, protein, vitamins, and minerals by way of fruits, vegetables, seeds, and nuts.

2.15.07 Common and Easy Recipes

The weekly list above and the alternates can be expanded to include a variety of other not too exotic dishes depending on available time for cooking and ingredients in the kitchen pantry. This added list includes beverages, desserts, dips, sauces, probiotics, salads, appetizers, breakfast, lunch, snacks, and desserts items. Recipe design must incorporate a complementary combination of as many vegetables as possible. Nuts and seeds should be included as toppings or inclusion materials in dumplings. As to the measures, a TBL is tablespoonful, tsp is teaspoonful, oz is 28.5 gram).

Beverages

A Cold Drink of Vegetable Stock For Vitamin A and C and Antioxidants

Ingredients: 1.00 TBL olive oil, two large chopped onions with skin on, 4 stalks of celery, 3 unpeeled coarsely chopped carrots, 2 coarsely chopped parsnips, 1 parsley sprig bunch of 10, 3 peppercorns, and 3 liters of water.

Preparation: Heat oil; add stir-fry vegetables just a little to make them crisp. Add all water and bring to boil. Simmer for one hour. Mash down the solids and strain. This can be frozen for three months for later use. Make drink on the rocks. antioxidants.

Nutrition: Twelve servings of a very low-calorie beverage. Each one-cup serving provides only 18 calories, no cholesterol and saturated fat, only 20 mg sodium, 2 grams carbohydrates, and 1 gram sugar.

A Brain Beverage of Hot Chocolate, Cinnamon, Peppermint, and Chili Powder

A cup of cocoa (hot chocolate) every alternate day is a great beverage for enhanced memory (Harvard University, Farzaneh A. Sorond); It promotes blood flow to the brain. Adding cinnamon to it helps moderates blood pressure.

Probiotic Raspberry Smoothie for folate, vitamin K, iron, magnesium, and zinc.

Ingredients: A very simple smoothie made from 1/2 cup low-fat milk, 3 TBL vanilla yogurt, 1/2 cup frozen raspberries, and optional skim milk.

Preparation: Combine all ingredients in a blender and puree to a desired consistency. It can be thinned by adding skim milk 1 TBL at a time.

Nutrition: I cup serving provides 210 calories, only 4.5 calories from 0.5 gram fat; no saturated fat and cholesterol; 85 mg sodium; and 45 grams total carbohydrates.

Probiotic Strawberry and Kiwi Smoothie for Vitamins C & K, Folate, and Choline

Ingredients: One 2.6 oz bag of frozen strawberries, 2 fresh kiwi, 1 oz strawberry yogurt, 1 tsp almond extract, and optional skim milk.

Preparation: Combine all ingredients in a blender and puree to a smooth consistency. It can be thinned by adding skim milk 1 TBL at a time.

Nutrition: 1 cup saturated fat and cholesterol-free serving provides 11 calories; 9.00 fat calories from 1 gram fat;32 mg sodium; 26 grams total carbohydrates; and 3 grams dietary fiber. This is a high-vitamin C smoothie.

Dips, Salsas, and Spreads

High-Antioxidant and -Phytonutrient Dips and Spreads of Artichoke and Bean

Ingredients: 19 oz white kidney beans, 14 oz artichoke, one fourth cup of extra-virgin olive oil, 3 TBL lemon juice, 3 cloves of quartered garlic, 1 tsp coarse salt, 1 tsp cayenne pepper, 1/4 tsp roasted red sweet pepper strips, 1/4 cup snipped basil, and 1/4 TBL sea or kosher salt.

Preparation: Use a food processor. Combine beans, artichoke, olive oil, lemon juice, garlic, salt, roasted red pepper, and cayenne pepper. Cover and process to a smooth paste. Transfer to serving bowl and chill for 24 hours.

Nutrition: This high-protein and high-fiber preparation makes four servings, each with 70 calories; 45 fat calories; 5 grams fat; 207 mg sodium; 8 grams carbohydrates; 3 grams fiber; 3 grams protein; and 18% % RDA of vitamin C . It is an ecellent source of vitamin K, folate, choline, iron, magnesium, and zinc.

Avocado and Edamami Spread for Vitamin K, folate, Zinc, Magnesium, Manganese, Zinc, Choline, and Omega-3 Fatty Acids.

This preparation yields 14 servings of 1 oz size, each with 6.4 gram good fat, 4 gram fiber, and 8.97 gram protein.

Ingredients: 16 oz edamami, 1 avocado, 1 clove of garlic, 1 TBL olive oil, 1 TBL fresh lime juice, and salt to taste. Two tsp of mustard paste is optional.

Preparation: Cook edamami in boiling water for 5 minutes, strain, and rinse with copious amount of cold water to stop cooking. Combine all ingredients and make the pureed spread in a food processor. Blend in mustard paste if you like. This is a flavorful, high-protein, and good-plant-fat dip with minerals and fiber. My wife chooses to add mint flavor to it.

Spiced Carrot Spread for 16,705 IU of Vitamin A and Added Power of Spices

Ingredients: 6 thinly sliced carrots, 1 clove of garlic, 1/2 tsp grated and peeled ginger, 1/2 tsp ground cumin, 1/2 tsp ground cinnamon, a pinch of cayenne pepper, 1 TBL tahini, 2 tsp lemon juice, salt and pepper to taste.

Preparation: Set a steamer basket in a saucepan in 2 inches of simmering water. Steam carrots for 6 minutes to a tender texture. Transfer to food processor along with garlic, cumin, cinnamon, cayenne pepper, tahini, lemon juice, and ginger. Season with salt and pepper. Process until smooth, 1 minute. Add up to 2 TBL water if necessary. As an option 1/2 cup of baked and mashed butternut squash can be added.

Nutrition: This saturated fat-free recipe makes four servings, each with 59 calories; 2 grams fat; 9 grams carbohydrates; 3 grams fiber; 2 grams protein. Butternut squash adds vitamins A, B complex, C, and mineral manganese.

Spiced Fruit Salsa for Vitamin K, Folate, and Choline (An Smoothie Equivalent)

Ingredients: 2 peeled and chopped large kiwifruits, 2 cups of fresh chopped strawberries, 2 minced scallions, 2 TBL brown sugar, 1/4 tsp cayenne pepper, and 1/3 cup lime juice.

Preparation: Combine all ingredients in a serving bowl. Refrigerate at least 1 hour. Serve with grilled seafood and poultry.

Nutrition: This fat-, cholesterol-, and sodium-free spiced salsa makes 10 half-cup servings, each with only 45 calories; 11 grams carbohydrates; 3 grams dietary fiber; 1 gram protein; and 7 grams sugar. In fact, this is a vitamin C salsa, with the health benefits of strawberries and scallions.

A Mayonnaise of White Beans, Greek Yogurt, and Sun-Dried Tomato

Ingredients: 15 oz white beans, 1/2 cup diced and dehydrated sun-dried tomato, 3/4 cup nonfat Greek yogurt, 2 TBL fresh grated Parmesan cheese, 1/4 cup chopped basil, salt and pepper to taste. This is a great replacement for mayonnaise.

Preparation: Add beans, sun-dried tomato, yogurt, and Parmesan cheese to the food processor and blend to creamy smoothness. Mix in basil; season with salt and pepper. Cover and refrigerate for 30 minutes before serving.

Nutrition: This fat-free preparation makes 16 servings, each of 2 TBL providing 35 calories; 55 mg sodium; 5 grams carbohydrates; 1 gram dietary fiber; 1 g sugar; and 3 grams protein. Also, it offers the benefits of high-protein, immuno-modulating peptides from cheese, probiotics, and eye health-promoting lycopene and lutein from tomatoes.

A Probiotic of Cabbage and Yogurt Slaw

Ingredients: 9 cups of medium green cabbage, 2 red bell peppers, 3 scallions, 2/3 cup Greek yogurt, 1 TBL cider vinegar, 1 TBL Dijon mustard, 2 tsp sugar, salt and pepper to taste.

Preparation: Toss together cabbage, bell pepper, and scallions in a large bowl. Whisk together yogurt, vinegar, mustard, and sugar. Season with salt and pepper in a small bowl. Pour dressing over greens. Toss to coat completely. Season to taste with salt and pepper. Refrigerate 20 minutes or up to two hours. This is a wonderful prebiotic fiber probiotic gut bacteria side dish.

Nutrition: Eight fat-free servings, each of 65 calories; 13 grams carbohydrates; 4 grams fiber; and 3 grams protein.

Soups

Asparagus and Scallion Soup with Almonds for Vitamins A, C, K, E, Folate, Choline, and Minerals magnesium and Zinc.

Ingredients: 1 and 1/4 cup sliced almonds, 2 medium sliced leeks, 6 thinly sliced scallions, 28 oz chicken or vegetable broth, 1/2 tsp dried thyme, salt and pepper to taste, 2 lb asparagus, 1 and 1/2 oz white beans, and 1 cup skim milk (optional).

Preparation: Place almonds in a saucepan over medium heat. Toast to golden brown color in 5 minutes. Set aside the nuts. Heat oil in the same pan, add leeks and scallions and cook for 5 minutes to tenderness. Add broth, skim milk, thyme, salt, and pepper and bring to boil. Add asparagus and beans. Bring to boil and then simmer for 15 minutes to soften vegetables. Cool and puree. Pour back into saucepan and heat to warm up. Serve in bowls garnished with scallions and toasted almonds.

Nutrition: Six servings, each providing 150 calories; 35 fat calories from 5 grams fat; 1 gram saturated fat; 290 mg sodium; 20 grams carbohydrates; 6 grams fiber; and 8 grams protein. This is a high-protein, high-fiber, high-folate, and high-magnesium soup. We should use it at least twice a week.

High-Fiber Spicy Black Bean Soup for Folate and Calcium, Magnesium, copper, and Zinc.

Ingredients: 1 lb dried black beans, soaked overnight and drained; 2 diced large yellow onions; 2 minced jalapeño peppers; 1 TBL virgin oil; 4 garlic cloves; 2 tsp ground cumin; and salt and pepper to taste.

Preparation: Use medium saucepan. Add beans, water to cover 2 inches, and one quarter each of onion and jalapeño, and bring to boil over high. Simmer for 45 minutes. Refrigerate and use it later or next day.

Use a heavy pot. Heat oil. Add garlic and rest of onion; season with salt and pepper. Cook for 10 minutes. Stir in all remaining jalapeño, cumin, beans, and cooking liquid. Simmer for 20 minutes. Add water if necessary while cooking. Add beans and puree. Serve garnished with chopped onions.

Nutrition: Four servings, each providing 336 calories; 5 grams fat; 1 gram saturated fat; 62 grams carbohydrates; 20 grams fiber; and 20 grams protein. This is a truly high-protein and high-fiber dish.

Thick Tomato Soup, a Concentrated Supplement of natural Nutrients

Ingredients: 1.25 oz diced celery, 1.25 oz diced onion, 16 oz diced carrot, 35 oz water, 5.5 corn bran fiber, 32 oz tomato juice, 14 oz chicken broth, 1 oz crushed tomatoes, half tsp oz extra-virgin olive oil, 1 tsp black pepper, 1 tsp oz salt, 1 tsp garlic powder, 1 tsp ground pepper, 2 tsp Worcestershire sauce, 1 tsp dried thyme, 2 tsp dried basil, and roasted red pepper puree and 2 TBL heavy cream optional for flavor and color. Red pepper is common in Indian recipes. This is a 6.5 lb recipe and 2 TBl heavy cream would not make much difference in nutrition per serving.

Preparation: Sweat the celery, onions, and carrots with the olive oil in saucepan. Add the chicken broth to the vegetables and simmer. Premix the corn-bran fiber with hot water using a blender, food processor, or immersion blender. Add corn-fiber slurry to the broth and vegetable mix. Add tomatoes, juice, Worcestershire sauce, ground black peppers, and all of the seasonings and continue to heat over medium heat. Once vegetables are tender and soup is heated throughout, use blender to puree until smooth. Place puréed soup over low heat and add the heavy cream; heat throughout. Garnish with basil or parsley and serve warm.

Nutrition: Use eight-fluid-oz serving that provides 100 calories; 54 fat calories from six grams fat; 25 mg cholesterol; 580 mg sodium; 8 grams carbohydrates; 3 grams dietary fiber; and 4 grams protein. This a high-sodium soup packed with protein and fiber.

High-Fiber Curried Sweet Potato and Lentil Soup

Ingredients: 2 TBL canola oil, 1 chopped medium onion, 3 cloves of garlic, 1 tsp fresh minced ginger, 2 TBL curry powder, 1 tsp salt, 1/2 tsp black pepper, 4 chopped plum tomatoes, 1 cup dry lentils, 1 quart vegetable broth, 14 oz can of light coconut milk, 1 lb half-inch chunks of sweet potatoes, 1 chopped zucchini, 1/2 cup cut green beans, 1/2 cup chopped cilantro or parsley.

Preparation: Heat oil in a medium-size pan over medium heat. Add onion and cook for 3 minutes to soft and translucent consistency. Add garlic and ginger and cook one more minute. Stir in curry powder, salt, and pepper and cook for 2 more minutes to proper color and fragrance. Stir in tomatoes, sweet potato chunks, and lentils, add vegetable broth and coconut milk, and bring to boil while partially closed. Reduce heat to simmering bubbles until lentils are soft in 15 minutes. Add stock or water for consistency. Cover and cook for 10 minutes. Stir in zucchini and green beans, adding more water for a good broth look. Cover and cook for 5 minutes to tenderness. Stir in cilantro; salt and pepper to taste.

Nutrition: Four servings, each of 1 cup that provides 446 calories; 15 grams fat; 6.5 grams saturated fat; 974 mg sodium; 63 grams carbohydrates; and 20 grams fiber. This is a high-fiber and high-vitamin A soup that also delivers 15% RDA of vitamin C.

Probiotic Cucumber Soup

Ingredients: 4 peeled and seeded small cucumbers, 2 cups Greek-style yogurt, 2 TBL lemon juice, 1/2 cup fresh-chopped mint, 1 clove of minced garlic, 1 TBL olive oil, and salt and pepper to taste.

Preparation: Add all ingredients to a food processor, puree for a minute, and pour into a container. Refrigerate for 3–4 hours. Serve with a garnish of minced dill.

Nutrition: Three servings of 1 cup each provide for 150 calories, including 45 calories from 5 grams fat; 0.5 gram saturated fat; 70 mg sodium; 11 grams carbohydrates; 2 grams fiber; 8 grams sugar; and 16 grams protein. This, in a sense, is high-protein Indian raiyata with Greek yogurt. This is a good way to increase daily vitamin K and molybdenum intake, along with anti-inflammatory and cancer-fighting cucurbitacins, lignans, and flavonoids.

Pea Soup for Vitamin A, K, Folate and Choline

Ingredients: 2 lb fresh or frozen peas, 1/2 cup water, half-and-half (optional), vegetable broth (optional), goat cheese bits (optional), and croutons (optional).

Preparation: Puree, filter, and simmer for 1 minute. Add half-and-half or cream for creaminess Dilute with water/vegetable broth. Goat cheese bits can also be added with or without croutons.

Nutrition: 8 servings of 1 cup each provide 132 calories, including 1 gram saturated fat; 433 mg sodium; % RDA of folate: 20%; % RDA of vitamin A: 18%; % RDA of vitamin C: 77%. Pea and asparagus soups can be used once a week for a rather complete methylation diet.

Carrot Soup for Vitamin A

Ingredients: 1.5 lb chopped carrots, 2 cups water, half-and-half (optional), and croutons (optional).

Preparation: Puree and filter. Simmer for 25 minutes. Can add half-and-half for creaminess. Can be served with or without croutons.

Nutrition: 8 servings of 1 cup each provide 77 calories with only 1 gram saturated fat; 484 mg sodium.

Salads

Asparagus Salad

Ingredients: 3/4 tsp olive oil, 3/4 lb asparagus, 1 TBL water, 1/2 lb sugar snap peas, 1 sliced scallion, 3/4 tsp low-sodium soy sauce, and 3/4 tsp honey.

Preparation: Heat oil in a pan over medium heat. Add asparagus and water. Cover and steam for 5 minutes. Add peas, scallion, soy sauce, and honey. Cover and cook for another 5 minutes. Season to taste with salt and pepper.

Nutrition: Four servings, each providing 34 calories, including 9 fat calories; 36 mg sodium; 5 grams carbohydrates; 2 grams fiber; and 2 grams protein. This is a high-folate salad to be used, if possible, twice a week.

President Clinton's Snow Pea Salad

Ingredients: 5 oz snow peas, 3 oz bean sprouts, 1/4 medium julienned red bell pepper, 1 TBL soy sauce, 2 tsp sesame oil, 1 TBL toasted sesame seed, salt to taste.

Preparation: Blanch snow peas in boiling water for 10 seconds; then quickly soak in ice water and pat the peas dry. Combine peas, sprouts, and red pepper; toss with soy sauce, sesame oil, and sesame seed. Salt to taste. Serve chilled.

Nutrition: Makes four cholesterol-free servings, each of 57 calories; 2 grams protein; 5 grams carbohydrates; 2 grams fiber; 3 grams fat (1 gram saturated fat); and 304 mg sodium.

Artichoke Salad with Baby Greens

Ingredients: 1 cup baby field greens, 6 cherry tomatoes halved, 4 oz artichoke hearts, 1TBL red wine vinegar, 2 tsp extra-virgin olive oil, 1 finely minced garlic clove, salt and freshly ground black pepper to taste, and 1/2 TBL grated Parmesan cheese.

Preparation: Arrange greens, tomatoes, and artichoke in a bowl. Make dressing in a separate bowl by whisking in red wine vinegar, olive oil, garlic, salt, and pepper and toss into the greens for making two servings. Top with Parmesan cheese. Preparation time: Less than 15 minutes.

Nutrition: 91 calories per serving, including 45 fat calories from 5 grams fat, containing only 1 gram saturated fat; 318 mg sodium; total 9 grams carbohydrates; 2 grams fiber; and 4 grams protein.

A High Nutrient Vegetable Salad

Ingredients—Pasta: 8 oz whole-wheat rotini noodle, 3 chopped medium tomatoes, 1 diced red pepper, 1 small yellow pepper, 1/2 cup minced parsley, 1 TBL minced fresh oregano, 1 diced cucumber, 1 can (15 oz) drained and rinsed chickpeas.

Ingredients—Vinaigrette: 3 TBL red wine vinegar, 1 TBL lemon juice, 1 tsp Dijon mustard, 2 and 1/2 TBL olive oil, and salt and pepper to taste.

Preparation: Combine the cooked pasta with tomatoes, red and yellow peppers, parsley, oregano, cucumber, and chickpeas. Combine the vinaigrette ingredients and mix. Toss it over pasta.

Nutrition: Six low-sodium and cholesterol-free servings, each providing 200 calories, including 65 calories from 7 grams fat, including 1 gram saturated fat; 120 mg sodium; 28 grams carbohydrates; 5 grams dietary fiber; 6 grams sugar; and 7 grams protein.

Lunch

Lunch of Wild Mushroom and Lentil Burger

Ingredients: 6 oz Shitake mushrooms, 15.5 oz rinsed and drained lentils, 1/4 cup whole-wheat bread crumbs, 1 large egg, 1/4 cup chopped celery, 1.5 TBL fresh thyme, 1 tsp Dijon mustard, 1 cup chopped onion, 4 oz mild cheese, 6 TBL yellow cornmeal, 3 tsp olive oil, 4 whole-wheat buns, 1/4 cup chopped roasted bell peppers, and 1/4 cup watercress.

Preparation: Heat oven to 400°F. Coarsely mash 3/4 of mushrooms and set aside. Add lentils, bread crumbs, egg, celery, thyme, roasted bell peppers, watercress, mustard, half of onion, and half of cheese. Pulse, and then form into patties. Coat both sides of patties with cornmeal. Heat 1 tsp oil and add remaining mushrooms and onion; heat to golden brown in about 5 minutes. Remove from pan. Add remaining oil to the pan and cook patties, turning once on each side. Transfer to baking sheet, top with remaining cheese, and bake for four minutes. Serve on buns.

Nutrition: Four servings, each providing 386 calories, including 125 fat calories from 13 grams fat; 5.5 grams saturated fat; 597 mg sodium; 51 grams carbohydrates; 12 grams fiber; 1 gram sugar; and 19 grams protein. This is a high-fiber and high-protein burger with mushroom and lentil nutrients.

A Lunch Food for Eye Health and Stress Reduction:

A butternut squash dish with rice contains three tablespoons olive oil, two garlic cloves, one small onion, one cup rice, one small butternut squash, one teaspoon paprika, one tablespoon maple syrup, four sage leaves, and one-half cup walnuts. To prepare the concoction, set oven to 400°F. In a saucepan, stir-fry garlic and onion to brownness in olive oil. Add rice, two cups water, salt, and pepper, and bring to boil. Simmer at low; stir-fry squash in oil. Add paprika, maple syrup, and salt, and roast for twenty minutes. Add walnuts to the cooked rice. The recipe adds the benefits of squash and walnuts to a common rice dish.

Nutrition: The recipe provides six servings, each providing 309 calories, thirteen grams fat, 45 g carbohydrates, 786 mg sodium, and three grams fiber. This is a rather high-sodium preparation.

President Clinton's Lunch of Herbed Quinoa with Green Onions

Ingredients: 1 cup quinoa, 2 cups vegetable stock, 1/2 cup disked cucumber, 1/2 cup diced tomatoes, 2 TBL diced red onion, 2 green onions finely sliced, 2 TBL chopped cilantro, 1 tsp chopped jalapeño, 3 TBL extra-virgin olive oil, and 1 TBL fresh lemon juice.

Preparation: Cook 1 cup of quinoa in 2 cups of vegetable stock, combine cooked quinoa with all other ingredients, toss well, and serve chilled.

Nutrition: Four cholesterol-free servings, each providing 268 calories; 34 grams carbohydrates; 13 grams fat including 2 grams saturated fat; 483 mg sodium; and 6 grams protein.

A Lunch of Veggie Burger

Ingredients: Tofu-4 Oz, Cremini mushroom- 1/2 lb, black pepper- 3/4 tsp, Kidney beans- 15 Oz, Coarse grated beet-1 cup, Almond or cashew chopped- 3/4 cup, Bread crumb- 1/3 cup, Queso blanco- 2 Oz, large eggs-2, mayonnaise- 2 TBL, Sliced scallion- 2, Garlic cloves-3, Paprika- 3/4 tsp, Crumbled tempeh-1 Oz, and Brown rice- 1/2 cup.

Preparation: Prepare oven at 425 Deg F. Cut tofu into 1/4" pieces. Place on baking sheet oiled both sides.Toss with salt and pepper. Transfer beans and beet on a separate sheet. Roast beans first for 15 minutes and then beet and tofy for 25 minutes. Grind in a food processor. Add bread crumb, cheese, and peprika. Pulse to mix well. Make six 1 inch thick patties. Grill 4-6 minutes each side. Can refrigerate for use during the week.

Nutrition Information: A 100 g serving delivers 177 calories, only 1.4 g fat, 400 mg sodium, 4.26 g fiber, 1.42 g sugar and 15.5 g protein along with B vitamins and trace minerals.

Lunch of High-Fiber Grilled Fruit Kebab of Pine Apple, Kiwi, Papaya, and Mango

Ingredients: 1/2 cup pineapple juice, 1 TBL brown sugar, juice of one lime, 1/2 tsp cinnamon, half a tsp allspice, and a pinch of clove.

Preparation: Soak wooden skewers in hot water for an hour. Heat the grill to medium. Combine basting-sauce ingredients of pineapple juice, brown sugar, lime juice, and cinnamon in a shallow bowl. Prepare the spice mixture of allspice and clove. Thread fruit cubes of kiwi, papaya, mango, and pineapple on the skewers. Sprinkle with spice. Grill and baste every few minutes for 10 minutes to brown color. Drizzle the remaining sauce over kebabs. Serve and enjoy.

Nutrition: Makes six cholesterol-free servings, each of 130 calories; only 5 fat calories; 0.5 gram fat, and only 0.1 gram saturated fat. 5 mg sodium; 33 grams carbohydrates; 4 grams fiber; 25 grams sugar; and 1 gram protein.

A Lunch of Couscous with Chickpeas, Dried Fruit, and Cilantro

Ingredients: 1/2 cup Water, 1/4 tsp ground allspice, 1 cup orange juice, 1/2 tsp salt, 1 cup whole-wheat couscous, 3 TBL olive oil, 1 sliced medium onion, 1 sliced green bell pepper, 3 cloves of minced garlic, 1 tsp curry powder, 1 can chickpeas, 15 oz sliced dried apricots, 1 and 1/2 cup sweetened cranberries, and 1 TBL cilantro.

Preparation: Combine water, allspice, half of the orange juice, and half of the salt in a saucepan. Heat at medium high and bring to boil. Add couscous and cook for 5 minutes. Remove from heat and let stand for 5 minutes.

Heat oil in a large nonstick frying pan over medium heat. Add onion, pepper, garlic, and curry powder. Cook while stirring 10 minutes. Add chickpeas, apricots, and cranberries, and cook while stirring. Pour in remaining orange juice and cook. Add cilantro and remaining salt. Serve over couscous.

Nutrition: Four servings of high-fiber and high-protein preparation, each of which provide 363 calories, including 76.5 fat calories from 8.5 grams fat, including 1 gram saturated fat; 320 mg sodium; 67 grams carbohydrates; 9 grams fiber; and 9 grams protein. A great lunch dish.

A Multigrain Lunch Heart-Healthy Toss of Sweet Potato and Edamami

Ingredients: 1/2 cup shelled edamami, 1/4 cup chopped onion, 1 cup mixed greens, 1 oz feta cheese, 1 medium sweet potato, salt and pepper, and 1 TBL vinegar.

Preparation: Boil edamami in water for 10 minutes. Drain and set aside. Heat 1 TBL vegetable oil in a pan; sauté onion and greens. Spread and flatten greens and cook at low heat. Add cheese and bind greens in bite size bits. Add chopped sweet potato, edamame, salt and pepper, and vinegar. Toss and mix. Serve warm.

Nutrition: Two servings each provide 200 calories, including 36 fat calories from 4 grams fat; 95 mg sodium; 47 grams carbohydrates; 1 gram fiber; and 3 grams protein.

Vegetable Mash

Sautéed Spinach with Garlic for Vitamins A, K, Folate, and Choline like Betaine

Ingredients: 16 oz baby spinach, 1 clove of garlic, and 1 TBL balsamic vinegar.

Preparation: Rinse spinach and add to skillet along with garlic. Cook on medium heat for 5 minutes. Sprinkle with drops of balsamic vinegar or lemon juice and serve.

Nutrition: This is a low-fat and cholesterol- and sugar-free preparation of four 1/4-cup servings, each providing 25 calories; 4 fat calories; 0.4 grams fat; 0.1 g saturated fat; 90 mg sodium; 4 grams carbohydrates; 3 grams fiber; and 3 grams protein.

A Multinutrient Mash of Sweet Potato Turnip with Sage Butter

Ingredients: 1/4 lb sweet potato, 4 oz turnip, 3 large cloves of garlic, 15 sage leaves, 1 TBL butter, 1/2 tsp salt, 1/2 tsp coarsely ground black pepper.

Preparation: In a medium saucepan, place sweet potato, turnip, garlic, and 6 leaves of sage and cover with water. Bring to boil. Cook at medium heat for 15 minutes to a tender soft texture. Drain and return vegetables to pan and cover. Heat butter to melt, and add remainder of sage. Let sage crackle to flavor for one minute. Pour sage butter over vegetables and mash. Stir in salt and pepper. Enjoy the nutritional benefits of sweet potato from vitamins A, C, B_6, choline, and cancer-fighting betaine.

Nutrition: Three servings, each serving with 88 calories; 4 grams fat; 3 grams saturated fat; 10 mg cholesterol; 224 mg sodium; 291 mg potassium; 12 grams carbohydrates; 2 grams fiber; and 1 gram protein.

Dinner

A Great Dinner of Cheesy Broccoli and Rice Casserole for Vitamins C, K, and Folate

Ingredients: Cooking spray, salt, 2.5 tsp olive oil, 1.25 cup quick-cooking brown rice, 4 cups vegetable or chicken broth, 1 can (12.5 oz) low-fat evaporated milk, 1 lb broccoli, one minced onion, 2 minced garlic cloves, 2/3 cup shredded cheddar cheese, a pinch of cayenne pepper, 1/4 tsp dry mustard, pepper to taste, and 3 TBL Romano cheese.

Preparation: Coat 9 X 12-inch casserole with cooking spray. Boil a large pot of water 1 tsp salt. Heat 1 tsp olive oil in a large Dutch oven; add dry rice and sauté for two minutes. Add broth and evaporated milk and bring to boil. Simmer for 20 minutes until rice is tender. Add broccoli to boiling water in the pot, turn heat off, and let stand for 2 minutes.

Preheat oven to 400°F. Heat the remaining oil in a large skillet, add onion, and sauté for three minutes, then add garlic and broccoli and sauté for 2 minutes. Add broccoli-onion mixture to cooked rice; add cheddar cheese, cayenne pepper, dry mustard, and pepper. Pour the mixture in the casserole and sprinkle with Romano cheese. Bake for 15 minutes until bubbly.

Nutrition: 8 servings of 1 cup each provides 250 calories, including 55 fat calories from 6 grams fat containing 2.3 grams saturated fat but no trans fat; 10 mg cholesterol; 430 mg sodium; 38 grams total carbohydrates; 4 grams dietary fiber; 9 grams sugar; and 14 grams protein.

2.15.08 Recipes by Great Chefs of the World

What follows is a select list of additionalrecipes of breakfast, lunch, snacks, appetizers, dinner, desserts, and beverages created by word's renounced chefs. The selection is based on both the nutrition and then the flavor and texture. One can always replace a compatible and complementary ingredients for a given season in a given region.

1. Tofu Breakfast

Ingredients	Nutrition Information/Serving	Preparation	Key Methylation Nutrients
Tofu blocks, 2-14 oz blocks Vegetable oil, 2 TBL Small Onion, 1 Small green pepper, 1 Small red pepper, 1 Coriander, 1/2 ts Cumin, 1/2 ts Turmeric, 1/2 ts Black bean, 1-15 oz can Chopped Cilantro, 1/4 cup Whole Wheat Tortilla, 4-6 inch	**Six servings** **Total Calories, 390** **Fat, 16 g** **Saturated Fat, 1.5** **Cholesterol, o mg** **Sodium, 620 mg** **Carbohydrate, 43** **Sugar, 5** **Fiber, 9** **Protein, 22**	1. Dry cut tofu in layers over paper towel and then mash. 2. Heat oil in a skillet at med heat, stir fry onion and peppers, add coriander and cumin. 3. Cook to fragrance and add tofu and turmeric 4. Add beans and cook for 4 minutes Garnish with cilantro and salsa and serve over tortillas.	**Complementary garnish: salsa, Chopped avocado, grated chedar cheese, sliced scallion, hot sauce for capasaicin, and tufu for isoflavones.**

2. John Besh's Southern Soup Au Pistou

Ingredients	Nutrition Information/Serving	Preparation	Key Methylation Nutrients
1. Carrot, French bean, red cabbage, button mushroom, and chopped kale, 1 cup each. 2. Chopped onion, 1/4 cup 3. Chopped garlic, 1 tsp 4. Moog sprouts 5. 3 Cups vegetable stock. 6. Salt and Pepper	**This is very low calorie methylation dish.** **It is equivalent to at least 1/3 rd the requirement of six servings of fruits and vegetables.**	1. Stir fry 1/4 cup chopped onion and 1 ts chopped garlic,. 2. Add all vegetable. sauté for 5 minutes. Add moong sprouts and sauté another 3 minutes. 3. Add vegetable stock, tomato sauce, season with salt and pepper, and season more to taste if necessary. 4. Serve with steamed rice, crackers, or noodles.	**Carrot for vitamin A, phytonutrients from cabbage, and unequalled methylation ingredient power of kale, and antioxidant power of onion and garlic are the key benefits of this soup.** **Moog sprouts add protein.**

3. Salad Recipe 01: Ferran Adria's Caesar Salad

Ingredients	Nutrition Informa-tion/Serving	Preparation	Key Methyla-tion Nutrients
Olive Oil, 4 TBL Bread, three slices Garlic, chopped, 1 clove Tofu, 10 oz Egg Yolk, 2 Sherry Vine-gar, 4 ts Sunflower oil, 6 TBL + 2 ts Parmesan Cheese, 1 1/2 Oz Salt and pep-per Romaine Lettuce, 2 medium	**Four Servings** **Calories, 451** **Fat, 38.7 g** **Sat Fat, 4.0 g** **Cholesterol, 108 mg** **Sodium, 304 mg** **Carbohydrate, 24.3 g** **Dietary Fiber, 7 g** **Sugar, 4.3 g** **Protein, 5.9 g**	1. Make croutons by stir frying bread chunks to a crispy/chewy texture. 2. For dressing, combine garlic and tofu in food processor and pulse to mince. Add egg yolk and mince. Add sherry vinegar and pulse to mince. Add half of parmesan cheese and mince a bit more. Season with salt and pepper. 3. Toss dressing and croutons on lettuce leaves	**Although fat cal-ories are below 30% of the total accompanied with high fiber and protein, one should like to reduce the portion and make six servings out of this salad prepa-ration.**

4. Fergus Henderson's Red Salad

Ingredients	Nutrition Information/Serving	Preparation	Key Methylation Nutrients
Raw beets, finely grated, 2 Red cabbaged, sliced fine, 1/4 Small red onion, 1 Dollops of cream Fraiche, 6 Bunch of Chervil, 2 Dressing: virgin olive oil, Balsamic Ginger, extra fine capers, salt and pepper	**Six Servings** **Calories, 190** **Fat, 16 g** **Sat Fat, 1.7** **Carbohydrate, 12.5 g** **Dietary Fiber, 3.5 g** **Sugar, 7.5** **Protein, 2.1**	1. Put together beats over red cabbage and red onion 2. The dressing of Balsamin vinegar, olive oil, cappers, salt, and black pepper intensifies the collor. Serve salad with cream fraiche or better simple probiotic yogurt and Chervil.	**Color of red onion, beets, and cabbage adds antioxidants.** **Beet provides betain, folate, magnesium, zinc, and copper.** **Onion provides allyl sulfides, quercetin, B$_6$, copper, magnesium, biotin, and fiber.** **Cabbage provides folate, vitamins A, C, and K.**

5. A Lunch of Thomas Keller's Stewed Winter Vegetables

Ingredients	Nutrition Information/Serving	Preparation	Key Methylation Nutrients
Medium Shallots, 8 Unsalted Butter, 2 1/2 TBL Parsnips cut to 2" length, 8 Large Turnips, 4 Large Leeks, 2 halved and cut Vegetable stock, 2 1/2 cup Thyme, 1 sprig Small red potato, 1/2 lb	Eight Servings Calories 240 Fat, 7 g Sat Fat, 1 g Cholesterol, 0.0 mg Sodium, 940 mg Carbohydrate 37 g Fiber, 6 g Sugar, 10 g Protein, 5 g	1. Bake the shallots on foil topped with 1/2 TBL butter in a preheated oven to 350 F for 30 minutes until tender, 2. Combine parsnips, turnips, carrots, leek, vegetable stock, thyme, and 2 TBL remaining butter. Bring to boil. Simmer at low heat for 20 minutes, add salt and pepper. Discard thyme sprigs. 3. In medv sauce pan, cook potatoes in boiling salt water for 10 minutes until tender. Cut in 2" cubes. 4. Add potatoes and roasted shallots to vegetable stew.	Red Turnip provides Omega- 3 fatty acid, choline, folate, vitamin C, and minerals calcium, iron, magnesium, and zinc. Leek is great source of vitamins A, K, B group folate, and choline. Parshnips deliver folate and minerals magnesium, zinc, copper, and manganese.

6. David Chang's Honey-Soy Glazed Crispy Mushroom

Ingredients	Nutrition Information/Serving	Preparation	Key Methylation Nutrients
1/2 cup Canola oil 1 # red turnip 1 # Radish 1/4 cup honey 2 TBL Soy sauce 1/2 # Swiss chord 2 TBL molasses 2 TBL water 6 large Shitake mushrooms 1/2 # Asian Rice Cracker	**Four Servings** **Calories, 98** **Fat, 7 g** **Cholesterol, 0.0 mg** **Sodium, 44 mg** **Carbohydrate, 7 g** **Dietary fiber, 2 g** **Sugar, 4 g** **Protein, 2.8 g**	1. Start with 1 TBL oil in the skillet and simmer. Add turnip and radish, cook over medium heat, add honey and cook over medium heat, thus glaze vegetables in 5 minutes. 2. Add soy sauce and cook for 5 minutes until syrupy, add lemon juice and cook another 3 minutes. 3. Cook at high and evaporate all water. 4. Whisk in molasses, water, and salt. Add Shitaki mushrroms. Add rice crackers and toss 5. Heat rest of the oil. Add coated mushrooms. Cook another 5 minutes. Top vegetables with mushroom and serve.	Red Turnip provides Omega- 3 fatty acid, choline, folate, vitamin C, and minerals calcium, iron, magnesium, and zinc. Swiss Chord: excellent source of vitamins A and K and mineral magnesium. Radish: good source of folate, choline, and magnesium. Shitake Mushroom: Source of folate, pantothenic acid, choline, and minerals magnesium, zinc, copper, and selenium.

7. Thomas Keller's Side Vegetable Gratin Recipe, a Snack

Ingredients	Nutrition Informa-tion/Serving	Preparation	Key Methyla-tion Nutrients
3 Roma tomatoes, sliced into 2 inches diameter Medium yellow squash, 1, cut into ¼ inch slices 1 Medium zucchini, 1 4" slices Japanese eggplant, 1 cut into ¼ inch slices Canola oil Coarsely chopped onions, 2 1/2 cups Garlic cloves, finely grated, 2 kosher salt Chopped thyme 1 TBL and 1 ts Extra virgin olive oil, 1/4 cup Freshly ground pepperFreshly grated Parmigiano-Reggiano, 1/2 cup Dried bread crumbs, 1/2 Cup	**Six Servings** **Calories, 330** **Fat, 20 g** **Sat Fat, 4 g** **Cholesterol, 10 mg** **Sodium, 625 mg** **Carbohydrate, 27 g** **Sugar, 4 g** **Dietary Fiber, 4 g** **Protein, 9 g**	1. Cook onion w/o browning with garlic seasoned with salt and pepper to translucent texture for 20 minutes at low heat. 2. Combine squash, zucchini, and egg plant in a large bowl and toss with olive oil and season with salt. 3. Drizzle tomato slices with olive oil and salt, combine bread crumb, parmesan cheese, and remainder of thyme. 4. Spread onion on the bottom of Gratin Dish. Layer the vegetables with zucchini on the outer and then move in with tomato and then egg plant each topped with parmesan cheese 5. Bake for 1 1/2 hour at 350 to tenderness. Remove from oven. Let stand for 10 minutes. Broil just before serving.	**A methylation dish that spells nutritional art,** **The favorite of our kitchen.** Benefits of tomato, eggplant, and zucchini: Lycopene, ferulic acid, anthocyanin flavonoid antioxidants, vitamins A, B vitamins, K, Choline, and minerals magnesium, iron, zinc, and copper. Browned breadcrumb adds texture and melted cheese adds protein nutrition.

8. Rene Redzepi's Kale, Red Pepper, and Tofu Snack

Ingredients	Nutrition Informa- tion/Serving	Preparation	Key Methyla- tion Nutrients
1 Bunch Kale 14 oz firm tofu 1 TBL soy sauce 1 TBL rice winw 1/4 C vegeta- ble stock 1 ts corn starch 1/4 ts salt 1 ts ground pepper 1/4 ts sugar 1 TBL canola oil 1 TBL minced garlic 1 TBL minced ginger 1 seeded ser- rano pepper 1 julianed red pepper 1 TBL dark sesame oil	4 Servings Sat Fat, 1 g Cholesterol, 0.0 g Sodium. 282 mg Carbohydrate, 14 g Sugar, 1 g Dietary Fiber, 3 g Protein, 12 g	Blanch kale in boiling water and dewater under paper towel. Cut tofu into dominos and de- water under paper towel. Combine soy sace, wine, vegetable stock,and corn starch. Combine salt, black pepper, and sugar. Stir fry tofu in canola oil. Add kale salt, sugar, and pepper. Add soy sauce mix and sesame oil. Stir fry 30 second Serve with grains or noodles.	Kale and vegeta- ble stock make this excellent methylation dish. Kale is an excel- lent source of vitamins A, C, K, folate, and minerals calcium, iron, magnesium, manganese, and zinc. Sesame oil adds vitamin E. Cano- la and sesame together provide for good plant fat. Stir fried bread crumbs can be added as a topping intead of grains or noodles.

9. Fergus Henderson's Spinach Dip

Ingredients	Nutrition Information/Serving	Preparation	Key Methylation Nutrients
Unsalted butter, 2 TBL Spinach , 1 lb Parmesan cheese, 2 oz Cream Fraiche, 2 TBL Dijon mustard, 1/2 ts Salt and pepper	Total Calories, 392 Fat Calories, 62.6 Cholesterol, 75.9 mg Sodium, 1041 mg (High !) Carbohydrate, 18.4 g Sugar, 0.2 g Fiber, 18.4 g Protein, 22.4 g	1. Melt butter on medium heat. 2. Cook spinach in four installments. 3. Stir in cheese, cream Fraiche and mustard. Mix and serve	This recipe may use 50/50 blend of spinach and kale. Can be served with sweet peas and edamami.

10. Eggplant Dip Recipe

Ingredients	Nutrition Information/Serving	Preparation	Key Methylation Nutrients
Olive oil-1/2 cup Eggplants -3 Medium red bell pepper-1 Canola oil-2 TBL Chooped onion-1/4 cup Feta cheese-1/2 Cup Roasted walnut-1/2 cup Red wine vinegar-2 TBL Paprika, 1/2 tsp Mint leaves-2 TBL Salt and pepper	Six servings Total Calories, Total fat, 20 g Sat Fat, 4 g Cholesterol, 75.9 mg Sodium, 200 mg (High !) Carbohydrate, 4 g Fiber, 1 g Protein, 2 g	1. Grill egg plant and red pepper, well oiled at 450 Deg F. Red pepper for 15 minutes and eggplant for a total of i hour 2. remove pepper stems. Scrap out the flesh of egg plant. 3. Blend two vegetables. Add salt. black pepper, and paprika. Add feta cheese and toasted walnut. Serve.	Ferulic acid and Anthocyanin flavonoids from egg plant is the key health benefit in addition to high fiber.

11. Vegetable Side Dish of Spinach Gratin

Ingredients	Nutrition Information/Serving	Preparation	Key Methylation Nutrients
Light butter, 3 TBL Finely chopped onion, 1 cup Flour, 1/4 cup Nutmeg, 1/4 tsp Milk 2%, 3 cups Chopped frozen spinach, 3 lb Squeezed and drained 1/c each of feta and cheddar cheeses	**4 Servings** **Calories, 287** **Fat, 19 g** **Sat Fat, 2.7 g** **Cholesterol, 87 mg** **Sodium, 625 mg** **Carbohydrate, 19 g** **Dietary Fiber, 3.5 g** **Protein, 12 g**	1. preheat oven to 345 Deg F 2. Melt butter in a sauté pan over medium heat, sauté onion about 12 minutes. Add flour and nutmeg. Cook 2 more minutes. Add milk and cook another 6 minutes. 3. Add spinach to the sauce. 4. Add 1/2 cup parmesan cheese, combine and season to taste. Can be feta or cheddar cheese. 5. Bake it all for 20 minutes.	**This recipe offers good supplies of vitamin A, C, B$_6$, B$_{12}$, calcium, and copper.**

12. Vegetable Appetizer Recipe

Ingredients	Nutrition Information/Serving	Preparation	Key Methylation Nutrients
Lettuce leaves, 16	Eight Servings	1. Arrange Lettuce leaves	This is a high chicken protein recipe.
Asian chili sauce, 1/2 cup	Total calories, 168	Keep chili sauce on the platter	Chicken can be replaced with fried tofu or Indian Panir or fried tofu.
Minched chicken thighs, 1 lb	Fat, 9.8 g	2. Mix chicken, scallion, soy sauce, and corn starch and marinate for 10 minutes.	
Minced scallion, 2	Sat Fat, 2 g		
Soy sauce, 2 TBL	Cholesterol, 37.2 mg	3. Heat oil in a skillet and stir fry mushroom. Add garlic, ginger, and chicken. Mix and cook for 5 minutes.	
Peanut oil, 2 TBL	Sodium, 848 mg		
Shitake mushrooms, 3 medium	Net Carbohtdrate, 8.1 g		
Garlic cloves, 2	Sugar, 0.7 g	Spoon on leaves and serve.	
Minced ginger, 1 ts	Fiber, 0.7 g		
Ground chopped fine, 1/4 cup	Protein, 11.6 g		

13. Vegetable Mash of Sweet Potato and Cauliflower

Ingredients	Nutrition Information/Serving	Preparation	Key Methylation Nutrients
1.5 lb sweet potato, 1" cubes 1/2 Head (1 1/4 lb) cauliflower 1/4 cup olive oil 3 fresh sage leaves 1 clove garlic, crushed Two TBL milk	**Four Servings** **Total calories, 140** **Fat, 7 g** **Sodium, 180 mg** **Carbohydrate, 19 g** **Fiber, 4 g** **Protein, 3 g**	1. Heat to simmering on high sweet potato in water with salt. Add cauliflower and simmer for 15 minutes. 2. Use another sauce pan, add oil, garlic, sage to golden color garlic. Discard sage leaves. 3. Puree sweet potato and cauliflower in batches. Add to it garlic and oil mixture, milk, and salt to taste. Combine well and serve.	A very good high fiber and high protein side dish. A 100 g serving supplies **Vitamin A, 19000 IU** Vitamin C, 83 mg; Vitamin K, 83 mcg Folate, 70 mcg; calcium, 85 mg Magnesium, 70 mg; manganese, 1.2 mg; Zinc, 0.8 mg

15. Vegetable Mash of Kale, Horseradish, and Potato

Ingredients	Nutrition Information/Serving	Preparation	Key Methylation Nutrients
2 lb gold potato cut in half. 1/4 cup butter 1/2 bunch kale w/o stem 1 1/2 green onions, sliced thin 1/4 cup low fat sour cream Twp TBL horse radish	**Four Servings** **Total calories per serving, 245** **Fat, 10 gram** **Sodium, 360 mg** **Carbohydrate, 32 g** **Fiber, 3 gram** **Protein, 7 gram**	1. Add potato to a salt water enough to cover and simmer for 25 minutes. 2. Separately in a sauce pan stir fry kale in butter with salt to taste for 2 minutes. 3. Mash potato, add kale, sour cream, and milk, and horse radish. Serve warm	A 300 g serving supplies **Vitamin A, 13,000 IU; vitamin C, 110 mg; vitamin K, 547 mcg; Folate, 85 mcg; B$_6$, 0.2 mg; Pantothenate, 1.1 mg; Choline, 44 mg; betaine, 0.6 mg;** **Calcium 90 mg; magnesium, 22 mg; zinc, 0.2 mg; and copper, 0.2 mg**

16. John Besh's Braised Kale for Lunch

Ingredients	Nutrition Information/Serving	Preparation	Key Methylation Nutrients
Extra-virgin olive oil, 1/3 cup Garlic cloves, very fine, chopped, 4 Chicken stock or low-sodium broth, 1 1/2 cup Kale, stems and inner ribs discarded, leaves coarsely chopped, 3 lb Salt and freshly ground pepper MAKE AHEAD The braised kale can be covered and refrigerated overnight. Reheat before serving.	**12 Servings** **A 3.5 oz or 100 g serving provides** **Calories, 38** **Total fat, 0.75 g** **Sodium, 23 mg** **Cholesterol, o mg** **Carbohydrate, 5.25 g** **Fiber, 2.25 g** **Protein, 1.5 g**	1. In a very large soup pot, heat the olive oil. Add the garlic and cook over moderately high heat, stirring, just until fragrant, about 30 seconds. Add the chicken or vegetable stock, then add the kale in large handfuls, letting it wilt slightly before adding more. Season with salt and pepper, cover and cook over moderate heat until the kale is tender, about 5 minutes. 2. Remove the lid and cook until the liquid has evaporated, about 3 minutes longer. Transfer to a bowl and serve.	**A great complement to Indian cuisine.** **Nutrition comes from stocks Kale.** **A 3.5 Oz serving supplies 15,367 IU of vitamin A, 815 mcg of vitamin K, 28 mcg of folate, 0.29 mg zinc, 0.29 mg of copper, and 0.75 mg of manganese.** **25 g broth which becomes part of each serving supplies 870 IU of vitamin A, 6 mcg of folate, and 4.5 mg of choline as added nutrient.**

17. Lemon Egg Plant Risotto

Ingredients	Nutrition Information/Serving	Preparation	Key Methylation Nutrients
1 pound eggplant (1 large or 2 small) [360] 2 tablespoons extra virgin olive oil 1 small onion, finely chopped (about 1/2 cup) 1 pound tomatoes, grated, or peeled, seeded and chopped 2 garlic cloves, minced 1 teaspoon fresh thyme leaves or 1/2 teaspoon dried thyme Salt to taste 250 grams (1 1/2 cups) arborio rice ½ cup dry white wine 6 cups vegetable stock or chicken stock Freshly ground pepper 1 ½ ounces Parmesan cheese, grated (1/3 cup) 1 grated lemon zest. 1 TBL Lemon Juic	4 to 6 Servings Calories 215 Fat, 7 g Cholesterol, 10 mg Sodium, 260 mg Carbohydrate, 40 g Dietary Fiber 6 g Protein, 8 g Plums, zuchini, and red pepper can be added and cooked with onion. Parmasan cheese can be increased to taste. Preparation Preheat the oven to 450 Deg F Bake egg plant on an oiled foil with lengthwise cut side down. Cut to the skin but not through. . Bake for 20 minutes. Egg plant is shriveled and collapsesd. Remove from the heat and allow to cool.	Fry onion in 1 tablespoon of the olive oil in a large, wide skillet. Cook to tenderness for 5 minutes. Add the garlic. Cook for 30 seconds while stirring. Stir in the tomatoes, thyme, diced eggplant and salt to taste. Cook tomato for 15 minutes while stirring. Simmer spiced vegetable stock for cooking rice. Heat the remaining olive oil . Pour in the rice, stir, and coat with oil.. Add the wine and stir until it is no longer visible. Stir in the tomato and eggplant mixture and cook, stirring, for about a minute. Combine well. Begin adding the simmering stock, a couple of ladlefuls at a time. The stock should just cover the rice, and should be bubbling.. Stir often and add next installment when you see that the stock has been absorbed by the rice. Add another ladleful. Repeat untill all stoock is used up. Add pepper, taste and adjust salt. Add finalr ladleful of stock to the rice. Add broiled eggplant flesh, lemon juice and lemon zest. Stir in the Parmesan and remove from the heat. The mixture should be creamy. Serve right away.	Ferulic Acid and anthocyanin from egg plant. Both tomato and egg plant have nicotine like alkaloids. Eggplant skin is full of fiber, potassium and magnesium and anthocyanin-flavonoid antioxidant. Vegetable stock is a great source of phytonutrients and trace minerals. Egg plant is known to reduce obesity, diabetes, and heart disease. Fiber, potassium, vitamin C, and B$_6$ are the key nutrients from egg plant. Polyphenols in egg plant are anticarcinogenic. Egg plant is very good source of potassium. Eggplant diet may reduce chanxces of breast cancer. Eggplant diet is known to reduce cholestero [361].

360   http://cancer.ucsf.edu/_docs/crc/nutrition_breast.pdf
361   http://ajcn.nutrition.org/content/81/2/380.full

18. Egg Plant Tagine or Stew

Six Servings (Source: Good Food Magazine, February 2004)			
Ingredients	Nutrition Informa- tion/Serving	Preparation	Key Methyla- tion Nutrients
Mustard oil, 1 TBL Large chopped onion, 1 Cloves of garlic, 3] Harissa, 1 TBL Cummin seed, 1 tsp Cinnamon, 1/2 tsp Vegetable Stock, 200 ml Chopped toma- to, 400 g Baby egg plants, 300 gram Lemon zest, 2 Butter (lima) beans, 390 g Couscous, 175 g Toasted al- mond, 40 g Yogurt with mint and garlic, 150 gram	Calories, 168- 300 Fat , 5.5 to 6.5 g Sat fat, 1.7 g Cholesterol, 5-6 mg Sodoim, 225 mg Carbohydrate, 30 g Fiber, 9.5 g Sugar, 6-19 g Protein, 5-10 g	1. Heat oil in a pan at medium high and cook onion. 2. Stir in Harissa (paprika and chili pepper in olive oil), cumin seed, and cin- namon and cook. 3. Add vegetable stock and tomato. 4. Add egg plant and lemon and cook for 20 minutes. 5. Add butter beans and warm through. 6. Cook couscous per package instruc- tions and stir in toasted almond. 7. Serve tagine on couscous.	Ferulic acid and anthocyanins from egg plant from . Vegetable stock has antioxidants and other methylation ingredients. Almond, tomato, lemon zest, and yogurt add to methylation value. Full RDA of vita- min C and good amounts of vita- mins A, B$_6$, calcium, copper, and folate,

Recipe for Greek Yogurt sauce: Blend in 1 cup of Greek Yogurt 1/2 a cup cilantro, 2 TBLs chopped mint, 1 TBL olive oil, 1 ts sugar, and garlic powder to taste and liking.
Vegetable stews are a great methylation dish. They can be served with rolls and bread.

19. Stuffed and Stir Fried Egg Plant

Four servings			
Ingredients	Nutrition Information/Serving	Preparation	Key Methylation Nutrients
8 Baby egg plants Onion, 1/2 Tamarind Paste, 1 tsp Mango powder, 1 tsp Red chilli powder, 1 tsp Funnel seed powder, 1/2 tsp Crushed garlic, 2 cloves Kalonji or onion seed, a pinch Coriander, 1 tsp	**Four Servings** **Calories 165** **Fat, 13 g** **Sat Fat, 1.8 g** **Cholesterol, 0.0 g** **Sodium, 20 mg** **Carbohydrate, 10 g** **Dietary Fiber, 5 g** **Sugar, 10 g** **Protein, 4 g** **Modify the stuffing with onion, carrots, and red peppers.**	1. Grind onion, add tamerind paste, and blend the two. 2. Wash and slit egg plants. 3. Add all spices. 4. Heat mustard oil in a pan. Fill egg plant between four slits. Cook with a cover for 20 minutes turning them over periodically every five minutes. 5. Serve with rice or couscous topped with cheese, or on pita bread.	**An excellent high fiber recipe.** **Antioxidant Ferulic acid and anthocyanins from egg plant.** **High vitamin C, vitamin A, and significant delivery of iron and calcium.**

20. Stuffed and Baked Egg Plant

Four Servings			
Ingredients	Nutrition Information/Serving	Preparation	Key Methylation Nutrients
Egg plants, 2 Mustard Oil, 2 TBL Cloves of Garlic, 2 Salt, 1 tsp Black pepper, 1/2 tsp Parmesan or Romano cheese, 1/2 cup 1 1/4 cup bread crumbs Large egg, 1 Chopped parsley, 1/3 cup Capers, 1 tsp Tomato sauce, 1 1/4 cup Basal leaves, 4	Four Servings Calories 350-390 Fat, 3.5 - 5 g Sat Fat, 0.4 g Cholesterol, 21 g Sodium, 1000 mg Carbohydrate, 38 g Dietary Fiber, 9-12 gSugar 15-16 Protein, 5-16 g Modify the stuffing with inion, carrots, and red peppers.	1. Preheat oven to 375 Deg F. 2. Scoop egg plants leaving some on the skin. 3. Chop and cook egg plant in water for 12 minutes. Add other ingredients reserving some cheese for topping. Blend and mix. 4. Fill the egg plant skin and add cheese topping. 5. Bake for 50 minutes 6. Slice widthwise and serve.	An excellent high fiber recipe. Antioxidant Ferulic acid and anthocyanins from egg plant. High vitamin C, vitamin A, and significant delivery of iron and calcium.

21. Thomas Keller's Glazed Carrot Dessert Modified

Ingredients	Nutrition information/Serving	Preparation	Key Methylation Nutrients
• Baby carrots, peeled, 1/2 lb • 1/4 cup walnut • (trimmed to 1 inch) • Unsalted butter, 1 TBL • Sugar, 1 TBL • Fresh thyme leaves, 1/2 ts • Fresh bay leaf, 1 • Black peppercorns, 5 • Kosher salt, 1/2 ts	Six Servings Three Servings Calories, 239 Fat, 3.7 g Sat Fat, 0.2 g Trans Fat, 0.0 Cholesterol, 0.0 **Sodium, 2 mg** **Carbohydrate, 27 g** **Dietary Fiber, 3.7 g** **Protein, 3.1 g**	1. To carrots in a single layer on the skillet, add enough water to cover, butter, sugar, thyme, bay leaf, and pepper corn. 2. Bring to boil, let simmer at low heat. Carrots are cooked and the glaze is almost finished. 3. Remove carrots. Reduce glaze to 2 TBL 4. Season carrots with salt and pepper and roll them in glaze.	**Great source of vitamin A.** **Good source of calcium, copper, zinc, iron, magnesium,and biotin.** **Add whey protein powder for extra protein.** **Thyme, pepper corn, bay leaf deliver antioxidants.**

22. My Wife Girija Shukla's Nutty Ginger Ball/ Bliss Balls/ Nut Laddu

Ingredients	Nutrition Information/Serving	Preparation	Key Methylation Nutrients
Almond, 1 cup Brazil nut, 1/4 cup Flax seed, 1/4 cup Walnut, 1 cup Pumpkin seed, 1/2 cup Sunflower seed, 1/2 cup Date, 1 cup; quick oat, 1/2 cup Fig, 1 cup Apricot, 1 cup Raisin, 1/2 cup Cacao, 4 tsp Coconut or roasted sesame seed Ginger, 4 tsp All spine, 3 tsp Cinnamon, 2 tsp	**One Ball is a serving of 45 grams.** **Calories, 90-142** **Fat, 3.7 -4.3 g** **Carbohydrate, 25- 27g** **Sugar, 3-5 g** **Protein, 2 - 3.1g** The recipe may include hazelnuts, melon seed, pistachio, and whey protein concentrate.	Roast all seeds and nuts including flax seeds. Blend all ingredients. Adjust Date and fig for proper rolling and binding. Make 1 and 1/2 " diameter balls. Use some peanut butter if you like	**Old Indian Traditions Spells Methylation Diet.** Called Sonthaura in India, it is mini methylation diet given to women during pre- and post pregnancy period, Calcium from Figs. Apricot delivers folate. Loaded with antioxidants, dietary fiber, complete protein, and omega-3 fatty acids,

22. Bruno Loubet's Modified Frozen Pea Snack

Ingredients	Nutrition Informa-tion/Serving	Preparation	Key Methyla-tion Nutrients
Frozen Peas, 1 lb Bread crumb, 2 Oz or more Whey protein Isolate Creamed and fried onion, 1 Eggs, 2 large Red chili flakes, 1/2 tsp Cumin powder, 1 tsp Coriander, 2 tsp Lemon Juice, 1 tsp Vegetable oil, 1 TBL Salt and pepper to taste	4 Servings alories 360 Fat, 23 gram Sat Fat, 7 g Trans Fat, o g Cholesterol, 260 mg Sodium, 680 mg Carbohydrate, 18 Dietary Fiber, 6 g Sugar, 18 g Protein, 18 g	1. Cook by boiling, pat dry, and puree peas. 2. Add creamed onion stir fried at medium heat with cumin seed and coriander and mix well. 3. Add lemon juice, bread crumb, whey protein isolate, and red chili flakes and mix again. 4. Grill 1 Oz mini pancake patties flattened to 1 cm thickness on both side at medium heat. Serve with Oolong tea.	Imagin a high fiber pea pancake with porched egg. High protein power comes from whey protein concentrate and eggs. Antioxidants come from red chili, coriander, cumin seeds, and black pepper. Finely chopped almond can be added to pea patty.

23. My Wife Girija Shukla's Ideal Pizza

Ingredients	Nutrition Information/Serving	Preparation	Key Methylation Nutrients
4 cups flour 1 ts sugar 2 package dry instant yeast 1 cup warm water Spices in cooked tomato , onion and spices (2 ts dry oregano, 3 TBL parsley, 2 ts cumin, 1 ts hot paprika, 1 bay leaf, 3/4 ts black pepper), and the mixture reduced. Toppings over tomato sause: blend of three cheeses, olives, mushrooms, chili pepper, and parsley.	**Calories, 350** **Fat, 10 g** **Trans Fat, 0 g** **Cholesterol 45 mg** **Sodium, 840 mg** **Carbohydrate, 36 g** **Dietary Fiber, 2** **Protein, 14 g** **The entire dough makes 8 crusts, each crust receives 1 cup tomato sauce and 1 oz cheese blend.**	1. Dough preparation is the key to crust volume, crispness, and texture, 2. Add a layer of tomato sauce. 3. Add a layer of mushroom, olives, and red chili pepper dices. 4. Add parmesan, provolone, and ricots cheese blend to cover all vegetables. 5. Keep oven ready for 15 minute in advance at 450 Deg F and bake for 30- 35 minutes until cheese begins to brown lightly.	**Antioxidants from spices and olive.** **A high protein diet** **This is a high protein methylation dish.** **One serving is 1/2 cup flour, 3.5 oz tomato, and 1 oz cheese blend.** **At 350 Calories, it is a light dinner or lunch item.**

Making tomato sauce: Heat a tbl of oilive oil, add all spices, stirr fry onions to brownness, add garlic powder, and 28 oz tomato, bring to boil with a little water, simmer and reduce to sauce like thickness

24. Mario Batali and Gordon Ramsey's Modified Herb Dumpling

Ingredients	Nutrition Informa-tion/Serving	Preparation	Key Methyla-tion Nutrients
Sweet potato, 1/2 lb Cauliflower, 1/4 lb Spinach and kale, 1/4 lb Parmesan cheese, grated 1/4 C Eggs, 2 All purpose flower, 1 cup Butter, 1/2 stick Black Coffee, 3/4 Oz Chives, 1 1/2 TBL Sour Cream, 2 TBL	**Six Servings** **Calories, 230** **Total Fat, 2.1 g** **Sat Fat, 0.5 g** **Cholesterol, 14.7 mg** **Sodium, 711 mg** **Total carbohy-drate, 40 g** **Dietary Fiber, 4 g** **Sugar, 6 g** **Protein, 13 g** A salt recipe.	1. Prepare oven at 400 Deg F 2. Bake sweet po-tato and cauliflow-er for 45 minutes. 3. Remove flesh, mash, and add cheese, eggs, nutmeg, salt, flour and mix to com-bine. Add chopped and stir fried spinach and kale. Use more flour to make non sticky dough. 4. Make 1 inch cuts of ribbon like dough dumplings. Boil them till they float. 5. Melt and brown butter in a pan. Add dumplings and expresso and coat well. 6. Serve with chives and sour cream.	**Sweet potato, spinach, and kale are good B vita-min and antioxi-dant suppliers.** **Cheese and eggs add protein power.**

Dumpling can be modified with respect to base mash (sweet potato or potato), mix of broiled vegetables like cauliflower, stir fried leafy vegetables, eggs, and type of cheese. Stirr frying of boiled dumpling dough pieces should be done with virgin olive oil and amount of added salt should be kept to a minimum. Chicken and sweet potato dumplings of one or the other kind are very common South American cousine.

25. Chips and salsa snacks as a General Item

Ingredients	Nutrition Information/Serving	Preparation	Key Methylation Nutrients
A zero cholesterol, transfat, and sugar every day Guacamoli or Avocado sace, present for centuries in the human food chain, has now become a great methylation food. It can be routinely modified for extra value. **Ingredients and Procedure:** Take two ripe avocado, cut and seed, and mash. Add to it 1/2 a teaspoonful salt and 1 tablespoonful lime choose to preserve and prevent browning, mis well and add two seeded and chopped chiles without stem, black pepper to taste and 1/2 ripe seeded and pulped out tomato. Refrigerate airtight to prevent browning. Mix and serve. This can also be prepared simply bu mixing one mased avocado with 1/4 cup salsa. Also it can be fortified with protein by mixing in and mashing cottage cheese and or mashed paste of soaked Brazilian and wall nuts. **Nutrition Information:** A two oz serving delivers 94 calories, 9 g fat, 1 g saturated fat, only 33 mg sodium, 5 g total carbohydrate, 3- 4 g dietary fiber, and 1-3 gram protein depending modifications with cottage or soaked nut paste. **NOTE:** Tomato for delivers lycopene and avocado for leutin			

In addition to the above 25 recipes and ideas on recipe design a few tables are appended below taken from my book "Our Genes Our Foods Oor Choices" including those on fiber rich foods (2.15.08), ORAC of various foods (2.15.09A), polyphenolic foods (2.15.09B, values from healthful foods and life choices (2.15.10), therapeutic values of food ingredients and our choices of life-style (2.15.11), and ingredients and mechanisms (2.15.12). Users of this book will find this appended information useful in designing their weekly methylation diet.

Consult for Nutrition Information: **http://www.cottonpatch.com/images/menu/cpc_nutritional.pdf**

2.15.08 Fiber-Rich Common Foods

Ingredient Amount Fiber, g Ingredient				Amount	Fiber, g
Raw oat bran	1 oz	12	Wheat berries	¼ cup	5
Raw wheat bran	1 oz	12	Wild rice	1 cup	3
Raw corn bran	1 oz	22	Brown rice	1 cup	4
Raw rice bran	1 oz	6	Bulgur	1 cup	8
All-Bran cereal	½ cup	10	Rye crackers/ wafers	1 oz	6
Fiber One chewy bars	1 bar	9	Cooked spaghetti	1 cup	6
Fiber from beans			Frozen green peas	1 cup	14
Cooked lima beans	1 cup	14	Cooked peas	1 cup	5
Adzuki beans	1 cup	17	Cooked Swiss chard	1 cup	4
Cooked broad beans	1 cup	9	Cooked beet greens	1 cup	4
Cooked black beans	1 cup	15	Cooked spinach	1 cup	4
Cooked garbanzo beans	1 cup	12	Cooked collard greens	1 cup	5
Cooked lentils	1 cup	16	Cooked mustard greens	1 cup	5
Cooked cranberry beans	1 cup	16	Cooked turnip	1 cup	5
Black turtle beans	1 cup	17	Fiber from nuts		
Kidney beans	1 cup	16	Almonds	1 oz	4
Navy beans	1 cup	19	Pistachios	1 oz	3
Pinto beans	1 cup	15	Sunflower seeds	¼ cup	3

Fiber from berries			Pumpkin seeds	½ cup	3
Raspberries	1 cup	8	Sesame seeds	¼ cup	4
Loganberries	1 cup	8	Cooked Hubbard squash	1 cup	7
Elderberries	1 cup	10	Zucchini squash	1 cup	3
Blackberries	1 cup	8	Acorn squash	1 cup	9
Fiber from grains			Kale	1 cup	3
Amaranth grain	¼ cup	6	Cauliflower	1 cup	5
Barley pearled	1 cup	6	Kohlrabi	1 cup	5
Buckwheat groats	1 cup	5	Savory cabbage	1 cup	4
Popcorn	3 cups	4	Broccoli	1 cup	5
Oats	½ cup	4	Brussels sprouts	1 cup	6
Dry rye flour	¼ cup	7	Red cabbage	1 cup	4
Quinoa	1 cup	5	Red potato	1	3
Teft grain flour	¼ cup	6	Sweet potato, fresh and skinned	1	4
Tricale flour	¼ cup	5			

Table 2.15.09A Oxygen Radical Absorbance Capacity (ORAC) of Antioxidants Present in Our Daily Foods

Common Foods as Source s of Antioxidants

Allium: from Garlic, leek, onion; Anthocyanins from egg plant, grape, berries; Beta-carotene: from pumpkin, mango, carrot; Vitamin C from Oranges, Kiwi, mango, berries; Vitamin E from Avocado, vegetable oils, and nuts; Copper from sea foods, nuts, legumes, and milk ; Catechins from Red wine and tea; Flavonoids from Tea, red wine, apples, onions; Indols from Broccoli, cabbage, cauliflower; Lignans from sesame and flax seeds, whole grains; Lutein from spinach like leafy greens and corn; Lycopene from Tomato, pink grapefruit; Manganese from nuts, sea foods, and milk ; Omega-3 Fatty acid from walnut; Polyphenols from Oregano and Thyme; Seleniumfrom Brazil nut, sea food, whole grains ; Zinc from nuts, milk, lean meat

Common Foods	Micromole in ORAC =Trolox Equivalent, TE per 100 grams
Sumac bran	312,400
Spices, cloves, ground	314,446
Cinnamon, ground	267,536
Oregano, dried	200,129
Turmeric, ground	159,277
Cocoa, dry powder, unsweetened	80,993
Unprocessed cocoa beans	28,000
Black pepper	27,168
Cinnamon, 1 tablespoonful	21,402
Pecan, 100 g	17,940
Raspberries, 1 cup	16,058
Oregano, 1 tablespoonful	16,010
Elderberries, 1 cup	14,697
Lentils, 1 cup	13,981
Red kidney beans	13,727
Turmeric, 1 tablespoonful	12,742
Chocolate, 30 grams	12,060
Pinto beans	11,864
Blueberry, Cherry, Cranberry, raw, 1 cup	9,584

Common Foods as Source s of Antioxidants

Allium: from Garlic, leek, onion; Anthocyanins from egg plant, grape, berries; Beta-carotene: from pumpkin, mango, carrot; Vitamin C from Oranges, Kiwi, mango, berries; Vitamin E from Avocado, vegetable oils, and nuts; Copper from sea foods, nuts, legumes, and milk ; Catechins from Red wine and tea; Flavonoids from Tea, red wine, apples, onions; Indols from Broccoli, cabbage, cauliflower; Lignans from sesame and flax seeds, whole grains; Lutein from spinach like leafy greens and corn; Lycopene from Tomato, pink grapefruit; Manganese from nuts, sea foods, and milk ; Omega-3 Fatty acid from walnut; Polyphenols from Oregano and Thyme; Seleniumfrom Brazil nut, sea food, whole grains ; Zinc from nuts, milk, lean meat

Common Foods	Micromole in ORAC =Trolox Equivalent, TE per 100 grams
Artichoke, cooked, 1 cup; Pistachio 100 g	7,904
Pomegranate juice 100%	5,923
Prune, 1/2 cup	7,291
Plum, dried	5,700
Black plum, 1	4,844
Red wine	5,693
Blueberries, raw, and anthocyanins, 1 cup	9,019
Sweet cherries, 1 cup	4,873
Apples, red, quircetin, and other polyphenols	5,900
Granny Smith, 1 apple	5,381
Watermelon, a great source of lycopene	3,800
Raisins	2,830
Blackberries, 1 cup	7,701
Strawberries, 1 cup	5,938
Pears, 1 medium	5,255
Pecans, 1 oz	5,095
Kale and spinach	1,700
Broccoli and Brussels sprouts	980

Note: Vitamin D function requires magnesium, magnesium and calcium control heartbeat. Magnesium relaxes and calcium helps contract muscles. Magnesium is critical to type 2 diabetes in relation to conversion of sugar to energy. It is critical to the energy process as a whole. Magnesium is next to potassium in concentration as a positively charged ion in our cells. Antioxidant enzymes glutathione peroxidase, superoxide dismutase, catalase, and coenzyme Q_{10} from sprouts can be routinely used to reduce oxidative stress.

Table 2.15.09B Polyphenols: Food Sources and Bioavailability

Foods	Serving size	Mg/Serving
Apigenin, cherry, g	100	16
Anthocyanins, egg plant, g	100	750
Catechin, Beans	100	80
Caffeic acid, Kiwi, g	100	60-100
Chlorogenic acid Cherry, g	100	18-115
Coumaric acid in plum, g	100	14-115
Cyanidin, blackberry	100	100-400
Daidzein, boiled soybean	100	75
Delphinidin, black grape, g	100	30-750
Epicatechin, Green tea, Black tea, apricot, cherry, g	100	30
Genistein, Miso, g	100	50
Ferulic acid in egg plant	100	60-66
Flavones, parsley, g	5	5
Flavones, orane juice	100	20-60
Flavonols, yellow onion, g	100	18-60
Chocolate, g	50	20
Gallic Acid, g black currant	100	4-13
Glycetin, Tempeh	100	40
Hesperetin, grapefruit juice, g	100	50
Hydroxybenzoic acid, g	100	8-27

Strawberry	200	4-10
Blueberry	100	200-220
Hydroxycinnamic acid, g blueberry	100	200-220
Isoflavone, Soy flour, g	75	100
Kaempferol, Leek, g	100	3-23
Luteolin, chili pepper, g	5	0.5
Malvidin, Cherry , g	100	35-450
Malvidin, red cabbage	100	25
Myricetin, blueberry, black tea, broccoli, g	100	4-10
Naringenin, lemon juice, g	100	30
Pelargonidin, black currant, g	100	130-400
Peonidin, blueberry , g	100	25-500
Protocatechuic acid, g	100	6-66
Quircetin, Curley Kale, g	100	30-60
Sinapic acid in apple , pear, chicory g	100	5-60
Artichoke	100	45
Coffee, ml	200	200

Health and Longevity by Antioxidants

Brazil nut is great source of antioxidant selenium. Blueberries prevent cancer and enhance immune system.

Dark green vegetables (leek, lettuce, kale) provide vitamins C, E, and A, calcium, magnesium, potassium, kaempferol for control of cancer and blood pressure.

Fish, colorful vegetables, and whole grains fight inflammation. Heart healthy and cancer preventing beans provide fiber, vitamin C, folate, calcium, ellagic acid, and selenium.

Fish, flax seed, and walnut are sources of Omega-3 fatty acids. Grapes provide anthocyanins, proanthocyanidins, vitamin C, and selenium.

Sweet potato, carrots, and squash are great sources of Vitamins A, C, B_6, K, and fiber.

Tea is ready source of anthocyanins, proanthocyanins, catechin, and epigallocatechin; fights cancer.

Whole grain provide fiber, zinc, selenium, and polyphenols; help fight cancer.

Anti-aging polyphenols like apigenin, baicalein, bromocriptine mesilate, chrysin, cyanidin 3 glucoside, delphinidin, diosmin, eriodictyol, fisetin, flavoxate, galangin, gossypetin, hesperetin, hesperidin, 3 hydroxyflavone; 6 hydroxyflavone, isokaempferide, isorhamnetin, kaempferol, luteolin, morin, myricetin, naringenin, pelargonidin, quercetin, resveratrol, rhamnetin, scutellarein, and wogonin found in our daily foods are of value to maintaing a long life. These molecules have been well identified and have chemical registry numbers associated with them.

Life expectancy rose from 59 years in 1925 to 79 years in 2015 and the increase is due to sanitation and availability of antibiotics against infections. What percentage gain is due to increased availability of antioxidants in US is not clear but Okinawa and Mediterranean diets make a better case in favor of antioxidants. I personally practiced mindfulness, what was talked about as **AKAAGRATAA** in India, when I was a junior high school young boy in India. Later here in USA I studied in 1971 Richard I. Hittleman's book on YOGA which appeared in 1964. This impacted heavily on me in terms of reinforcing the old Eastern values, values that are the corner stone of alternative medicine today all over the world. Looking more critically at longevity enhancing factors I find that many of them are tied to antioxidants. The list has grown to include rapamycin as inhibitor of mTOR gene, resveratrol that controls stress and enhances mitochondrial function, activation of telomerase production, production of GD 11 gene responsible for bone morphogenesis, and production of Klotho hormone for mineral metabolism.

Controlling osteoporosis, chronic pain, the health of our skin, freedom from diabetes, heart health, and cancer control are directly related to health of mitochondria and thus the long life. Antioxidants from fruits, vegetables, seeds, nuts, and whole grains are clearly a longevity nutrient. Daily cancer fighting fruits and vegetables of Table 2.15.12 are critically important in our day to day nutrition.

Table 2.15.10 A Comparison of Health-Promoting Nutrients and lifestyle choices

Disease	Mechanism of Action	Curative Foods
Osteoporosis Mitochondrial DNA may be involved in male osteoporosis.	Prevent inflammation Reduce prostaglandins and COX-2 activity. Permits proper collagen formation. Bosvellia extract (Bosvellic acid) switches off pro-inflammatory cytokines. Vitamin B_6 prevents homocysteine formation. Bosvellia extract (Bosvellic acid), black pepper, and turmeric are good food cures.	Green vegetables, roasted nut snacks, snacks of seeds of pumpkin and sunflower, and omega-3 fatty acids from flaxseed, walnuts, black pepper, turmeric, black currant, ginger, oranges, sweet potatoes, and prunes. Nutrients are B_6, folic acid, vitamin K, vitamin D, coenzyme Q_{10}, boron, calcium, selenium, magnesium, and zinc.
Pain-free life Mitochondria are involved in inflammation and neuropathy.	Glutamine, Flavonoids (apricots, avocadoes),omega-3 fatty acids, vitamin D, glutathione, tryptophan; calcium-to-magnesium ratio of 600:300 mg per day; chromium, selenium, and zinc can help reduce pain. So can lack of anxiety and a stress-free life, meditation, yoga, and exercise.	High-glutamine foods (cabbage, beets, beef, chicken, fish, beans, and dairy products) contribute to gamma amino butyric acid—a pain inhibitory neurotransmitter. Trace minerals of chromium from garlic and onion, zinc from pumpkin seed, and selenium from Brazil nuts are involved in elastin formation.

Disease	Mechanism of Action	Curative Foods
Skin beauty simply means healthy mitochondria.	Vitamin D is a beauty vitamin. Vitamins A, B complex, C, D, E, and K, choline, minerals copper, selenium, and zinc, and DMAE (dimethyl aminoethanol) are good for skin and overall health. The objective is to prevent DNA damage, reduce stress, and maintain the estrogen-progesterone ratio. Also, a good night's sleep is good for skin health.	Zinc from mustard and pumpkin seed, selenium and copper from sunflower seeds and Brazil nuts, and chromium from garlic and onion are great for skin health, and so are phytoceramides 3 and 6 and bromelain from pineapple. Reducing stress by exercise and meditation also helps. Genes p53 and Satb1 are involved in chromatin remodeling and gene expression.
Diabetes-free life. 1% of all diabetes is due to mutations in mitochondrial genes.	Betatropin hormone therapy is on the horizon. Glutamic acid decarboxylase encoded by two genes is seen by immune cells as an antigen; the T-cells with autoantibody begin to destroy beta cells. Gene therapy may become possible in this case.	Control sugar intake. Consume omega-3 fatty acids, foods containing chromium, B vitamins, vitamins D, C, E, and K, chromium, selenium, zinc, and antioxidant vitamins C and E.

Disease	Mechanism of Action	Curative Foods
Mitochondria are critical to heart health.	Foods containing natural statins (gugal in India, red rice yeast in Japan), coenzyme Q_{10}, phytosterols, omega-3 fatty acids, and prebiotic dietary fiber reduce risks of cardiovascular diseases. Prevention of dense small LDL particles and keeping homocysteine below 15 micromoles/liter is a medical need. Test it periodically.	Maintain the health of 2.5 trillion red blood cells. Get enough exercise. Do yoga. We need 6 molecules of oxygen for every molecule of glucose we burn in our cells by exercise and yoga. More research is needed about genes governing cholesterol receptors, genes behind homocysteine metabolism, and low oxygen-tolerant robust CA3 neurons of the hippocampus.

Disease	Mechanism of Action	Curative Foods
Dysfunctional mitochondria cause cancer.	Protect against DNA damage by a full complement of methylation nutrients. Consume niacin, vitamin C, folic acid, protein, vitamins A, B_6, and B_{12}, carotenoids, D, E, and K_2. Consume antioxidants, leutin, lycopene, kaempherol, and 3, 3 diindolylmethane from kale, endive, spinach, cauliflower, and broccoli, and minerals selenium and zinc. Use low-calorie diet.	Use twice the daily recommended allowance of antioxidants; use common fruits, dark green vegetables, and tomato products for leutin and lycopene. Minerals selenium and zinc from tree nuts and seeds of pumpkin and sunflowers must be part of the anticarcinogenic dietary arsenal. Consume anticarcinogenic Gouda and Emmentaler cheeses.

Disease	Mechanism of Action	Curative Foods
Healthy mito-chondria enhance longevity	Out of 44 genes that can go wrong as we age, 12 are involved in growth, metab-olism, and fat and cholesterol processing. Alpha-synuclein gene, IGF gene, telomerase gene, FOXO 3 gene that upregulates genes, and daf2 gene are very important in this regard. The antiaging mol-ecule dimethyl aminoethanol (DMAE) is an antioxidant present in anchovies and sardines. Neu-rotransmitter acetylcholine is involved in heart function, breathing, and sleep.	DMAE methylates choline to DNA; it can go across the blood-brain barrier. Other key nutrients are B_6, B_9, B_{12}, amino acids arginine, tryptophan, tyrosine, miner-als magnesium, selenium, zinc, and antioxidant ubiquinine. Also needed are ribose, 3-phenyl-3-acet-amineindol, high proteins, and high antioxidants. Dimethyl aminoeth-anol works with neurotransmitter acetylcholine. Don't allow stress to shorten telomere.

Beyond antioxidants we have the life style factors including mindfulness, exercise, sleep, stress control, and spiritual connectivity that have positive implications in maintaining long life. Emerging new gene and enzyme therapies may come to augment our health, quality of life, and life extension. The details, to the extent that we know them, are listed in Table 2.15.11.

Table 2.15.11 A Comparison of Health-Promoting Therapies and Lifestyle Choices		
Gene therapy	Mature technology has yet to evolve.	Possible germ-line and somatic gene therapies are in the making.
Enzyme therapy	Low-lactose milk treated with lactase is already sold.	Sprouted grains and legumes are other routine sources of enzymes.
Vitamin D	Vitamin D is a blessing for beauty and skin health.	Vitamin D is a multifunctional steroidal anti-inflammatory hormone. It is necessary for bone and heart health and protection from infections.
Antioxidants	Antioxidants manage electrons. The redox potential of hydroxyl is + 0.23 volt, of hydrogen peroxide is + 0.36, and of superoxide is + 0.07 volt. Thus, different antioxidants are suited for dealing with different radicals.	Whereas enzyme antioxidants such as superoxide dismutase, catalase, and glutathione peroxidase prevent initial free-radical attack, vitamin C, vitamin E, glutathione, and coenzyme Q_{10} repair oxidizing radicals. Vitamin C cooperates with vitamin E, and it actually repairs and recycles vitamin E.

Exercise	Consume high-arginine proteins for nitric oxide. Exercise for more ubiquitin and brain-derived neurotrophic factor. Manage hypothalamic response by exercise, which can potentially affect DNA methylation of 7,663 genes and thus promote gene expression. It can prevent resistance of insulin and leptin. It prevents even Alzheimer's disease. Exercise promotes genes PGC-1a, DPK4, PPAR δ, and CIDE.	The genetics of exercise is different for different people. Exercise can change blood flow, gene expression, activity of nitric oxide synthase from arginine, serotonin transfer protein 5HTT, and mutated genes in white fat cells for small fat globules. Common foods that reduce the number of white fat cells are not known. Exercise can burn white fat cells off.
Meditation	Meditation works with the parietal lobe and increases production of nitric oxide and GABA (gamma amino butyric acid). It reduces stress and thus influences gene expression.	Can help with modulation of homeostasis, helps renew cells, and helps control of somatic nervous system.
Stress	Causes imbalance of calcium, sodium, and potassium ions; it damages cells, DNA, and the immune system. It shortens telomere. ATF3 gene, expressed in the central nervous system, is silenced by stress.	Reduce stress by adaptogenic foods, exercise, meditation, and yoga. Cortisol, serotonin transporter gene, and neuropeptide Y (NPY) induce corticoprotein-releasing hormone in response to stress.
Sleep	Deals with brain and chronobiology	Consume foods high in tryptophan for serotonin production.

Belief and faith	Ubiquitin generates telomerase and influences gene expression for a good immune system. Consume methylation foods for cell membranes.	Belief is critical to neuro-biology and physiology; faith deals with cells and not DNA, though. Epigenetic effects can be inheritable.

Our health depends on how well our body manages the cycles of cell division. We run into cancer if they can't stop dividing because of poor cell to cell communication. In the process of division, the nutrients have to accumulate because the genome has to double before splitting into two along with splitting of other organelles, cytoplasm, cell membrane , and the nucleus. Take mouth and skin cells for an example. **Mouth and skin cells are dividing constantly and we have a few million of them dying every minute.** Appropriate nutrients by type and amount are essential.

The idea of vaccines, interleukin-2 and α cytokines , monoclonal antibodies, and checkpoint inhibitors comes to play only when we already have run into cancer. A better idea is to stop it from happening by anti-angiogenic cruciferacea vegetables containing isothiocyanates, methyl sulfide, and diallyl sulfides, caffeine, and cucurmin from turmeric. So six servings of fruits and vegetables per day delivered by designed recipes makes sense for cancer prevention.

Following is a list of cancer fighting nutraceuticals from many a common foods. We can choose high dose polyphenol antioxidant recipes using common fruit or vegetable below (mg/g).

Kiwi, for caffeic acid- 330, aubergine (egg plant) for ferulic acid- 33, anthocyanins- 412, cyanidin from blackberry- 110, flavonol from yellow onion- 55, flavones from parsley- 82.5, and isoflavone from soy flour-82

Table 2.15.12 Cancer Fighting Foods	
Common Food	**Ingredients and Mechanisms**
Aragula	Myrosinase enzyme and glucosinolate
Asparagus	Glutathione, β-carotene, vitamin C, and Nacetyl-cysteine
Avocado	glutathione, vitamin E, and vitamin C.

Blueberries	Glutathione, vitamin E, and vitamin C.
Broccoli	Sulphoraphane and repair of damaged DNA
Brussels sprout	High ORAC phytonutrients
Cabbage	Glucosinolates
Carrots	Falcarinol on top of β-carotene and vitamin A.
Celery	Eight different anti-carcinogens
Cherries	Perillyl alcohol
Coffee	Caffeine
Dark Chocolate	Flavonoid antioxidants
Fish Eggs	Great source of DHA and EPA omega-3 fatty acids
Garlic	Allicin is a potent anti-carcinogen
Green Tea	Urokinase, catechins, and bvitamin C
Horseradish	10 times more glucosinolate than in cruciferors vegetables
Kale	β-carotene and vitamin C in kale are ten times higher than in broccoli
Onions	Quircetin, a flavonoid
Raspberries	High ellagic acid content
Rosehips	Proanthocyanins and vitamin E.
Salmon	Omega-3 fatty acids and astaxanthin
Shitaki Mushroom	Betaglucans
Sweet Potato	β-carotene, vitamin C
Tomato	**Lycopene, β-carotene**, and vitamin C.
Turmeric	**Cucurmine, a powerful anti-carcinogen**
Watercress	**phenethyl isothiocyanate (PEITC), β-carotene and lutein**

Inflammation simply means "cells in trouble" and therefore means of self-protection in full advance. Poor replication or copying of DNA of cell is even worse. We need to stop it. Foods preserve stem cells and keep us in constant rejuvenation? One million molecular leisions although only 0.000165% of total base pairs, can cause significant DNA damage and harmful mutations.

We know antioxidants are biological saviors. Foods can cure diseases and prevent pain (table 2.15.10), life style choices can make us healthy (table 2.15.11), and evidence is gathering to show that foods fight cancer (tabl1 2.15.12). Foods help us methylate our genes and soon we will make therapeutic genes for ourselves. But we will still have to depend on omega-3 fatty acids, essential amino acids, and vitamins from external sources. In other words we are not fully evolved yet.

Our cells control and balance metabolic pathways by following molecular traffic through various pathways and by sensing concentration of nutrients and metabolites. The calorie restricted daily methylation diet matters. Enzymes that DNA encodes can make hydrogen peroxide break into water and oxygen in seconds by lowering activation energy from 76 to 30 KJ/mole and increasing the volume ratio of reaction 10^8 fold. Enzymes change the "orientation in space" of electrons and protons involved in these reactions. Food affects other processes of antagonism, inhibition, and activation. Life is a reduction-oxidation process and antioxidants and free radicals deal with our existence as a living organism.

Major Research Institutions

Denver Naturopathic Clinic
Linus Pauling Institute, Oregon State University
Institute of Functional Medicine
Center for Mind -Body Medicine
Massachusetts Institute of Technology
NYU Langone Medical Center
The united Mitochondrial Disease Foundation
Foundation for mitochondrial Medicine
The mitochondrial and Metabolic Disease Center, UC San Diego.

3

Different organs have different numbers, size, shape, and structural features of mitochondria in our body. Collagen allover the body and mitochondria are very connected [362].

Mitochondria are behind all vital signs and strength and serious physiological failures of vital organs[363] ,[364], [365] ,[366] *including multiple organ failures, congestive heart failure, sepsis, and night blindness. This can happen due to nutrient dificiency or bacterial and viral infections. Diseases of the eye are most affected by mitochondrial dysfunction.*

In final analysis, vital signs and function of vital organs depend on electrons, protons, ions on and working through the geometries and topologies of proteins designed either by nuclear or mitochondrial genes. Shape of proteins is very critical in biology. To keep the best of order, electron shuttling nutrients CoEnzyme Q_{10} and Pyrroloquiniline Quinone(PQQ) *are essential mitochondrial foods in addition to B vitamins and trace minerals of iron, sulfur, copper, and molybdenum, selenium and zinc.* All such minerals must be part of daily methylation diet in order to *maintain vital signs by keeping the mitochondria of vital organs healthy. Coenzyme Q_{10} and PQQ are well known drug like nutrients and so are other vitamin antioxidants like beta-carotene and vitamins A, D,E, and K present in our foods of fruits, vegetables, seeds, nuts, and whole grains. What matters is the variety presnted*

---

362 http://www.ncbi.nlm.nih.gov/pmc/articles/PMC3940501/
363 http://www.ncbi.nlm.nih.gov/pmc/articles/PMC3224479/
364 http://icu-metabolism.se/Attachments/p48-50_Olav_Rooyackers%20low.pdf
365 http://www.ncbi.nlm.nih.gov/pubmed/19751827
366 http://www.medschool.lsuhsc.edu/pediatrics/docs/130519%20Primer%20Mitochondrial%20Disease.pdf

rather explicitly by color, composition, freshness, ansate of ripening as indicators of quality and possible absence of free radicals which may be present in rancid foods.

Chapter 3
Vital Signs and Vital Organs

"Fever is a mighty engine which nature brings into the world for conquest of her enemies." –Thomas Sydenham 1666.

Foods we eat support the health of mitochondria incells of our vital organs of brain, heart, lung, liver, kidney, and muscles. Our organs are routine users of mitochondrial power and behind all vital signs is the power of mitochondria. This organelle in everyone of our cells with exception of red blood cells controls and runs our life. Vital signs are indicators of the autonomy of our brain-body relationships when we are well and healthy. Abnormal signs means we are abnormal and sick. Vital signs of heart rate, blood pressure, rate of breathing, oxygen saturation of blood, temperature, pain, cancer, and even sensory perceptions are controlled by the brain. The autonomic nervous system does its best to keep vital signs in a reasonable range but things do go wrong because of poor and probiotic deficient dietary habit and lack of exercise that can cause inflammations, poor immune system, and bacterial or viral infections.

Stable vital signs indicate optimum mitochondrial performance. Mitochondria proliferate for meeting increasing energy demand by the heart, muscle, and brain cells. Foodborne bacterial pathogens interfere with mitochondrial dynamics and destabilize vital signs [367]. The defense and health of all cells in our body depends on mitochondrial performance [368]. This chapter describes vital signs for an average person so he or she can use them as a guidelines for proper maintenance of good health and wellness. The

367   http://www.pnas.org/content/110/40/16003.abstract
368   http://www.pnas.org/content/110/40/16003.abstract

very idea of personal genomics and personal diet will be terribly incomplete without personal monitoring of vital signs.

Our Vital Signs

Mitochondrial function underlies all vital signs including brain activity and pain and dysfunctions associated with routine impulses. This is the major reason why this chapter not only has 11 citations on vital signs but it is also supplemented with 10 citations on mitochondrial dynamics and health, 3 citations on mitochondria and mind, 2 citation on origin of mitochondria, 14 citations on nerve conduction, 4 citations on mitochondrial diseases, 8 citations on relevant mitochondrial mutations and diseases, 3 citations on immunity, 7 citations on blood pressure examinations, 2 citation on foods for mitochondrial health, 2 citations on liver function, 4 citations on inflammation, 3 citations on pulmonary function, 13 citations on multiple sclerosis, 2 citations on stress, and one citation each on eye disease, steathohepatitis, energy expenditure by central nervous system, neurodegenerative diseases, microbiome and health, autosomal mutation, autophagy, autism, antioxidant gene therapy, mitochondrial DNA damage, mitochondrial gene coding, nitrous oxide, reading of human brain, and assisting our enzyme systems. In addition, there are appropriate website URL citations specific to a given topic section by section throughout the chapter.

A young physician during his apprenticeship at a hospital can live with potassium of 2.8. hemoglobin of 9.8, and billirubin of 4.5 but he can't live with bad numbers on vital signs because he knows that his patient is not doing well. Take fever for example. The physician has to find the cause of fever, treat the cause of fever, and see that the fever goes away. Same way breathing must keep acid-base balance and appropriate gas exchange for the patient's health. The physician knows that the autonomic nervous system is a wonder in biology and that it will do its best to compensate for a range of human body derangements. It will keep vital signs stable and the patient alive as long as the mitochondria in brain, heart, lung, liver, and kidney cells are doing their job at an optimum. Let us begin this chapter with a belief that our body is a car and the mitochondria in cells of vital organs are the engines that run and control the cellular processes. Fatigue itself is low cardiac output due to poor mitochondrial function. Inefficient mitochondria means reduced programmed death of cells in our organs letting cancer cells have a free reign. Poor vital signs indicate damaged or dysfunctional mitochondria as indicated below in the block by the list of organs and demand on mitochondrial performance in their cells.

Poor Mitochondrial Function: Poor Supplies of ATP To Critical Organs Causes

Brain: Seizures, stroke, dementia, and migraines.

Ear: Hearing loss

Liver: Failure of biochemical factory.

Eyes: Sight has a very high energy demand

Heart: Poor energy causes congestive heart failure

Skeletal Muscle: weakness, fatigue, myopathy, neuropathy

Colon: Obstructions

Pancreas: Failure of insulin production and secretion of enzymes

Kidney: filtration rates goes down

Immune cells: killing of pathogens is inefficient and the bacteria take over.

The figure below provide added functional description.

Mitochondria in Vital Organs	
	Protein regulates the movement of mito- chondria in brain cells. Maintain Synaptic function and resting potential. Neurons can't func- tion without proper energy supply. Energy requirement of different neurons varies. Intermittent fasting and exercise are good for mitochondria
	Myelinated auditory axon fiber.
	Oxygen consumtion and ATP production is high for Heart con- traction.

Mitochondria of Vital Organs

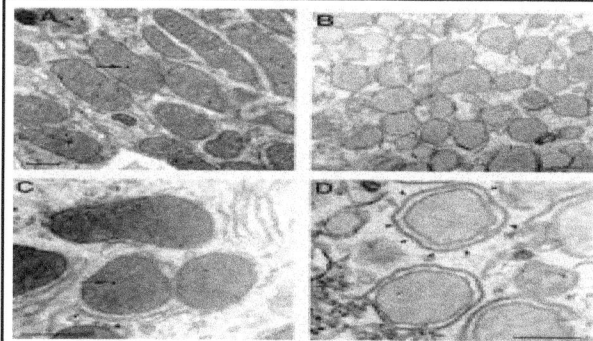

A very high number and total surface afforded by liver mitochondria

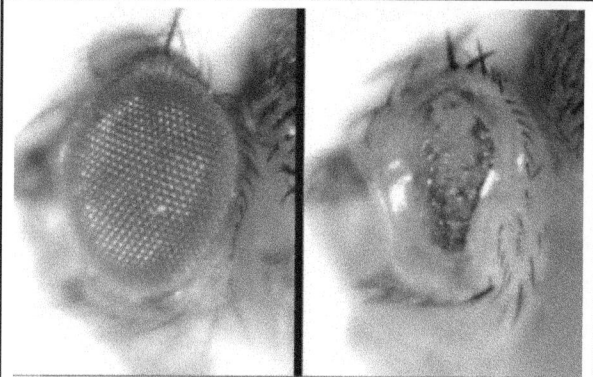

Mitochondria on the left eye is almost destroyed by apoptosis.

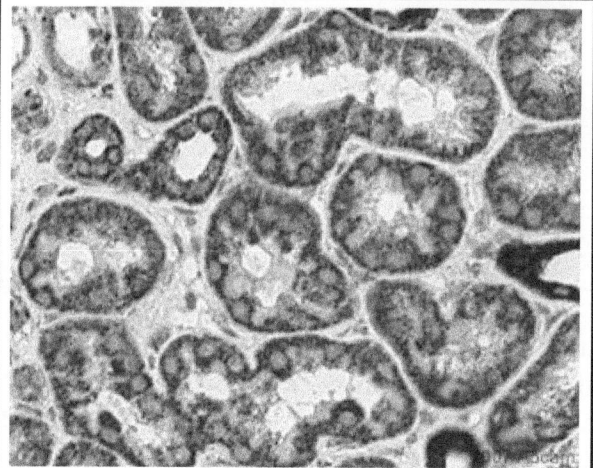

Mitochondria play a key role in renal diseases.

Mitochondria of Vital Organs	
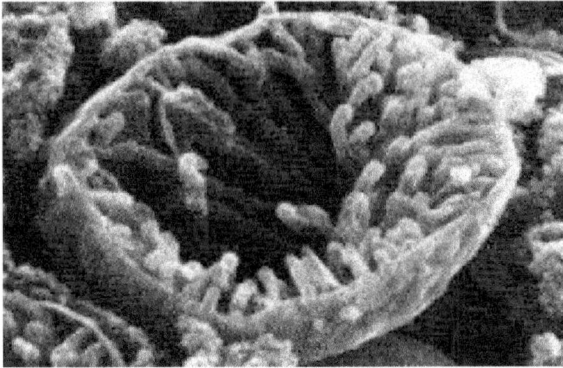	Pancreatic mitochondria have functions of insulin, glucagon, carbonate and and enzyme production.
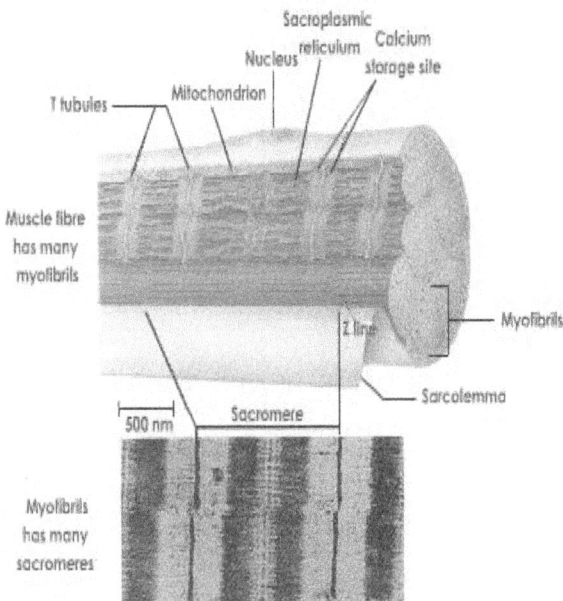	Skeletal muscles require a lot of energy and Type II diabetics suffer from dysfunctional muscle mitochondria

Vital signs of heart rate or pulse, respiration or breath per minute, temperature, blood pressure, pulse oximetry or oxygen saturation in blood, and pain are common physiological statistics recorded by the nurses and physicians. There is a great deal of chemistry behind such statistics [369]. Additional signs of stress, blood glucose, and shortness of breath should be checked even at home.

---

369   http://www.elsevieradvantage.com/samplechapters/9781455701506/9781455701506.pdf

Immune Cell Mitochondrial Function

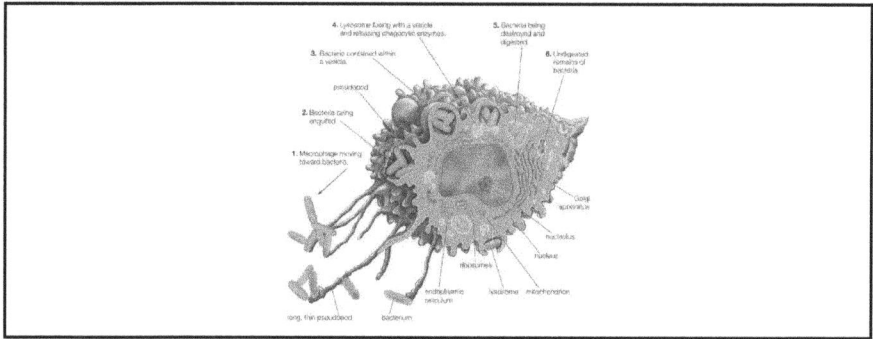

Immune cells grab and digest bacteria and other pathogens. Behind this function are active and functional mitochondria. Good heath simply means well functioning mitochondria without damage to their DNA and the mitochondrial DNA from our mother's egg should not be faulty to begin with.

Table 3.01 Normal Range of Vital Signs			
	Infant	**Teens**	**Adults**
Heart Rate/Minute	100- 160	70-120	
Respiration: Breath/ minute	30-60	20-30	
Blood Pressure, mm mercury	65-95	110-135	120-80
Prehypertensive			140-90
Hypertensive			150-90
Temperature	98.6	98.6	98.6
	97.4-99.6	97.4-99.6	97.4-99.6
Pulse Oximetery, %			> 96

Table 3.01 gives a range of data on vital signs. All vital signs depend on age, gender, stress, exercise and physical activity, metabolism, fever, and certain medications specific to individuals. All vital organs function by mitochondria [370],[371]. Mitochondrial degradation in case of intensive care unit patients can

---

370   http://icu-metabolism.se/Attachments/p48-50_Olav_Rooyackers%20low.pdf
371   http://link.springer.com/chapter/10.1007%2F978-3-642-18081-1_32#

be the cause of multiple organ failure. A case in point is the best of perfusion techniques of delivering blood to capillaries. If it doesn't work in cases of septic shock, the mitochondria are not getting enough oxygen through the circulating blood. As a matter of fact, mitochondria are behind homeostasis, making of axons and dendrites, myelination of nerves, neuropathy in general, neurotransmission, Parkin's disease, programmed cell death, optic atrophy, and their own dynamics, fusion, and mobility. They are involved in every disease and in molecular events at every synapse of our nervous system. Let us try to understand vital signs organ by organ as indicators of our health.

3.01 Functions of Heart

3.01.01 Heart Rate

Mitochondrial function is a must for healthy heart. Heart is a pump and it requires constant supply of energy as ATP. As such heart mitochondria are gates of life and death [372]. Every heart muscle cell has mitochondria ready to produce ATP on demand and the arrangement of 5000 heart mitochondria in heart cells is unique. A change in their shape by-and-in-itself is an indicator of function.

Pulse or heart rate is read by monitoring expansion of radial artery at the wrist. Taking pulse simply means counting beating of the heart per minute. The physician does it by his/her stethoscope by counting heart beat. Since heart relies heavily on mitochondrial function, its output depends on the rate it beats and volume of blood pumped out per stroke [373],[374]. An average person consumes 5000 milliliters of blood per beat containing 20% oxygen of which 32 percent goes to the muscle cells [375]. **This calculates to 320 ml oxygen extracted from the blood per minute.** Given an average of 75 beats per minute, there is 5000/75 = 66 milliliters per stroke which can be increased to 100 milliliters by increasing heart rate by a simple aerobic exercise. Since one mole of oxygen makes six moles of ATP. Given 22,400 milliliters per mole of any gas, 320 milliliter of oxygen is 320/22,400 = 0.14 mole of oxygen or 0.0857 mole or 5 X 10^{22} molecules of ATP made per

---

372   http://cardiovascres.oxfordjournals.org/content/77/2/334.full
373   http://www.ncbi.nlm.nih.gov/pubmed/553325
374   http://www.annualreviews.org/doi/abs/10.1146/annurev.ph.41.030179.002413
375   http://web.viu.ca/conwayg/ZNOTE/Biol067_ATPExerciseLAB.pdf

minute. That is 10 billion trillion of energy molecule that the mitochondria needs to produce every minute, of which heart consumes a good portion.

Heat rate (HR) is number of contractions or beats per minute recorded as bpm. *Even more important is Heart Rate Variability (HRV) or time gap between two beats. High HRV under relaxed and unloaded conditions indicates stress free good health and low HRV indicates fatigue and stress.* In technical terms HRV indicates beat-to-beat dynamic alterations due to stress and aging process [376]. This phenomenon, as we know by our minute by minute experience, is rhythmic. *A low gap between beats suggests reduced activity in the vagal center of our brain. As a matter of fact HRV measures the vagal input into cardiac rhythm.* In simple terms ECG (electrocardiogram) tells the story of heart to brain connection [377].

Since mitochondria are behind HR and HRV, they are targeted for combating heart diseases due to poor blood flow (Ischemia) [378]. We need to do our best to improve heart mitochondrial health by

1. Aerobic exercise that can increase moles of oxygen consumed for production of energy molecule ATP by additional 66% of resting use level. One mole of oxygen is 15.9994 grams in a liter of blood.

2. App Cardiio, a MIT invention, can be installed on a smart phone for routine measuring of blood flow dependent scattered light which related to heart rate. The application maintains a monthly summary of heart rate, fitness, and even life expectancy.

3.01.02 Blood Pressure

Mitochondria influence blood pressure by way of over active renin-angiotensin system and reduction of heart rate variability [379]. The ventricle contracts or squeezes to apply pressure and squirt blood through the arteries. *An ideal 120 mm blood pressure is 133 Pascals (2.4 psi or 16,000 Newtons per square meter).* This phenomenon is related to effective open diameter of the artery and even a small amount of arterial occlusion can cause havoc. Actually, a 20% reduction in radius under conditions of arteriosclerosis can raise the blood pressure to 293 mm and 100 cm^3/min blood flow at 120mm can drop to 41 cm^3 per minute. We pass out if the blood doesn't get to

---

376   htt http://www.heartmath.org/research/research-home/heart-rate-variability.htmlp://www.macses.
      ucsf.edu/research/allostatic/heartrate.php
377   http://www.heartmath.org/research/research-home/heart-rate-variability.html
378   http://circres.ahajournals.org/content/111/9/1222.full
379   http://www.hindawi.com/journals/ijhy/2013/136028/

the brain. We know that vasodilators work by increasing the radius of the artery. Just a 19% increase can double the blood flow making us feel better. Blood pressure readings represent **systolic blood pressure corresponding to maximum heart contraction or squeeze** creating a pressure to 120 mm. An ideal diastolic blood pressure is 80 mm or below.

Functioning mitochondria are necessary for energy and power generation for the heart [380] and poor mitochondrial output is the main reason for heart failure. *Although the role of mitochondria in heart cell function has yet to be fully understood [381], new research reveals that blood pressure and cholesterol levels are affected by mutations of mitochondrial DNA [382].* It appears that all aspects of metabolic syndrome, an epidemic in the United States, are attributable to mutations in mitochondrial DNA. Metabolic aspects of this epidemic include cholesterol, LDL, HDL, triglyceride, insulin resistance, and obesity. Hypertension per se in aging populations is also caused by mutations in mitochondria [383].

There is no doubt that exercise and proper diet of restricted calories, low refined sugar, and low sodium allow for better heart health via multiple mechanisms. Low cholesterol foods, antioxidants, and proper intake of vitamins and minerals is a long-term prevention against cardiovascular diseases. Cutting down sodium and refined sugars (glucose via corn syrup, high fructose which is glucose and fructose say by 50% can definitely lower blood pressure. This is why the current FDA recommendation for daily refined sugar intake is less than 20 g.

A blood glucose at 100 mg/deciliter means 0.1% sugar in the blood. My entire circulating blood of 7 liters thus has 7 grams of sugar. If this were to double to 14 grams because I overate and didn't do any exercise, the blood pressure shall definitely rise causing headache, nausea, blurred vision, blood in urine, and even irregular heartbeats.

A good range of blood sugar is 60-100 mg/deciliter. A level below 60 is also dangerous. *A level above 140 mg/deciliter can cause nerve cell damage, pancreatic beta-cell death, and cardiovascular diseases [384].* Seeing the physician regularly and keeping a good record of the following three types of blood glucose is a great health control strategy.

---

380   http://www.ncbi.nlm.nih.gov/pubmed/19347572
381   http://www.ncbi.nlm.nih.gov/pubmed/553325
382   http://www.sciencedaily.com/releases/2004/10/041022105304.htm
383   http://www.spandidos-publications.com/10.3892/ijmm.2013.1459
384   http://www.phlaunt.com/diabetes/14045678.php

Fasting Blood Glucose: A blood test that requires you to fast for at least 8 hours. The test determines your basal glucose level without food.

Glucose Tolerance Test: A blood test that requires consuming sugar solution 1-2 hours before testing. It is a measure of how body manages glucose.

Hemoglobin A1C: A blood test that determines your average glucose level over a period of 2-3 months. Health care providers use these results in order to evaluate the overall glucose control in people with diabetes. High glucose build up in case of diabetics simply means that glucose doesn't get to the cells where mitochondria can use it for producing energy. Instead, it stays in the blood and accumulates to dangerous levels.

3.02 Functions of Lung

3.02.01 Respiration or Rate of Breathing

It is mitochontria that breathe. Actually, they breathe protons with the help of oxygen that reduces itself into water by picking up electrons and protons. Mitochondria in our cells consume oxygen and maintain and regulate the redox state of lungs. Breathing rate depends on how often the brain tells the body to breathe. ***Normal respiratory or breathing rate of 12-16 per minute is good for proper oxygen delivery and an optimal concentration of carbon dioxide.*** An easy way to measure breathing rate is to count chest expansion per minute. While there is no easy way of measuring mitochondrial respiration in-vivo, oxygen level and acidification of tissue can be measured. Too little CO_2 in exhalation is a good indication of blood being acidic if the kidneys are functioning fine and acid byproducts are eliminated.

Medulla oblongata, the lowest most part of the brain stem, controls respiration rate which depends on rate of ATP production [385]. A breathing rate higher than 20 per minute for an adult can be due to fever, dehydration, asthma, COPD (chronic Obstructive Pulmonary Disease), hyperventilation due to stress, infections, and lung cancer. **High breathing rate is a serious health problem.** While apnea is a temporary loss of respiration, a blue color indicates low oxygen supply. Slow breathing means that not enough

385   http://www.ncbi.nlm.nih.gov/pmc/articles/PMC3076726/

carbon dioxide is cleared causing blood pH to fall. On the other hand, hyperventilation causes alkaline blood. *Brain maintains a balance by regulating respiration on one hand the kidney functions on the other.*

Aerobic exercises strengthen heart, lower pulse rate, lower body fat, increase energy, and lower low density lipoprotein (LDL), the bad cholesterol. Exercise is very helpful in maintaining good vital signs and in preserving our body's autonomy.

3.02.02 Pulse Oximetry

Pulse oximetry relates to the journey of oxygen from lungs to every cell of our body. *The surface -active lining of the mammalian lung is literally a mass of mitochondria [386].* Mitochondrial density and number in alveolar cells vary and epithelial cell mitochondria are sufficiently motile [387], [388]. Density differences are regulated and can be up to five fold.

Oximetry reveals saturation of hemoglobin with oxygen. A 100 percent level corresponds to 400 oxygen molecules per hemoglobin molecule. It is 70% when a molecule of hemoglobin carries only 360 molecules of oxygen. A good range is 95-99%. A few deep breath quickly raises percent oxygen saturation if there are enough hemoglobin molecules, say around 11-12% in the blood. A less than 95% oxygen saturation reading indicates potential problems.

The level of mitochondrial NADH concentration is the bellwether of the health of and oxygen delivery to tissues and organs [389] such as brain, heart, liver, kidney, pancreas, and the rest. Mitochondrial function puts an upper limit to use of oxygen [390]. When we feel dizzy once a while getting up from sleep in the morning, the culprit is oxygen in poor supply below 320 milliliter per minute.

---

386   http://www.sciencemag.org/content/137/3532/750.abstract
387   http://www.fasebj.org/cgi/content/meeting_abstract/25/1_MeetingAbstracts/865.8
388   http://www.atsjournals.org/doi/abs/10.1164/ajrccm-conference.2011.183.1_MeetingAbstracts. A2536
389   http://www.ncbi.nlm.nih.gov/pubmed/16594157
390   http://www.unm.edu/~lkravitz/Article%20folder/limitations.html

3.03 Temperature

Human body maintains a constant temperature. When we shiver, we produce heat to maintain temperature. Every electron that is transferred over the electron transport chain releases some energy as heat. Also the proton gradient across the inner mitochondrial membrane is regulated to produce heat when needed.

The thermostat for body temperature is the hypothalamus in the brain. It controls temperature within 1-2 Degrees F by managing heat produced and heat lost. Heat is produced by muscle contraction, digestion of food, and breaking down of nutrients, fever, and stress. Heat loss happens via urine, feces, exhaled vapor, perspiration, and radiation from our body.

A major cause of high temperature is bacterial or viral infection. Other causes can be heart stroke, drugs, and damage to central nervous system. A high temperature often indicates infection though. It is mild grade if between 99-101.4, serious if greater than 105.8, and literally fatal if greater than 109 Degree F.

Basal metabolism increases by 7% per degree of temperature rise. We feel chills when hypothalamus is set at high temperature maximizing involuntary muscle contraction. We perspire when hypothalamus lowers the temperature setting.

Fever mechanism is physiologically defensive in that immune cells produce **pyrogens** , proteins produced by white blood cells, that tell hypothalamus to feel cold and, therefore, generate heat. Pyrogenes inhibit heat sensing neurons and stimulate cold sensing neurons. The biological purpose is to raise the body temperature so that the invading bacteria and virus do not grow [391]. They love to grow at 98.6, the normal body temperature and stop growing or grow slowly at higher temperatures

Mitochondria are connected to autonomous nervous system that controls our vital signs including temperature and they go in overdrive in order to defend us against bacteria and viruses [392]. A lot changes as we gain years and age. It is difficult to control temperature for older people and some times temperature may not increase even when they are suffering from infection. There is often a risk of overheating or hyperthermia and decreased sweating. Much of it is because of poor health of mitochondria as we age.

---

391   http://www.britannica.com/EBchecked/topic/205674/fever
392   http://link.springer.com/chapter/10.1007%2F978-3-642-18081-1_32#page-1

3.04 Pain, the fifth vital sign

Mitochondria hold a great promise in pain treatment therapies [393]. Mitochondrial fission is related to painful neuropathies. It appears that the physiological functioning of mitochondria may contribute to induction of chronic pain. *The relative oxygen species produced in mitochondria may be involved in transduction of pain perception*. The mitochondrial energy generating system, reactive oxygen species generation, mitochondrial permeability transition pore, pathways of cell death and calcium mobilization within the cell may play roles in neuropathic pain inflammation but we understand very little about it today [394]. A few new findings are encouraging and worth paying attention to.

Pain is attributable to mitochondrial function. Glial cell mitochondria, other than mitochondrial diseases per se [395], in the brain are involved in pain modulation [396], [397] and mitochondria in general play key role in pathogenesis of chronic pain [398], [399]. Plasma membrane calcium ATPase and mitochondria seem to be main regulators of pre-synaptic calcium signaling [400].

Primary pain nociceptors involved in connections with second order pain neurons in dorsal horn of the spinal cord convey peripheral pain signals to central nervous system and the plasticity of these synapses contributes to intense feeling of pain.

Pattern recognition receptors (PRR_s) see pathogen associated molecular patterns ($PAMM_s$) and damage associated molecular patterns ($DAMP_s$). They begin to act like a pathogenic bacteria in causing systemic inflammation because of an inability to differentiate a pathogen from a damage [401].

3.05 Cancer Diagnostics

As a huge multicellular organism with 10 trillion cells we live by killing tired and week cells and by rejuvenating them each day. In case of a human adult, 50 to 60 billion of these cells die each day but by an ingenious and robust

393   http://painresearchforum.org/news/9570-make-way-mitochondria
394   http://www.ncbi.nlm.nih.gov/pubmed/24151337
395   http://www.umdf.org/site/c.8qKOJ0MvF7LUG/b.7934627/k.3711/What_is_Mitochondrial_Disease.
       htm
396   http://www.mitopain.com/publications/
397   http://www.mitopain.com/publications/
398   http://www.ncbi.nlm.nih.gov/pubmed/24151337
399   http://www.ncbi.nlm.nih.gov/pubmed/24151337
400   http://www.ncbi.nlm.nih.gov/pubmed/23381900
401   http://www.nature.com/scitable/topicpage/mitochondria-and-the-immune-response-14266967

biochemical program. There are genes behind the works of shrinking the cell, condensing the cytoplasmic liquid in the cell, fragmentation of the envelope of nucleus containing DNA, growth of irregular protrusions on the cell's membrane, breaking apart of the cells, and carrying away and disposal of dead cells by phagocytes. This set of essential activities is influenced by inflammation, autoimmune problems, and bacterial or viral infections. The result is "immortal cancer cells" when mitochondria have gone wrong and inefficient. Obviously mitochondria do fail to manage the lifecycle of cells in our body causing us to succumbm to cancer.

Mitochondria thus cause cancer because of deviations from their common functions [402]. The problem is mutation of mitochondrial genome leading to an altered state of metabolism [403], [404]. The alterations may include method and extent of energy production, maintenance of redox equilibrium, calcium imbalance, and programmed death and renewal of regular cells.

Formation and growth of tumor cells has a very complex biology and there is no single diagnostic test for cancer. Nonetheless common signs of early phase of cancer can be poor digestion, toxins, blood pressure imbalance, and adrenal exhaustion. Cancer can affect the whole body in relatively advanced stages . The physician begins with examination of cells under the microscope and may elect to do biopsy and examine the cells of affected organs. Additional tests can be about specific proteins and even DNA. Although not all tumors are cancerous, a fast growing malignant tumor can spread all over the body. An understanding of what is involved in cancer diagnosis and what to do post diagnosis is a necessity for all cancer patients.

The mucous membrane of bronchia, the two branches of air tube, are inflamed and have become spasmodic. We cough and put out phlegm because the cells of mucous membrane have become thick enough to shut off airways and we breathe with difficulty. Behind this difficulty in breathing is poor functioning of mitochondria [405]. In case of pneumonia, which is infection of the lung by a bacteria causing inflammation of air sacs, the real problem is impaired mitochondrial function [406]. In case of lung cancer the uncontrolled growth of cancer cells doesn't allow proper oxygenation

402   http://www.ncbi.nlm.nih.gov/pubmed/20206201
403   htthttp://www.nature.com/nrc/posters/mitochondria/index.htmlp://www.nature.com/onc/journal/v25/n34/full/1209589a.html

404   http://www.nature.com/nrc/posters/mitochondria/index.html
405   http://www.umdf.org/atf/cf/%7B858ACD34-ECC3-472A-8794-39B92E103561%7D/Metabolic%20Precautions%20and%20ER%20Letter.pdf

406   http://www.davidwheldon.co.uk/supplement_rationale.html

for mitochondrial function and, therefore a high breathing rate. Infectious diseases and cancers can be indirect causes of mitochondrial dysfunction.

Blood and urine tests are often performed for complete blood count (CBC), glucose, electrolytes, enzymes, hormones, blood urea nitrogen, and fats. Other tests include imaging by ultrasound, MRI, and CT Scan and tests for tumor markers, and endoscopic examination. Description of few important tests that are becoming common for cancer evaluation is described below.

Prostatic Acid phosphatase (PAP) is a glycoprotein enzyme present in semen. It is produced by the prostate gland. Its concentration increases beyond 2.1 nanogram/ml in patients with prostate cancer.

Prostate Specific Antigen (PSA) is a protein found to be high in blood samples of prostate cancer patients. A test reading of 4.00 nanogram/ml is normal. The test has become controversial because of false positives. There is a belief though that a low level of free PSA is a good marker for prostate cancer.

Alpha-Fetoprotein (AFP) encoded by AFP gene present on chromosome 4 (4q25) is a kind of serum albumin. It is an indicator of liver cancer and neural tube defect. An accumulation of 500 nanogram per millileter of blood is downright dangerous.

Carcinoembryonic Antigen (CEA) is a tumor marker test for cancers of colon, rectum, and pancreas [407]. This glycoprotein is not present in the blood of adults but its presence helps detect cancer, evaluate effects of surgery or chemotherapy, and monitor possible return of cancers. The cut off level is 5 nanogram/ml of blood.

Human Chronic Gonadotropin is small glycoprotein hormone produced by fertilized egg and placenta in pregnant women. It serves a marker of testicular cancer in men and uterine cancer in non-pregnant women if present above 5000 IU/ml.

---

407   http://www.apims.net/Volumes/Vol7-4/Carcinogenic%20Embryonic%20Antigen%20Levels%20 in%20Colorectal%20Carcinoma%20and%20its%20Correlation%20with%20Stage%20of%20Disease.pdf

Lactate Dehydrogenase is an enzyme protein present in heart, liver, muscle, kidney, and brain cells. It is a respiratory biochemical in breakdown of glucose to pyruvic acid and then in low oxygen conditions to lactic acid. However, if present in higher than 300 IU/l, it is a good indicator of tissue damage and cancer, leukemia, heart attack, lung cancer, and anemia.

Neurospecific Enolase (NSE) is a test for an enzyme that is involved in respiration. NSE converts phosphoglycerate to phospoenol pyruvate. It is a good indicator of lung lesions and cancers of pancreas and intestine if present in levels above 100 nanogram/liter [408].

CA 27-29 A blood test for breast cancer antigen.

CA 15-3 (MUC1) is a breast cancer test for a glycoprotein antigen.

CA 19-0 is an antigen test for pancreatic cancer.

Our daily diet can help prevent and stop reoccurrence of cancer(s) because it has the intrinsic value of empowering mitochondria. Cancer per se is much beyond mitochondrial effects on our vital signs but it no doubt relates to mitochondrial functions [409]. Organ by organ, mitochondria represent the physiological state of our cells. Emotional distress is actually the sixth vital sign in case of cancer.

3.06 Sensory Perceptions

We feel pain and pleasure by mitochondria in our cells. The brain gets the idea of crisp and crunchy texture on one hand and filth and stink on the other. Visual, auditory, olfactory and smell, taste, and touch somato-sensory receptors sense with high sensitivity and mitochondria are involved in sensory neuronal death and survival[410]. Mitochondria are abundant at the peripheral terminals of sensory nerves and excessive oxidative stress and accumulated reactive oxygen species affect receptors. Mitochondrial dysfunction can be traced to be cause of all inflammatory diseases [411].

---

408   https://www.questdiagnostics.com/testcenter/testguide.action?dc=TH_NSE

409   http://www.nature.com/nrc/posters/mitochondria/index.html
410   http://www.ncbi.nlm.nih.gov/pubmed/22923263
411   http://www.ncbi.nlm.nih.gov/pubmed/23444014

Our eyes are the most complex sensory organ [412]. It is very much like building an artwork [413]. Mitochondria manage calcium in our cells, levels of 300-600 nanomole in the darkness of night opposed to only 30-50 nanomole during the day time. A light activated proton pump generates proton motive force (PMF) in the mitochondria [414] and thus we see by proton motive force.

We run into hearing loss because of free radicals that mitochondria produce under loads of noise [415]. Hearing loss is attributable to defective mitochondrial DNA [416]. It is mitochondria that make us smell and perceive by calcium signaling [417]. Mitochondrial dynamics, ion transport and ion control, and the very neuronal activity in these regards is yet in early phases of research. A greater understanding can cure many malfunctions and diseases [418]. All muscle diseases are most likely due to mitochondrial malfunctioning [419]. Loss of motor nerve feeling at the extremities is now known to be a mutated mitochondrial DNA [420].

Our cells loose power when mitochondria degrade and degraded mitochondria cause diseases of Alzheimer's, autism, cancer, cardiovascular illness, Parkinson's disease, and type II diabetes [421]. Mitochondria trigger apoptosis (cell death) and manage our cell's lifecycle.

Krebs cycle, what I call the electron mill, operates within mitochondria. A high test for PHI or phosphohexoisomerase test means poor Krebs cycle and poor mitochondrial functioning. Other vital signs may be urinary continence and kidney, end-tidal $CO2$ (graphical measurement of concentration or partial pressure of carbon dioxide), stool examination, emotional stress, blood glucose, shortness of breath, gait speed, and menstrual cycle [422], [423].

Vital signs tell us about the function of mitochondria and mitochondrial functions describe our cellular physiology. Sum total of all that goes on in our body is also depicted clearly by our emotions. Our emotions are normal only when vital signs are normal and aptly controlled by mitochondria.

---

412   http://webvision.med.utah.edu/book/part-ii-anatomy-and-physiology-of-the-retina/photoreceptors/
413   http://www.emergentmind.org/PDF_files.htm/receptor0702.pdf
414   http://www.nature.com/srep/2013/130409/srep01635/full/srep01635.html
415   http://www.ncbi.nlm.nih.gov/pubmed/23361190
416   ht http://www.ncbi.nlm.nih.gov/pubmed/22446879tp://brain.oxfordjournals.org/content/123/1/82. long
417   http://www.ncbi.nlm.nih.gov/pubmed/1715612
418   http://www.plosbiology.org/article/info%3Adoi%2F10.1371%2Fjournal.pbio.1001755
419   http://mda.org/disease/mitochondrial-myopathies/overview
420   http://www.plosone.org/article/info%3Adoi%2F10.1371%2Fjournal.pone.0086340
421   http://www.ncbi.nlm.nih.gov/pmc/articles/PMC2920932/
422   http://ccn.aacnjournals.org/content/23/4/83.full
423   http://ccn.aacnjournals.org/content/23/4/83.full

The remedy is to consume methylation diet which eliminates high glycemic sugars from diet and supplies all B vitamins and trace minerals for well functioning mitochondria. We should use above average RDA of antioxidants, omega-3 fatty acids, and even conjugated linoleic acid as we advance in years.

Electron transport in the inner mitochondrial membrane coupled with proton motive force for production of energy molecule ATP is the key in order to meet varying energy demands of various vital organs. We are oxygen dependent beings. We breathe, oxygen saturates the blood over a large surface area in the lung, the heart gets the oxygenated blood for copious energy production, and pumps it to all cells in our body. On its way to the cells, the blood collects nutrient- digest from small intestine, and delivers both energy source glucose and glucose burning oxygen pretty much at the same time. As liver, our metabolic factory, and various other cells work, they produce mitochondrial waste products which are filtered out by the kidneys. Our vital organs thus are brain, lung, heart, liver, and kidney and vital signs are indicators of the health of these organs. Bacterial and viral infections have different effects but related to mitochondrial dysfunction.

We can now, thanks to nuclear explosion during World War II, find out as to when a cell was created by Carbon[14] dating[424]. *Cells in our body have a "time-stamp". Throughout our life time, the brain cells live the longest, cardiopulmonary systems co-develop [425], heart cells renew, lung cells regenerate every 8 days, liver cells renew every 220 days, and kidney cells renew in 286 days.* Functioning under extreme acidic and alkaline conditions, the digestive system's cells last hardly for a week to two. Bladder cells can last up to 66 days [426].

Vital signs that our physicians record more often have to do with our heart and lung function. The two together control supply of oxygenated blood to each and every cell in our body. Blood pressure and pulse relate to heart and oxygen concentration related to lung. Temperature is an indicator of infection. Included in this chapter are discussions about brain, liver, kidney, pancreas, and muscles because all these organs function by mitochondrial activity and there are tests indicative of vitality.

We have 200 types of cells in various organs and, as pointed out earlier, 50 billion of them die and regenerate each day. With opportunities of daily

---

424   http://www.nih.gov/researchmatters/april2009/04132009heartcells.htm
425   http://www.sciencedaily.com/releases/2013/07/130721161714.htm
426   http://www.fountainmagazine.com/Issue/detail/The-Human-Being-in-Numbers-Last-Lesson-for-Peter

creation of cells, there are problems of daily disposal as waste. *Vitality of our organs depends on how efficient this system of daily birth and death is.* **Many a practical programs are evolving in understanding our vital signs at major US universities**[427],[428] , [429]. For instance Worcester Polytechnique Institute is designing smart phone applications for vital signs[430]. Part of us dies every day and part of us is born every day. Mitochondria are the key because they govern this daily cycle of birth and death. Vital signs give us a measure of this governance that may soon be available on an Apple's watch on our wrist.

Our Vital Organs

3.07 The Brain

The brain uses relatively high amount of energy. *About 25% of basal metabolic energy is devoted to sustaining the electrical charge or action potential by our brain cells or neurons.* To put in perspective, it is the electric field outside the skull that is measured by electroenchepalographs. Therefore, brain health relates to its electrial activity. We have 30 billion neurons and there are 10,000 mitochondria in each one of them producing energy from glucose. They need twice as much energy compared to other body cells because they work as an organized community (as a grid or network) and depend on knowing each other as closely as possible. They wire each other, insulate their fibers, and constantly communicate at an appropriate speed.

A broken myelin in case of a multiple sclerosis patient means slow communication because glial cells can't do their job under conditions of deficiency of amino acids, vitamins and other micronutrient. Amino acids that act as neurotransmitters such as gamma aminobutyric acid, glutamate, serotonin, N-methyl D-aspartate (NMDA) and norneonephrine are involved in depolarization (electrical change) and key protein complexes are involved in sodium channels. **All such processes of transmission alone consumes**

---

427   https://ufhealth.org/vital-signs-children
428   ht http://www.sciencedaily.com/releases/2011/10/111006113622.htmtp://vitalsigns.bangordaily-news.com/
429   http://changetheequation.org/sites/default/files/vital-pdfs/TX-CTEq-vital-signs.pdf
430   ht http://www.scientificamerican.com/article/reading-paper-screens/tp://www.sciencedaily.com/releases/2011/10/111006113622.htm

10 percent of total body energy [431]. Migraine, sensory loss, poor memory, dementia, seizures, and stroke like episodes can occur at any stage of mitochondrial disease when basal ganglia, thalamus, and cerebellum are affected (Fig. 3.07). The effects may be for a minute or for a month. Magnetic resonance imaging can show regions of elevated lactic acid concentrations under various conditions of mitochondrial malfunction.

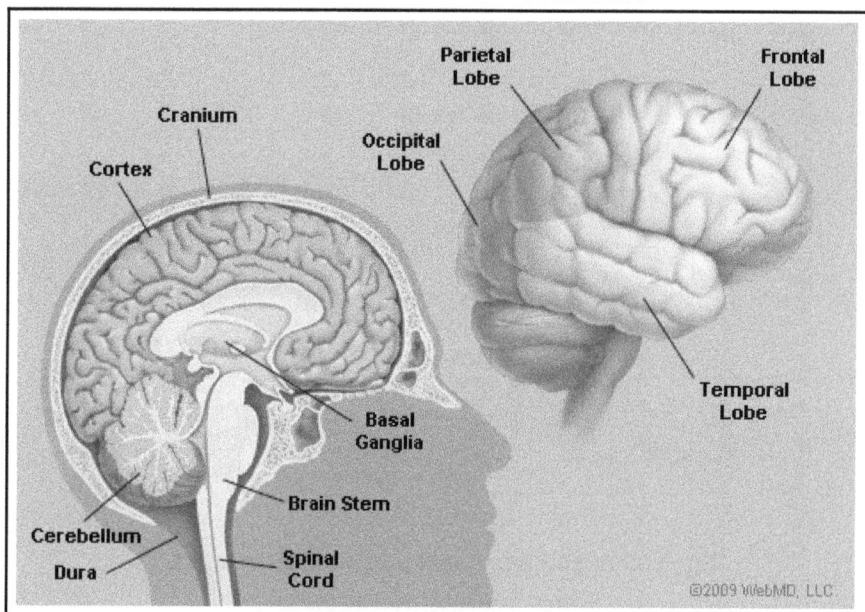

Fig. 3.07 Anatomy of human brain.

Source: National Institute of Health

Chewing, swallowing, secreting enzymes, peristalsis, and active transport of nutrients require ATP. Therefore, our second brain (the enteric nervous system) that regulates digestion uses ATP energy for inhibitory neurotransmission (neuron to smooth muscle), sensory mediation, and transduction of sensory stimuli [432]. *Actually, stomach cells exchange protons by spending considerable energy to make a stomach juice of pH 2.0 or below* [433]. Mitochondrial failure can be disastrous to brains, heart, lung, liver, kidney, and the digestive system.

---

431   http://www.fi.edu/learn/brain/carbs.html
432   http://www.ncbi.nlm.nih.gov/pubmed/12934708
433   http://www.madsci.org/posts/archives/1998-10/909609313.Bc.r.html

3.08 The Heart

My defibrillator implant (Fig. 3.08) always reminds me that metabolically active tissues of sinoatrial and atrioventricular nodes in my heart keep conducting electricity all the time because of mitochondria in them. Heart muscles are very vulnerable to mitochondrial diseases. This is why an electrocardiogram check up should be taken seriously.

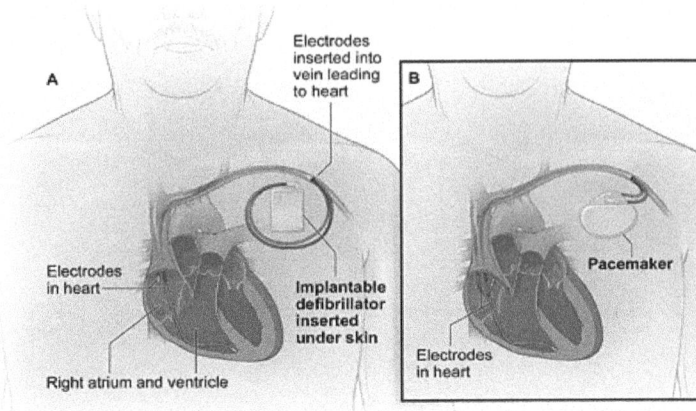

Fig. 3.08 Defibrillator electrode inserted in heart.
Source: National Heart Institute

The degree of oxidative phosphorylation or production of ATP energy depends on number and volume of mitochondria. Mitochondria for ATP production are critical to heart cell survival. Each human heart cell may contain 5,000 to 10,000 mitochondria for almost instant power supply [434]. As the gate of life and death, heart cells contain 60 mg of mitochondrial protein[435],[436]. **The high energy requirement corresponds to the work of pumping 1.38 gallons of blood per minute or 2000 gallons per day.** In addition, mitochondria monitor growth factors, oxygen, Reactive Oxygen Species, DNA damage, potassium channel protein, and calcium homeostasis.

Overconsumption of salt in excess of 2300 mg/day increases blood pressure. The consumers in Western societies with abundant processed

---

434   http://www.heartmdinstitute.com/anti-aging/ageless-body/at-the-cellular-level/393-love-your-mito-chondria
435   http://www.annualreviews.org/doi/abs/10.1146/annurev.ph.47.030185.003241?journalCode=physi-ol
436   hhttp://www.ncbi.nlm.nih.gov/pubmed/21614449ttp://cardiovascres.oxfordjournals.org/con-tent/77/2/334.long

foods have very little control over it and that is a serious problem [437]. A high blood pressure forces mitochondria to higher gear. Chronic fatigue syndrome results from low cardiac output due to mitochondria dysfunction and poor ATP production. Coenzyme Q_{10} supplement helps by effective shuttling of electrons in the electron transport chain.

3.09 The Lung

Lung is an organ that delivers oxygen to the blood (Fig. 3.09). It delivers 3.7 liters of net oxygen per minute to the blood that eventually goes to the cells and their mitochondria. Human lung cells have mitochondria that respond to level of oxygen that we breathe and volume/density of lung cell mitochondria is directly related to oxygen consumption [438]. Lung cell mitochondria become progressively dysfunctional as we age and antioxidants like melatonin protect lung mitochondria from aging[439]. We must sleep well for this effect. ***Mitochondrial DNA is central to managing cytotoxic exposure of lung cells [440].*** Our daily dose of antioxidants should almost double as we begin to enjoy life after our 60th birth day.

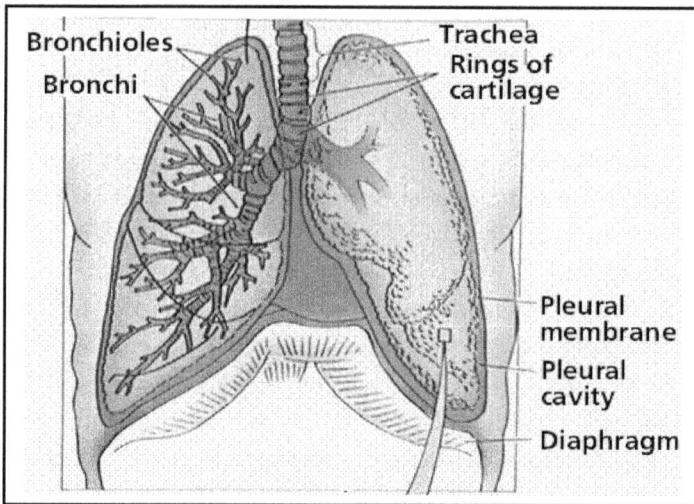

Fig. 3.09 Anatomy of Lung.
Source: National Institute of Health

---

437   http://www.cdc.gov/mmwr/preview/mmwrhtml/mm61e0207a1.htm
438   http://www.ncbi.nlm.nih.gov/pubmed/1141087
439   http://www.ncbi.nlm.nih.gov/pubmed/21614449
440   http://ajplung.physiology.org/content/306/11/L962

Smoking is a very serious risk factor in human health. Cigarette smoking damages lung mitochondria causing low energy production and even death of lung cells [441]. Also, smoking depletes antioxidant glutathione that prevents free radical formation [442]. There occurs more mitochondrial damage resulting in lung cancer because of continued smoking [443]. Dysfunction of lung mitochondria can cause asthma, COPD (chronic obstructive pulmonary disease), cystic fibrosis, and cancer [444] and there is high risk of respiratory damages because of mitochondrial dysfunctions [445]. Exposure to acrolein that comes of frying oils in the kitchen or restaurants can cause mitochondrial damage[446]. Lung health is important in terms of net normal oxygen intake of 3.7 liters per minute which calculates to 11,000 liters or 388 cubic feet of air (3.7 liters of oxygen) intake per day. The mitochondria regulate this intake.

3.10 The Kidneys

We have two kidney, each the size of our fist. Fig. 3.10 shows the anatomical details of one of them. With a million nephrons in each, the kidneys filter 45 gallons of blood per day. This acounts to filtering all blood every half an hour under pressure through glomerular capillaries. The filtrate is water, ions, glucose, and proteins of molecular weight below 30,000. Our entire blood of 7-8 liters gets filtered 20-25 times per day producing 1.5 to 2.0 liter urine as waste. **Functions of kidney other than filtration include production of erythropoietin for manufacture of red blood cells, renin for controlling blood pressure, and vitamin D activation for control of calcium.** All this requires energy producing mitochondria and kidneys fail when their mitochondria fail[447].

Given up to 6 micromole of oxygen consumption per minute and 6 moles of ATP produced per mole of oxygen, **our kidneys use up to 36 millimoles of ATP per minute per Kilogram body weight or about 18-19 grams of ATP [448].** Metabolic support of renal sodium pump which is a transmembrane enzyme ATPase is dedicated to acid-baseand electrolyte balance [449]. The epithelial

441   http://www.trdrp.org/fundedresearch/grant_page.php?grant_id=5323
442   http://www.immunehealthscience.com/what-depletes-glutathione.html
443   http://journals.sfu.ca/rncsb/index.php/csbj/article/view/csbj.201303019/333
444   http://www.ncbi.nlm.nih.gov/pubmed/23978003
445   http://www.mitochondrialncg.nhs.uk/documents/Respiratory_Guidelines_2011.pdf
446   http://www.ncbi.nlm.nih.gov/pubmed/24056970
447   http://adc.bmj.com/content/78/4/387.full.pdf
448   http://www.annualreviews.org/doi/abs/10.1146/annurev.ph.48.030186.000301
449   http://hyperphysics.phy-astr.gsu.edu/hbase/biology/nakpump.html

cell surface is packed with microvilli that make a border like structure for resorption and sensing of flow. Cytoplasm is loaded with mitochondria for transport of sodium ions out of tubules. This too requires ATP energy.

Reduced mitochondrial function is behind many diabetes related diseases [450] **and Diabetic kidney (ESRD) disease in particular is due to poor functioning of mitochondria** [451], [452], [453]. **Glomerular blood hydrostatic pressure (GBHP) of 75 mm is opposed by the back pressure in the renal tubule and the osmotic pressure of the blood** [454]. **The difference of 25 mm is what determines the filtration rate. This depends on mitochondrial activity and tubular cells of kidney require steady supply of ATP energy.**

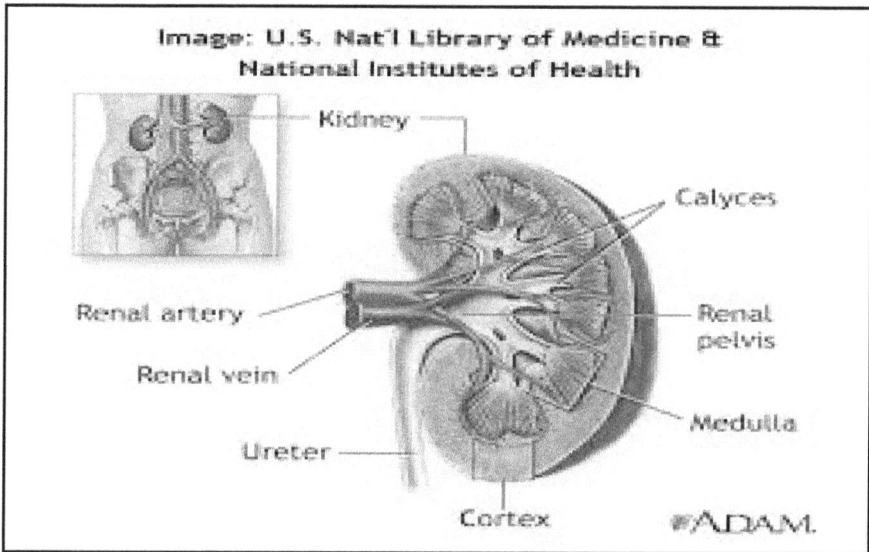

Fig. 3.10 Anatomy of kidney.

Source: National Heart Institute

Mitochondrial diseases cause loss of amino acid and electrolytes in the urine. Ubiquinol or reduced form of coenzyme Q_{10} improves functions [455] of kidney because of its antioxidant effect [456].

450   http://www.sciencedaily.com/releases/2013/10/131010204758.htm
451   http://www.ncbi.nlm.nih.gov/pubmed/23949796
452   http://adc.bmj.com/content/78/4/387.full
453   http://www.nature.com/nrneph/journal/v1/n2/full/ncpneph0031.html
454   http://faculty.ucc.edu/biology-potter/kidney.htm
455   http://www.ncbi.nlm.nih.gov/pubmed/20878200
456   http://ubiquinol.org/clinical-studies

3.11 The Liver

Liver, our body's biochemical factory, has immense energy demand and it uses amost 50% of basal metabolic energy (Fig. 3.11).

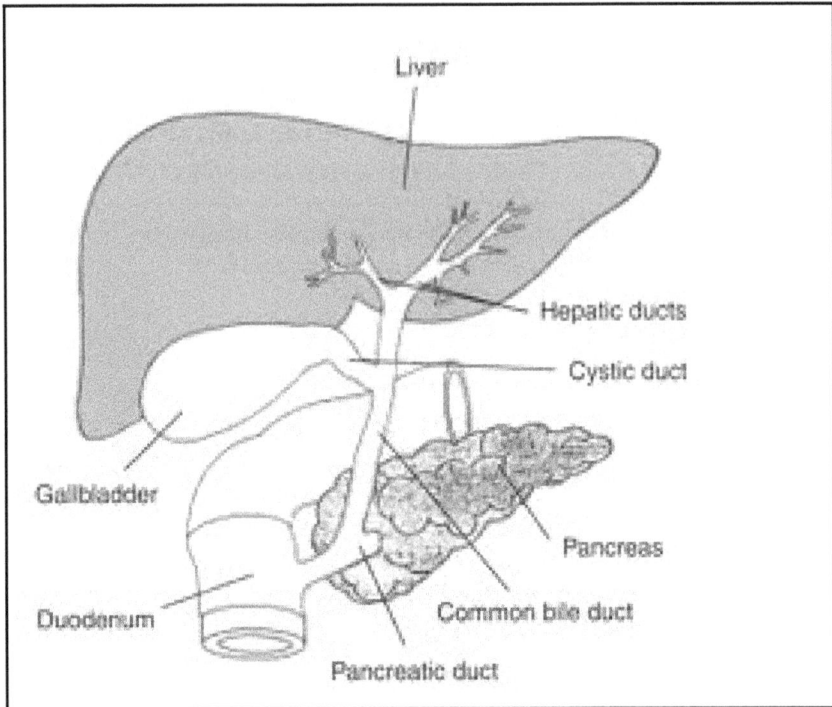

Fig. 3.11 Liver and associated organs.

Sources: National Heart Institute

Number of mitochondria per cell in the liver can be more than 10,000. The volume of a liver cell has been estimated to be 5000 μm³ with a membrane area of 110,000 μm² [457]. This gives a surface to volume ratio of 20 and renders it very efficient in running our daily metabolism and detoxification [458]. Glycogen metabolism per se in liver demands high ATP production by mitochondria [459].

A key function of liver is to control blood glucose. Defects in production

---

457   http://highered.mcgraw-hill.com/sites/0072919183/student_view0/chapter3/thinking_scientifically. html

458   http://www.autismspeaks.org/science/science-news/mitochondrial-disorder-more-common-expected-asd

459   http://www.biomedcentral.com/content/pdf/1743-7075-8-38.pdf

of glucose from proteins and fats is attributable to problems with electron transport chain in inner membrane of mitochondria. A mitochondrial dysfunction can cause deficiency of enzyme pyruvate decarboxylase. There can be deficiencies of acetyl-CoA dehydrogenase and carnitine palmitoyltransferase also.

Liver diseases can be due to both mutations in nuclear DNA and deletions or duplications of mitochondrial DNA. **Prolonged fasting can also cause lactic acidosis and elevated blood ammonia** and drastic changes in mitochondrial functions and signals can cause too many unexpected chronic diseases [460].

3.12 The Pancreas

Pancreas is a factory that produces master hormone insulin, many digestive enzymes, and sodium bicarbonate in order to neutralize acidity of stomach juice. **It is a mixed gland that produces both endocrine and exocrine secretions**[461] . **Obviously malfunctioning mitochondria in pancreatic cells cause many types of health havocs.** Ability of pancreatic cells to consume oxygen goes down and so does the potential across the inner mitochondrial membrane causing low ATP production [462]. Both type 1 and type 2 diabetes are due to malfunctioning mitochondria in beta cells of pancreas. KRAS mitochondrial gene mutations are known to be behind pancreatic cancer [463]. Naturally pancreatic mitochondria are targets for treatment of pancreatic cancer [464]. Protein in daily methylation diet must deliver proper RDA of all essential amino acids.

Take a good look at pancreases in Fig. 3.12. This six inches long mixed gland sitting across the back of the abdomen behind the stomach has very high volume and membrane area. Pancreatic cells have a volume of 1,000 μm^3 and a total membrane area of 13,000 μm^2. The surface to volume ratio of 13 for a rather smaller but very active organ of pancrease is a little more than half of liver, a much larger organ, whose ratio is 20.

460   http://www.ncbi.nlm.nih.gov/pubmed/21269263
461   http://classes.midlandstech.edu/carterp/Courses/bio211/chap16/chap16.htm
462   http://mrb.niddk.nih.gov/sherman/Utah/Utahchap.pdf
463   http://www.nature.com/nature/journal/vaop/ncurrent/full/nature13611.html
464   http://www.nature.com/nrclinonc/journal/v11/n10/full/nrclinonc.2014.143.html

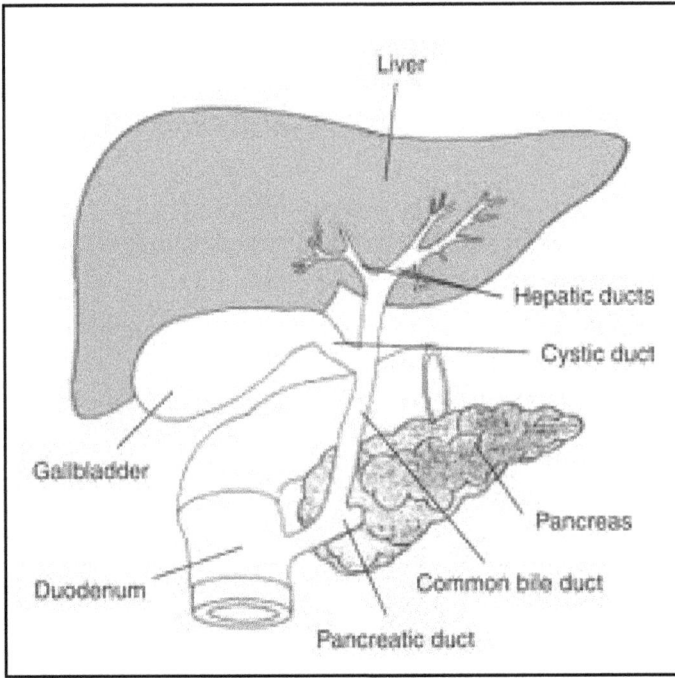

Fig. 3.12 The pancreas.

Source: National Institute of Health.

Beta cells of pancreas make digestive enzymes and master hormone insulin [465], A cells make hormone glucagon [466], and D cells make somatostatin [467]. MELAS (mitochondrial encephalomyopathy, lactic acidosis, and stroke like syndrome) results due to a defective mitochondrial genes where base guanidine is substituted by adenine. sadly more than 1% of patients with adult-onset diabetes mellitus may have MELAS [468].

High cysteine diet by way of whey protein concentrate may be helpful in reducing pancreatic cancer incidence [469]. Cancer Research UK suggests use of enzyme supplements [470]. American cancer society guidelines [471] emphasize the following.

---

465   https://www.umassmed.edu/uploadedFiles/otm2/Ready_to_sign/05-18%20Ref.pdf
466   https://www.inkling.com/read/endocrinology-jameson-de-groot-6th/chapter-35/biosynthesis-of-pan-creatic
467   http://mcb.berkeley.edu/courses/mcb135e/pancreas.html
468   http://www.ncbi.nlm.nih.gov/pubmed/7554321
469   http://www.ncbi.nlm.nih.gov/pubmed/8669840
470   http://www.cancerresearchuk.org/about-cancer/type/pancreatic-cancer/living/diet-and-pancreat-ic-cancer
471   http://pathology.jhu.edu/pancreas/TreatmentNutrition.php?area=tr

1.   Exercise.
2.   Optimum weight.
3.   Very low fat and and almost no meat .
4.   High consumption of fruits, vegetables, and whole grains.

3.13 The Muscles

Muscle cells may have 4000 mitochondria for effective locomotion that demands frequent burst of energy[472]. Energy production on quick demand needs a large number of mitochondria [473]. Weakness of muscles including those of eyelids and cramping of large and small muscles are the first symptom of mitochondrial disease (Fig. 3.13). Clinically enzyme creatine kinase level go as high as 10,000 U/liter. Poor motility of esophagus, stomach, and intestine can cause unbearable morbidity. Anorexia and weight loss happen in case of MEALAS (mitochondrial encephalopathy, lactic acidosis, and stroke like) syndrome and anorexia nervosa like MNGIE (myoneurogenic gastrointestinal encephalopathy) diseases. The patient simply avoids foods, actually anorexia nervosa itself can cause mitochondrial failure.

Protein PPAR Alpha works in hippocampus for processing memory. This relates to liver function of burning belly fat. If the liver overworks, there is not enough PPAR alpha left for hippocampus for memory function causing dementia [474] and Alzheimer's disease[475].

---

472   http://juvenon.com/jhj/vol1no04.htm
473   http://www.hindawi.com/journals/jar/2012/194821/
474   http://www.rush.edu/webapps/MEDREL/servlet/NewsRelease?id=1726
475   http://www.sciencedaily.com/releases/2013/10/131009100620.htm

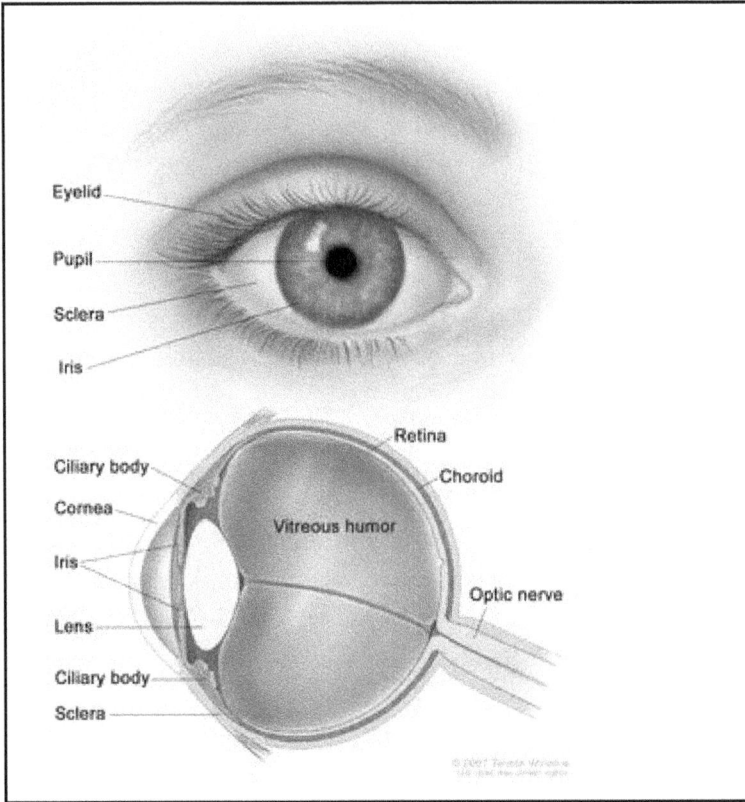

Fig. 3.13 Eyelid musculature,
Source: National Institute of Health

There are reference citations at the end of this chapter for our readers who want to learn more about general anatomy of vital organs, general biology and physiology of brain, lung, heart, liver, and kidney. Reference topics on diagnostic procedures, value of annual physical examinations, tracing mitochondrial connections, role of stress in mitochondrial diseases, mitochondrial mobility and transport, and mitochondrial mutations are included .

Mitochondrial performance depends not only on its own DNA but also on the nuclear DNA. This performance goes much more beyond simple energy production and covers calcium transport, sensing of growth factors, sensing and signaling of oxygen level and level of reactive oxygen species, DNA damage recognition, and cytotoxic exposures.

Behind it all is a large area of untapped knowledge and practical understanding that major research institutions in the world are focused on. We have had hardly 26 years of experience beginning 1988 on research devoted to mitochondrial diseases. We now know that disorders of central nervous system, eye and vision, Type II diabetes, heart diseases, kidney problems, skeletal muscles, and fast aging process depend on mitochondrial gene. Much more applied and clinical works on mitochondrial biology are coming in rather rapidly for routine health care.

3.14 Methylation Diet for Healthy Organs

Soon examination of vital signs and day to day performance of our vital organs will hopefully give us a better picture of our health. In the mean time a methylation diet is our best friend. Proper intake of methylation diet rich in N-acety-l-aspartate, coenzyme Q_{10}, vitamins C, E, and B complex is strongly advised for healthy mitochondria that underlie our routine health. Important to this discussion are a few noteworthy developments.

3.14.01 THe Portable Ultrasound Imaging Devise:

A smartphone size ultrasound imaging device will soon become the stethescope of 21st century for diagnosing problems of heart failure, fluid in the lungs, and other organs including galstones, bulged aorta, blood clot, and enlarged prostate. A leading center of research is Ultrasound Institute of University of South Carolina Medical School.

3.14.02 Twenty Minute Pathogen Testing:

Ultra fast detection of bacterial pathogens will soon come about by nanotechnology. A gold nanowire imbedded in a silicon chip by virtue of its siky hill dome like shape will be able to electrically detect more than 1000 bactrial pathogenic antigens in trillions of molecules in a blood sample. The sensitivity comes both from negatively charged DNA-ruthenium metal complex on one hand and the the smooth hills of nano-gold with smooth surface capable of accomodating 5 target DNA molecules. This research at Xangenic in Toronto complemets to gold nanosphere technology for detecting cancer cell DNA at the Northwestern University, SlipChip Wireless technology (microfluidic device called **SlipChip**, a cell phone camera, and cloud computing) capable of quantifying nucleic acids developed at the California Institute of Technology, and HIV detection technology developed at Colombia University [476]. We live by our DNA, we can detect diseases by watching DNA, and we do die by DNA gone amuck.

3.14.03 The Misfolded Prions:

Understanding of Prions (the misfolded small infectious particles of proteins) like beta-amyloid in case of Alzheimer, α-Synclein in case of Parkinson's diseases, and protein particles of Huntington disease. Most of these neurological diseases are result of very small misfolded shape of the protein particles [477]. Proteins that run our brain function and communication can ruin it when misshapen [478].

Included below is the list of major research institutions that our readers can consult for timely research on clinical and routine ailments that affect our vital organs including skin and stomach with large and small intestine. Those described in this chapter are the ones we could not live too long without in good function. The research centers listed below offer plenty of information on them in regard to periodic testing directed to health maintenance.

Major Research Centers

Addiction Technology Transfer Center Network, University of Missouri.

Adelphi University, Center for Health Innovation

CDC. Vital Signs: Prevalence, treatment, and control of hypertension — United States, 1999–2002 and 2005–2008. MMWR 2011;60:103–8.

---

476   http://engineering.columbia.edu/smartphone-finger-prick-15-minutes-diagnosis%E2%80%-94done-0
477   http://www.scientificamerican.com/article/what-is-a-prion-specifica/
478   http://memory.ucsf.edu/cjd/overview/prions

Dartmouth Medicine

Cleveland Clinic

National Public Health Institute

UCLA Clinical and Translational Science Institute

University of California, School of Medicine, San Diego, CA

US Department of Health and Human Services, Health research and Quality

Worcester Polytechnique Institute

Adelphi University Center for Health Innovation.

Assessment Technologies Institute: Nursing Education.

Clear bridge Vital Signs, National University of Singapore.

Indiana University

Medline Plus.

Oregon Clinical and translational Research Institute.

United Mitochondria Foundation.

University of Rochester Medical Center.

University of California, LA Health.

4

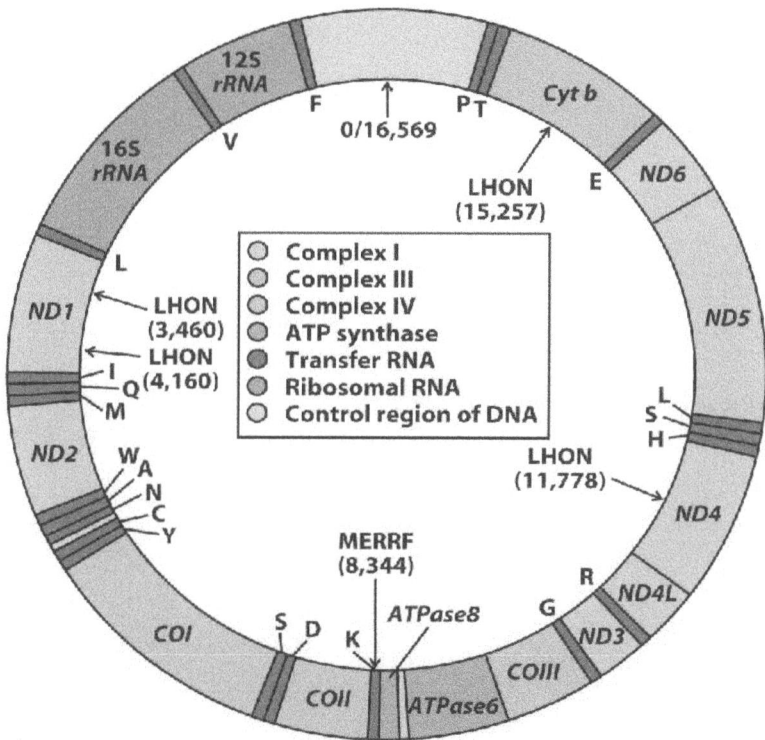

Mutated Mitochondrial Genes Cause Many Difficult to cure Diseases

Non-germ line somatic mutations related to cancer (p53 deletion, pry deletion, PTEN deletion, cyclin E amplification to name a few) □□ □□□□□ □□□□□□ *our life time. We need to stabilize our mitochondrial and nuclear genes, prevent somatic mitochondrial gene mutations, and manage routine gene expression for a disease free life by methylation diet. Overuse* *of antibiotics causes mitochondrial fatigue and dysfunction. Methylation diet high in Coenzyme Q_{10} and PQQ help mitochondrial biogenesis and function. These nutrients can do timely epigenetic reprogramming. Although many diseases due to defective mitochondrial genes are difficult to cure, methylation diet is now known to revert chronic problems of diabetes, cardiovascular diseases, and cancer. LHON and MERRF gene locations are indicated above.*

Chapter 4
Mitochondrial Diseases

Quantum effects of electrons, protons, photons, and ions seem to underlie our health and longevity.

Triveni P. Shukla

Myriads of reactions and functions in our cells in various organs depend on stable and healthy mitochondria free of mutated genes. Can defects of mitochondrial genes be edited and corrected by nutrients in our foods routinely? Can nutrients alone regulate the complex control of nuclear and mitochondrial genomes and gene expression for optimal operation of chemical energy (ATP) production? Can genes of cytochrome b and cytochrome C be stabilized and induced on demand for full expression? Is mitochondrial gene therapy the only plausible answer? The answer is a cautionary yes but at least a ecade away.

Methylation diet high in antioxidants via fruits, vegetables, and whole grain can no doubt help us manage mitochondrial dysfunction to a large degree and we need to consume, as a matter of daily dietary regimen, essential amino acids, essential fatty acids, conjugated isoprenoid food molecules like omega-3 and omega-6 fatty acid, isoprenoid antioxidants such as quinones , flavones, and anthocyanidins, and all vitamins and trace minerals necessary for making of heme b proteins like hemoglobin and myoglobin and the rest of metalloproteins. The isoprenoid units in cholesterol, beta-carotene, vitamins D, E, K , coenzyme Q_{10}, and PQQ are there for their unique electronic properties [479]. Supplied with good nutrients, mitochondrial biobatteries in our vital organs may permit electron flow, energy production, and antiinflammatory effects in order to avoid chronic diseases. Mitochondrial DNA damage occurs due to mutation or deletion on one hand and oxidative damage due to free radicals on the other. Overuse of antibiotics also causes mitochondrial dysfunction which can be minimized by proper intake of antioxidants like N-Acety-l-Cysteine, PQQ, and coenzyme Q_{10}. The health of mitochondria is essential for preventing diabetes type II, cardiovascular diseases, and many types of cancer. A methylation diet rich in omega-3 fatty acids and fat soluble vitamins keeps mitochondria stable and functional. These molecules of life have been around through out our evolution.

The Patient and the Physician

4.01 My Physicians and I

Let me speak for myself and say that my interactions with attending physicians have always been less than complete at least up to the age of 62 years. They never brought up health implications of mitochondria during my visits to their offices or in my hospital room. Why doesn't a physician talk to his/her patients about the mighty mitochondria, the electron and proton manager in our cells by whose function we live and by whose dysfunction we die? This is a bit troubling because of its direct implication in problems of chronic stress, over weightness, obesity, diabetes, congestive heart failures, and cancer. I should like to advise readers of this book to interact with their physicians willfully in sufficient detail just to find out if their health problems are connected to their daily diet, the dietary deficiencies in particular, and mitochondrial dysfunction.

The diagnosis, the tests, the clinical evidence, the happy prognosis, and all the rest should be part of the doctor-patient interaction. My wife and I began interacting in this manner some three years ago but only after getting to face problems of my heart attack and my wife's multiple myeloma cancer. Unfortunately this happeneded in our late sixties.

---

479   http://www.bioinfo.org.cn/book/biochemistry/chapt09/bio3.htm

Damage to Nuclear and Mitochondrial DNA

Let us begin with axiomatic truths in human biology. Number one is that oxygen we breathe in, water we drink, and foods we eat are processed by mitochondria in our cells for power productions. This is the organelle responsible for running Krebs cycle for electron abstraction from foods we eat and transporting them for reducing oxygen we breat. Number two is that mitochondria are responsible for much of signaling and body-brain wide communication. Number three is that they direct birth and death of our cells. Number four and the most important is the fact that mitochondria operate with their own 37 genes in close coordination with genes in our cell's nucleus. Their dysfunction of ATP or power production alone determines fatigue, alertness, and capacity of vital organs to do what they are supposed to do. **Free radicals are produced off the electron transport chain less than 20 nanometers away from unprotected mitochondrial genes making them prone to mutation and we know that oxidative damage of mitochondrial DNA cause difficult to cure diseases.** Any existing mutations of nuclear genes make the situation even worse.

Let us think of us human beings a walking nano-factory. Every cell with the exception of red blood cell is a factory where many hundreds or even thousands of mitochondria process electrons and protons to produce chemical energy ATP. Our brain, liver, muscles, heart, eyes, and tongue use much of this energy second by second of our life. Naturally mitochondria gone wrong can make us tired, weak, and neuro-muscularly sick. They are known to be the cause of many diseases including asthma, lung disease, hypertension, dysfunction of coronary artery, depression, bipolar disorder, Alzheimer's disease, Parkinson's disease, type II diabetes, and cancer. Mitochondrial dysfunction seems to cause autism, spectrum disorder[480] , and type II diabetes [481], [482], [483].

Mitochondrial diseases and neurological disorders are caused by many nutrient deficiencies including iron and sulfur proteins of electron transport

---

480   h http://www.ncbi.nlm.nih.gov/pubmed/19650713ttp://www.nature.com/pr/journal/v69/n5-2/full/pr9201192a.html

481   http://www.ncbi.nlm.nih.gov/pubmed/19650713
482   http://diabetes.diabetesjournals.org/content/53/suppl_1/S103.full
483   http://circres.ahajournals.org/content/102/4/401.full

chain [484], [485]. The chart of functions of mitochondrial nutrients (table 2.04.02) offers a list of nutrient and disease relationships. Many of these diseases are linked to our daily diet.

We need to combine our knowledge on biology of mitochondria with that of therapeutic nutrition in examining nutrient function with respect to health and population of mitochondrial in our cells. A proper B vitamin mix including folate and high intake of antioxidants coenzyme Q_{10} and pyrroloquinoline quinone can help manage mitochondrial diseases [486]. I should list a few key functional nutrients that have been part of our evolution: DHA involved in brain function [487], vitamin D and evolution of color of skin [488], B_{12} and evolution of our brain [489], FMN, a B_2 or riboflavin derivative and energy production by electron transport chain, Vitamins C and E along with enzymes superoxide dismutase and catalase are free radical quenching molecules present very early in evolution, and vitamins A, D, E, K, and flavoproteins are all important in energy production by our cell's mitochondria [490]. Diabetics suffer a lot because of problems in energy production and homeostasis. An obvious connection of mitochondria with diabetes, which is a metabolic disease, is specially relevant to a major portion of population in all industrialized nations on the globe.

This chapter cites 14 references on defects of mitochondrial DNA, 11 on mitochondrial diseases in general, 5 on problems of electron transfer chain, 10 on various diseases including multiple sclerosis and diabetes, and 4 on specific cases of cancer. There are 24 citations on mitochondrial diseases, 15 citations on mitochondrial gene mutation, and 1 each on hepatic disorder, transfer RNA mutation, cytochrome C deficiency, obesity and type II diabetes, methylation and cancer, and multiple sclerosis. In addition, the chapter is referenced topic by topic and theme by theme with appropriate and critical website references, the URL_s. Current research does document the mighty power of our immortal mitochondria.

484   http://www.stevenhamley.com.au/2012/01/mitochondrial-dysfunction.html
485   http://drlwilson.com/Articles/MITOCHONDRIAL.htm
486   http://www.ncbi.nlm.nih.gov/pmc/articles/PMC3561461/
487   http://www.ncbi.nlm.nih.gov/pmc/articles/PMC3257695/
488   http://www.nasw.org/article/vitamin-d-levels-determined-how-human-skin-color-evolved
489   http://www.livescience.com/24875-meat-human-brain.html
490   http://entomology.unl.edu/ent801/vitamins.html

Diseases of Mitochondrial DNA
4.02 Diseases of Mitochondrial DNA

Mitochondria produce 90% of all body energy and their dysfunction can cause diseases and even death of our cells [491]. Many problems happen to our brain and muscles because they literally depend on mitochondria for on demand instant energy supply [492]. Organs that are affected rather quickly are eyes, heart, liver, ear, and gastrointestinal tract. Diseases of autism, Parkinson's, Alzheimer's, Lou Gehrig's, muscular dystrophy, and chronic fatigue are problems of power failure in our body because the mitochondria have either gone dysfunctional or are working slowly or inefficiently. Their numbers may be reduced also. In case of Leigh's disease, whose occurrence is only in 0.002% of US population, the "power blackout" has been found to be literally fatal. There can occur calcium overload and instant neuronal death [493].

Mitochondria represent an extremely complex enzyme system run by more than 37 mitochondrial and about 963 nuclear genes. Mitochondrial diseases can affect brain, heart, and the muscle. Fortunately only 0.03% people succumb to them any time during their life time. Early diagnosis, although difficult, includes brain imaging, muscle biopsy, and laboratory evaluations supported further by clinical, biochemical, and genetic characterization and tests.

Although a majority of diseases are neuromuscular in nature, mitochondrial dysfunction is known to be responsible for type II diabetes, chronic fatigue, fibermyalgia, and tumor cell modification. Symptoms can be poor growth, loss of muscle coordination, muscle weakness, visual problems, hearing problems, heart disease, kidney disease, gastrointestinal disorder, respiratory disorder, autonomic disorders, neurological problems, and dementia. Mitochondrial DNA is known to be responsible for these diseases in up to 15% cases and the overall inheritance pattern is unique and complicated [494].

---

491   http://rarediseases.info.nih.gov/files/White_Paper_v3_8_FinalCGedits.pdf
492   http://rarediseasesnetwork.epi.usf.edu/namdc/learnmore/index.htm
493   http://www.ncbi.nlm.nih.gov/pubmed/14749273
494   http://www.ncbi.nlm.nih.gov/books/NBK1224/

4.03 Mitochondria and Immune System

White blood cells make our Immune System and all of them have mitochondria [495]. There are five types of them: Monocytes and lymphocytes are *agranular* and neutrophiles, basophiles, and eosinophiles are *granular*. **Neutrophyles, the bacterial slayers and destroyers, are most numerous. Eosinophiles kill parasitic worms by toxins. Histamine and heparin producing basophiles respond to inflammation. B lymphocytes produce antibodies and the T type lymphocytes literally kill bacteria.** Collectively they make our immune system. Natural killer cells reorganize around tumer cells and their mitochondria produce power on demand to destroy the stressed out cells [496].

On an average there can be 20-30 mitochondria in immune cells of an average 14.4 microns diameter with a total volume of 1,563.4 cubic micron [497]. White blood cells have high concentration of lysozyme, the enzyme they need to defeat and devour invading bacteria and virus alive. They have been isolated from white blood cells and observed to exhibit extra-mitochondrial control by free calcium [498].

Reactive Oxygen Species (ROS) fire up the natural killer T cells of our immune system [499]. They are intimately involved in antibacterial and antiviral immunity. They can also be a threat to our existence [500] though. T cells have potassium channel K_v 1.3 proteins in their inner membrane [501]. A cascade of biochemical events including DNA replication, RNA and protein synthesis, and ATP production follow for defense right after a bacterial attack [502]. The invading bacterial antigens trigger this sequence of events. **Surprisingly T cells have the power even to kill themselves and proliferate when the need arises and there are specific genes for this purpose [503].**

Our fighting immune cells need best of protection from oxidative damage by high antioxidant methylation diet so that they are ever ready and alert for our body's defense [504]. Please review immune boosting foods for mitochondrial health in Table 2.04.02. There is no doubt that a well designed methylation diet can balance and boost our immunity.

---

495   http://www.ncbi.nlm.nih.gov/pubmed/20367054
496   http://www.ncbi.nlm.nih.gov/pubmed/19038287
497   http://cancerres.aacrjournals.org/content/2/9/655.full.pdf
498   http://www.ncbi.nlm.nih.gov/pmc/articles/PMC1158169/
499   https://www.cell.com/immunity/abstract/S1074-7613(13)00060-5
500   http://www.nature.com/scitable/topicpage/mitochondria-and-the-immune-response-14266967
501   http://www.jbc.org/content/280/13/12790
502   http://www.jleukbio.org/content/46/2/128.full.pdf
503   http://www.jimmunol.org/content/182/7/4046.full
504   http://www.ncbi.nlm.nih.gov/pubmed/11382196

4.04 Mitochondria and Our Second Genome of Gut Bacteria

The close relationship among cells in our body and the bacteria in our intestine is the corner stone of our evolution. Probiotics that inhabit our intestine and the endosymbiotic mitochondria have common ancestry [505]. As a matter of fact the electron and proton processing mitochondria in our cells were once upon a time a bacteria. Our gut bacteria, the probiotic symbionts, are essential to our digestive health and immune system. They convert lignans in high omega-3 flax seed we consume into hormone modulating compounds and produce **immune factor bacteriocin**. Also, they produce vitamin B complex and B_{12}, detoxify pesticides and xenobiotic chemicals like bisphenol-A from plastics, produce short chain fatty acids, and enhance our immune system. The genes of the probiotic bacteria are very material to our health as a supplement to our genome.

Methylation foods containing phytosterols, phospholipids, and B vitamins protect our long-term health by supporting mitochondrial function [506]. Probiotics may play a definite role in mitochondrial energy production and intracellular calcium ion concentration [507].

4.05 Major Mitochondrial diseases

Mitochondrial Disease Foundation [508] lists many mitochondrial diseases that are caused by a faulty mitochondrial DNA [509], [510], [511]. This section is devoted to a few that can be diagnosed accurately and for which therapies are being sought after today.

---

505   http://www.nleducation.co.uk/news/tocotrienols-probiotics-and-phosphoglycolipids-a-perfect-pre-scription-for-the-liver/
506   http://ntfactor.com/ClinicalTrials/tabid/99/TagID/12/PID/465/global/yes/Default.aspx
507   https://www.academia.edu/5631068/Influence_of_Probiotics_and_a_Novel_Probiotic_Product_on_Mitochondrial_Energetics_and_Calcium_Signal_Dynamics
508   http://www.umdf.org/site/c.8qKOJ0MvF7LUG/b.7934629/k.4C9B/Types_of_Mitochondrial_Disease.htm
509   http://www.ncbi.nlm.nih.gov/pmc/articles/PMC1762815/
510   http://www.med.unc.edu/neurology/files/documents/child-teaching-pdf/Mitochondrial%20Re-view%20DiMaro%2005.pdf
511   http://www.emdn-mitonet.co.uk/PDF/COHEN701MitoAdults.pdf

Chronic Diseases

4.05.01 Diabetes Mellitus and Deafness

The media reminds us daily of the problems of over weightness, obesity, and diabetes. Hypertension, high cholesterol, diabetes, coronary heart disease, stroke, gall bladder problems, osteoarthritis, sleep apnea, and cancers of breast, colon, and endometrium are health problems associated with weight. Furthermore, we are told that diabetes has its connection with our pancreas, the enzyme factory dedicated to daily digestion. But the more obvious problem is consumption of too many calories eaten 32% of the times away from home rather irregularly. A few scary examples are a 340 calories perfect margarita (Applebee's), 440 calories green tea frappachino (Starbucks), 540 calories carrot walnut muffin (Au Bon Pai), 610 calories vegetarian lettuce wrap (P.F. Chang's), and 1,080 calories pecan crusted chicken salad (TGI Fridays). This world's 30% of 7.2 billion people are obese and the excess weight causes 5% of global death. A single way to deal with the problem is nutrient dense but portion controlled and calorie restricted daily methylation food at home or away from home.

World Health organization, based on its global obesity data, tells us that Body Mass Index is out of control in most industrialized countries. Actually, it is often above the normal range of 18.5 to 23. Populations above a BMI of 30, characteristic of obesity, are at great risk. BMI is body fat measured indirectly as pound weight of fat divided by height in inches. We need to keep it about 20-22. While a BMI of 29 is bad news, 29% body fat may be just fine and healthy. That is how indirect and not close to reality BMI is. You and I may have same weight and height but different percentage of fat. **A better test is DEXA scan by X-Ray that the physicians can order for confirmation and better interpretation of BMI data.** There are serious consequences of misuse of BMI data. Misuse of BMI data by insurance companies and even employers is a widely discussed problem. They blindly use the data to declare that one is stressed out. Technically the problem has its root in mitochondrial function.

Mitochondria produce ATP, regulate energy expenditure, and affect fat and glucose metabolism [512]. Fat cells maintain a delicate balance in these regards. Obesity is loss of this balance [513]. *It is the altered mitochondria in overweight and obese populations that lead to a chain of metabolic problems leading to obesity, high blood pressure, leptin resistance, insulin resistance, kidney disease, and poor eye health.* Obese people have smaller and fewer mitochondria that may be degenerated to a point of reduced electron transfer activity [514], [515]. Scientists are finding out a brain signal that turns unhealthy white fat cells into brown fat cells [516]. A drug based on the science of brown fat soon be in the market for reducing excess body fat. In case of Type I Diabetes stem cells have been developed that respond to sugar in lab and also in human cells [517]. **Although a few years away, stem cell therapy may be a boon to Type I patients [518], [519], [520].**

A simple calorie restricted diet can restore mitochondrial biogenesis and capacity [521]. Exercise that boosts PGC-1Alpha, a master activator and integrator of energy metabolism by boosting appropriate genes is very helpful. Brown seaweed (algae) containing fucoxanthin in our routine diet is known to enhance PGC-1Alpha activity for weight control [522], [523]. Clinical trials were done at Hokkaido University, Japan. An RDA for this carotenoid xanthophyl is recommended to be 150 mcg, although FDA in the US has no prescribed RDA. Commercial fucoxanthin is extracted by carbon dioxide critical fluid extraction process [524]. Better and more reliable cure will come from genome editing and rewriting the genes as advances in genomic medicine become more common place therapeutics [525], [526], [527].

Obesity is a state of low pH and high hydrogen ion (proton) concentration when we don't get enough light. We gain weight and get fat if there is less energy as "electrons". The pH of body fluids is low, magnetic flux in mitochondria is low and magnetism is degraded, temperature is high,

512   http://www.ncbi.nlm.nih.gov/pubmed/20585248
513   http://brn.sagepub.com/content/10/4/356.abstract
514   http://www.juvenon.com/obesity-examining-the-role-of-the-mitochondria-313/
515   http://www.ncbi.nlm.nih.gov/pubmed/20585248
516   http://www.sciencedaily.com/releases/2014/10/141016085652.htm
517   http://www.cirm.ca.gov/our-progress/type-1-diabetes-fact-sheet
518   http://hsci.harvard.edu/news/stem-cells-billions-human-insulin-producing-cells
519   http://www.nature.com/nrendo/journal/v6/n3/full/nrendo.2009.274.html
520   http://www.technologyreview.com/featuredstory/535036/a-pancreas-in-a-capsule/
521   http://www.ncbi.nlm.nih.gov/pubmed/17108241
522   http://www.ncbi.nlm.nih.gov/pmc/articles/PMC3944525/
523   http://www.ncbi.nlm.nih.gov/pubmed/21475918
524   http://pubs.acs.org/doi/abs/10.1021/jf400740p
525   http://www.technologyreview.com/review/524451/genome-surgery/
526   http://www.sciencedaily.com/releases/2014/10/141020090436.htm
527   http://www.genome.gov/27541912

and inflammation manifests. Leptin resistance takes over because satiety hormone doesn't work. Each fat cell produces leptin that accumulates exponentially and resistance sets in [528], [529]. The Iron-Sulfur clusters in electron transport enzyme system loose capacity to let electrons tunnel because iron radii expand and transfer steps are more than 14 Angstrom apart. This causes Leptin resistance which is symptomatic of inability of electrons to tunnel through enzyme complexes in the inner membrane of mitochondria [530], [531]. Leptin receptors know how to connect to Iron-Sulfur clusters but not much can be done if theren't enough of them.

Circadian signaling also goes faulty and electrons from foods are not used properly [532]. The diabetics have rather low Electron Paramagnetic Resonance signal. Cold Thermogenesis works directly on mitochondria and its entangled electrons and the magnetic fields. Chromium increases electrical resistance and stimulates magnetic flux. Actually, chromium, a transition metal, as an antiferromagnetic helps type II diabetics because it helps electron tunneling [533]. The D shell electron of chromium do the trick in glucose metabolism by interacting energetically with the iron-sulfur clusters. Underlying technology is now commonplace. For instance antiferromagnets in solid state electronics are used to form spin-valves that are magnetic sensors. The hard drive in our computer is an even more common example.

Thermogenesis is important in weight reduction and control. In cold, electron transport is uncoupled. Infra-red radiation is produced as heat and mitochondrial proteins fold. Free fatty acids help uncoupling and production of infra-red radiation. We are more magnetic when cold.

It is hot when we have inflammation. Protons are in excess and infra-red radiation is produced as heat. There is swelling and electric and magnetic fields are low. Temperature is high and electron and protons are less entangled. They are behaving more like particles. Cold thermogenesis, coordinated and conditioned by environment, increases electric magnetic field of mitochondria, slows electrons down, and increases magnetic sense meaning more of mitochondria are magnetized, and more oxygen is used. **Magnetism orders electron flow.** Proper weight then comes from thermogenesis and leptin.

---

528   http://link.springer.com/article/10.1007/s00018-004-4432-1#page-1
529   http://www.ncbi.nlm.nih.gov/pubmed/17937601
530   http://www.ncbi.nlm.nih.gov/pmc/articles/PMC3122475/
531   http://www.ncbi.nlm.nih.gov/pmc/articles/PMC3080324/
532   http://www.northwestern.edu/newscenter/stories/2005/04/obesity.html
533   http://www.pnas.org/content/103/44/16212.full

Actually, leptin receptors are vital to weight control because they account for light harvesting by mitochondria [534],[535].

We know that exercise generates free radicals. Exercise, a good night sleep, and exposure to sunlight at noon helps reduce and maintain weight.

4.05.03 Cardiovascular Diseases

Let us begin by thinking of heart as pump that generates its own power by 5000 mitochondria in each of its 3 billion muscle cells. Think of mitochondria as an organelle that strokes the heart. Muscle cells connected to intercalated discs with protein tunnels conduct current (action potentials) for 70 contractions of heart per minute. The cells, the discs, and the myofibrils create a structure that eliminates any resistance to conduction and a superbly coordinated contraction pumps 5 liters of blood each minute.

Heart is a machine that functions in fractions of milliamps and millivolt range and heart cells are electrically coupled. Sinoatrial node in the upper right atrium generates 70-80 action potentials per minute. **Even at 0.25 milliamps, there is a flow of at least 2 trillion electrons and ions per second.** Cardiac muscles are very complex and heterogeneous in terms of morphology, pacemaking activity, and potential configuration and conduction [536]. **Pace maker cells in sinoatrial node with 40% of their volume as mitochondria are a drug delivery device where drug is a bunch of electrons and then electricity is electron flow per second.** The range of potential difference is between - 94 millivolt to + 30 millivolt. Discovery of this knowledge on the mechanics of electrical function of hear won Dr. Einthoven a Nobel Prize in 1924. Although heart regulates its beats, beats per minute and strength of heart muscle is controlled by parasympathetic (increase) and sympathetic (decrease) systems of autonomous nervous system.

For every heart activity there is a gene. Six of them have been identified as cause heart diseases: MTHFD1L, PSRC1, MIA3, SMAD3, CDKN2A/CDKN2B, and CXCL12 genes [537]. Genes that cause cytochrome C deficiency can affect heart function for reasons of poor energy supply and mitochondrial gene defects cause dysfunction of ischemic heart failure [538]. Heart muscle problem originates from a mutated mitochondrial DNA and cardiovascular risk factors

534   http://www.jbc.org/content/272/10/6093
535   http://ghr.nlm.nih.gov/condition/leptin-receptor-deficiency
536   http://cardiovascres.oxfordjournals.org/content/47/4/658
537   http://www.webmd.com/heart-disease/news/20070718/6-heart-disease-genes-found
538   http://circ.ahajournals.org/content/91/4/1266.full

and diseases are often due to mitochondrial damage and dysfunction resulting in oxidative and nitrosooxidative stresses [539], [540]. For these reasons, mitochondrial functions are chosen therapeutic target in drug discovery and development [541]. They control numerous key function: the pacemaker cells that generate electric current, conducting cells that spread the pacemaker signal, and the contractile cells that actually do the mechanical pumping; heart health is maintained by supply of energy pretty much on demand and supplies of calcium and electron carrier NADH. Maintaining calcium homeostasis and producing of ATP for energy are very critical functions[542]. Calcium stimulates Krebs Cycle, NADH redox potential, and finally ATP production.

Problems due to mitochondrial dysfunction and damage can now be diagnosed and possible treatments are available [543], [544]. We should like to prevent and treat heart problems by our daily diet. Actually, coenzyme Q_{10} is often prescribed to heart patients. Methylation diets designed with apples for quircetin, spinach and kale for folate or vitamin B_9; beef and sardines for routine delivery of coenzyme Q_{10}, avocado for L-carnitine, tomato for lycopene, walnut and spinach for magnesium, blueberries for polyphenols, and wine and grapes for resveratrol with planned regularity can improve heart health. Coenzyme Q_{10}, carnitine, magnesium, alpha-lipoic acid (broccoli and spinach), vitamin C, melatonin (tart cherries), and resveratrol are key heart nutrients. Alpha-lipoic acid is a very useful antioxidant for mitochondria because it is soluble in water and fat; it can prevent damages in both water and fat soluble cellular components.

4.05.04 Mitochondrial DNA and Cancer

Mitochondria, the Bacterial endosymbiont in our cell, is key to our daily living, our health, and our longevity [545]. The genes in mitochondrial genome have to be translated and expressed into proteins that are part of the electron transport system for energy production. It is difficult to research on defective mitochondrial gene expression because of their coordination

---

539   http://www.ncbi.nlm.nih.gov/pubmed/15855047
540   http://www.ncbi.nlm.nih.gov/pubmed/15855047
541   http://content.onlinejacc.org/article.aspx?articleid=1481177
542   http://www.ncbi.nlm.nih.gov/pubmed/22399426
543   http://www.springer.com/medicine/cardiology/book/978-1-4614-4598-2
544   http://www.biomed.unipd.it/en/research-old/research-groups/mitochondrial-dysfunction-and-cardi-
       ac-diseases/
545   http://www.hindawi.com/journals/bmri/2010/737385/

with many nuclear genes. We do know, however, that poor respiration, excessive production of reactive oxygen species and resultant oxidative stress, fast aging, and many neurological diseases are due to mitochondrial gene dysfunction [546]. There is growing evidence that mitochondrial DNA mutations and deletions are involved in cancer although the mechanism is not known [547], [548,549]. Lung cancer is a case in point [550]. Case studies of other cancers, aging and longevity, sudden infantile death syndrome, and many neurodegenerative diseases are reported extensively[551].

Cancer alters the nanomechanical properties of a healthy cell. Cancer cells are less stiff and are capable of changing their cytoskeleton. Cancer appears to be a disease of coherent electrical polar states (vibrations) and endogenous electromagnetic field and dysfunctional energy production by mitochondria leads to cancer [552]. There ensues disregulated signaling, proliferation, migration, and tissue organization. Endogenous electromagnetic field generation by microtubules in the cell is disrupted when cancer cells take over[553]. There are a number of approaches to diagnosis and potential cure of cancer.

- Diagnosis: Nanodetection and amplification of electromagnetic differences between healthy and cancer cells.

- Photodynamic Therapy: Wavelength specific activation of a photosensitizer molecule that may kill cancer cell .

- Blocking of voltage gated N_a^+channels of excitable cancer cells [554].

Mitochondrial reactive oxygen species can be targeted therapeutically to treat cancer [555]. An over expression of gene for superoxide dismutase

546 http://mcb.asm.org/content/26/13/4818
547 http://www.nature.com/onc/journal/v25/n34/abs/1209604a.html
548 http://www.nature.com/cr/journal/v19/n7/full/cr200969a.html
549 http://www.ncbi.nlm.nih.gov/pmc/articles/PMC1867534/p://www.nature.com/nrg/journal/v6/n5/full/nrg1606.html
550
551 http://www.scitechnol.com/roles-of-mitochondrial-dna-changes-on-cancer-initiation-and-progression-CzML.php?article_id=373
552 http://www.vitatec.com/docs/referenz-vitalfeld/pokorny-2008.pdf
553 http://www.hindawi.com/journals/tswj/2013/195028/
554 http://scitechnol.com/biophysics-of-cancer-cellular-excitability-celex-hypothesis-of-metastasis-j7fz.php?article_id=1931
555 http://www.jhoonline.org/content/6/1/19

production is an ideal target [556]. Cancer is a mitochondrial disease and mitochondria in our cells are good therapeutic targets[557].

4.05.05 Diseases of Old Age

All diseases of the old age have often to do with our mind, memory, and mental acuity. We need to keep our neocortex, basal ganglia, hippocampus, and amygdala healthy with good foods. Let us briefly examine why.

Cortex is a bundled layer of cells of the outer brain, the home for long-term memories of events such as the high school pom, spring breaks, images of town of birth and growth. Underneath it are structures of basal ganglia and cerebellum responsible for procedural memories of how to brush teeth, how to play tennis, and how to do carpentry in the garage. Further below is hippocamus responsible for short-term memories like remembering names, directions to places, and last week's wedding. Amygdala is our center of emotion that must be activated for vivid memories. To keep them all healthy for filing information in the brain we need to consume sufficient omega-3 fatty acid DHA, a lot of leafy greens for B vitamins, at least five servings of snacks of seeds and nuts every week, antioxidant loaded blueberries, and olive oil for monounsaturated fat.

Mitochondrial dysfunction can cause many psychiatric disorders including mood disorders, autism, Huntington's disease, hyperactivity, Parkinson's disease, dementia and Alzheimer's disease, schizophrenia, depression, and bipolar disorder[558], [559], [560], [561], [562]. It is a very dynamic organelle in our cells and its impairment is related to birth and death of cells, movement and geometry of enzyme proteins, fidelity of mitochondrial quality control functions, synaptic plasticity, cellular resilience, dimensions and polarity of nerve cells, rate and timing of power (ATP) production, and metabolic disorders in general.

There are no reliable nutrition and exercise based therapies to treat mitochondrial diseases at the present [563] but positive results are accumulating

---

556   http:/ http://www.ncbi.nlm.nih.gov/pmc/articles/PMC3587793//www.sciencemag.org/content/263/5150/1128.abstract

557   http://www.ncbi.nlm.nih.gov/pmc/articles/PMC3587793/
558   http://www.ncbi.nlm.nih.gov/pubmed/19664343
559   http://www.nature.com/mp/journal/v6/n6/full/4000926a.html
560   http://www.ncbi.nlm.nih.gov/pubmed/22735187
561   http://www.sciencedirect.com/science/article/pii/S0925443909001653
562   http://www.jbc.org/content/288/5/3070.abstract
563   http://www.ncbi.nlm.nih.gov/pubmed/12394637

as to therapeutic values of intervention by nutritional cofactors such as coenzyme Q, vitamins B complex, C, E, K, and lipoic acid [564], [565]. Mitochondrial dysfunctions affect our digestive tract, eyes, heart, liver, kidneys, and skeletal muscles and a balanced methylation diet can do no harm but good.

Alzheimer's Disease

Alzheimer's disease presents the most common form of dementia characterized by memory loss. Other symptoms may include mood swing, poor judgment, misplacing items, and getting lost. Memory, language, and thinking simply begin to vanish [566].

Mitochondria are the major contributor to Alzheimer's disease as they deteriorate during our senior years [567]. We can now see in Petridish as to how the disease develops. This may help discovering new and effective drugs in the near future [568].

A NMDA receptor antagonist NAMENDA works well. Other drugs such as Aricept, Reminyl, and Cognix have been around for a while but the best preventive is a life-long methylation diet. Alzheimer's disease is for sure linked to mitochondrial damage [569], [570].

A heart healthy natural protein diet, physical activity, and social and cognitive stimulation can be very helpful in preventing Alzheimer's diseases. *Antioxidant nutrients and vitamins E and C must be included in the diet up to twice the normal RDA [571].*

Parkinson's Disease

Parkinson's disease is a neurological disorder due to loss of motor nerves in the brain as a result of mutation in mitochondrial genes. Brain cells begin to fail communicating well. There is a loss of dopamine production because of

564   http://www.ncbi.nlm.nih.gov/pubmed/12891154
565   http://biochemgen.ucsd.edu/mmdc/ep-15-16.pdf
566   http://www.medicalnewstoday.com/articles/142214.php
567   http://www.ncbi.nlm.nih.gov/pubmed/20442494
568   http://www.nia.nih.gov/alzheimers/announcements/2014/10/groundbreaking-alzheimers-model-pe-tri-dish-points-amyloid-disease
569   http://www.sciencedaily.com/releases/2009/04/090402143453.htm
570   http://www.clinlife.com/lpg/1351?gclid=CK-PgKfNq70CFYZcMgodVGYADQ
571   http://www.medscape.com/viewarticle/466037

degeneration of nerve cells that produce it [572], [573], [574], [575]. Over production of free radicals because of defective complex I of electron transport chain causes DNA and protein damage [576] resulting in not enough energy availability in time in places where it is needed in the brain, protein phosphorylation is compromised, abnormal proteins and neurological toxins accumulate, and calcium is no longer properly regulated. Pre- and post synaptic transport fails and communication stops . The very quality control function of mitochondria goes out of control because their morphological, biochemical, and physiological integrity is destroyed [577]. **In simple language we can say that nerves cells for locomotion die [578].**

Major symptom are weakness, trembling, uncontrolled movement that results from problems in axonal transport and loss of communication in brain cells. Treatments today include administration of dopamine antagonists and coenzyme Q_{10}.

Huntington's Disease

This inherited disease devastates young people in the age group of 30-40 years. The disease is caused by breakdown and wasting away of native brain cells in certain regions. The mitochondria simply melt down [579], [580], [581]. The result is loss of movement, thinking, learning and cognition, difficulty in swallowing, speaking, and controlling voluntary movements [582]. Muscles become rigid, eye movement slows down, and gait and pasture is impaired. Patients lose ability to organize, systematize thoughts, act and think well, and to know how to control their behavior.

Although there is no sure cure, proper nutrition in terms of avoidance of coffee, cheese and other dairy foods, and trans fat is useful. Reduced calorie

---

572   http://mitochondrialdiseases.org/parkinsons/
573   http://www.ncbi.nlm.nih.gov/pubmed/22735187
574   http://www.lef.org/protocols/neurological/parkinsons-disease/page-01
575   http://www.sciencedirect.com/science/article/pii/S0925443909001963
576   http://www.jneurosci.org/content/26/19/5256.short
577   http://perspectivesinmedicine.cshlp.org/content/2/2/a009332.full
578   http://www.sciencedaily.com/releases/2011/11/111110142104.htm
579   http://www.ninds.nih.gov/news_and_events/news_articles/mitos_fragmented_in_HD.htm
580   http://www.sciencedirect.com/science/article/pii/S0925443909001653
581   http://www.mayoclinic.org/diseases-conditions/huntingtons-disease/basics/definition/con-20030685
582   http://www.ncbi.nlm.nih.gov/pubmed/19682570

diets of fruits, vegetables, and whole grain products can improve memory and improve immune system [583], [584], [585], [586]. Regular exercise is of great help.

Depression

Depression, schizophrenia, and bipolar disorder are mitochondrial diseases[587]. Mitochondrial dysfunction plays a major role in pathophysiology of depression, stress, and anxiety [588], [589]. Low ATP production leads to lack of energy and fatigue , inability to concentrate, and weak immune system. Serotonin deficiency, inflammation, and depression seem to be interrelated[590]. Let us also note that the happy hormone serotonin is often of only dubious benefit. It induces release of stress hormone cortisol, causes irregular heartbeat, can cause appendicitis and inflammation of the intestine. Depending on high doses of serotonin against depression is known to back fire.

Schizophrenia

Schizophrenia is also a disease of mitochondrial dysfunction due to poor mitochondrial gene expression, poor rate of ATP production, altered cerebral energy metabolism, and involvement of dopamine in both hypo and hyper cycles in schizophrenia [591], [592]. Genes do not get decoded for protein production. Poor synaptic plasticity [593], poor signaling and gene expression [594], and mitochondrial gene mutations [595] are considered to be involved. Much more has to be learned about schezophrenia.

583   http://www.hdsa.org/images/content/1/2/12996.pdf
584   http://www.futuremedicine.com/doi/pdf/10.2217/nmt.11.69
585   http://www.futuremedicine.com/doi/abs/10.2217/nmt.11.69
586   http://www.mayoclinic.org/diseases-conditions/huntingtons-disease/basics/lifestyle-home-reme-
       dies/con-20030685
587   http://www.mitoaction.org/blog/psychiatric-disorders-mitochondrial-disease
588   http://www.nature.com/tp/journal/v4/n6/full/tp201444a.html
589   http://psych.lf1.cuni.cz/zf/publikace/b005.pdf
590   http://www.ncbi.nlm.nih.gov/pubmed/20691744
591   http://www.ncbi.nlm.nih.gov/pubmed/12472879
592   http://www.nature.com/mp/journal/v9/n7/full/4001532a.html
593   http://www.ncbi.nlm.nih.gov/pubmed/15006492
594   http://link.springer.com/article/10.1007%2Fs10059-012-2284-3#page-1
595   http://www.academicjournals.org/article/article1379934667_Chandra%20and%20Manatt.pdf

Bipolar Disorder

Mitochondrial function is the key to controlling bipolar disorder [596]. We can examine in-vivo brain chemistry by magnetic resonance spectroscopy and imaging [597]. The disease is because of loss of ATP production (bioenergetic controls) and neurochemistry of phospholipid metabolism. It is a disease of energy metabolism [598] and specific causes are changed morphology of mitochondria, increase in DNA mutation, poor regulation of protein production for electron transport chain and ATP production, and low brain pH. Naturally mitochondria are the drug target in all above disorders including those of mood. The objective is to link hormonal, metabolic, and signaling pathways.

A methylation diet in all these cases has to be designed carefully for antioxidants by emphasis on fruits and vegetables, for probiotics for gut health, and an optimum tryptophan intake. Too much serotonin is not all that good in case of these disorders. A commitment to regular breathing exercises can be greatly helpful in managing them.

4.05.07 Multiple Sclerosis

MS is a neuronal response to inflammation (axons gone wrong) controlled by defective nuclear and mitochondrial DNA. Unfortunately MS is both an autoimmune and neurological disease. The causes could be genetic, viral, autoimmunity, demethylation of DNA, mitochondrial dysfunction, free radical production, too much nitric oxide, ionic imbalance due to poor cellular clearance, and final loss of axons [599, 600, 601, 602].

Females of northern European heritage are more prone to multiple sclerosis. For a long time multiple sclerosis has been considered as a chronic inflammatory disease of the central white matter causing demethylation disorders. Myelin antigens in response to unknown causes are also considered to be the cause of autoimmunity problems. It appears to be a neuro-degenerative disorder caused mitochondrial dysfunction [603] including DNA defects, poor DNA repair, poor gene expression, faulty mitochondrial enzyme

---

596   http://www.plosone.org/article/info%3Adoi%2F10.1371%2Fjournal.pone.0004913
597   http://www.nature.com/mp/journal/v10/n10/full/4001711a.html
598   http://www.sciencedirect.com/science/article/pii/S0736574810003801
599   http://link.springer.com/article/10.1007%2Fs11011-012-9277-y#page-1
600   http://cmmg.biosci.wayne.edu/mitomed/index.php
601   http://journal.frontiersin.org/Journal/10.3389/fphys.2013.00169/abstract
602   http://cbr.meduniwien.ac.at/fileadmin/db_files/pub_art_177.pdf
603   http://www.ncbi.nlm.nih.gov/pmc/articles/PMC2790545/

system, and excessive stress due to free radical generation. The chromosomes involved are 5p13, 10p15, and 16 that regulate interleukin 2 and 7. Also, known is the fact that human leucocyte antigens (HLA), the class II factor in particular, underlie this potential autoimmunity problem.

Genetics of multiple sclerosis is complex and it involves many genes. Common symptoms are episodic occurrence of chronic excessive fatigue, spasm, and paralysis of muscles. Low vitamin D and oxidative stress are part of MS etiology.

Multiple sclerosis has celiac like symptoms and gluten protein avoidance is necessary. Gamma amino butyric acid can offset the deleterious effects of high glutamate and N-methyl D-aspartate that cause pain and even depression. Also, consuming sulfur containing amino acids like glutathione, N Acetylcysteine, taurine, and methionine and avoiding monosodium glutamate and artificial sweetener Aspartame can be of help. Good quality proteins like egg white must be part of diet for managing levels of serotonin and norepinephrinine. Foods for gamma aminobutyric Acid are yogurt, Korean Kimchi, tea, fermented foods, and germinated brown rice. We should keep in mind that GABA is an inhibitory neurotransmitter and its deficiency causes havoc on our brain [604]. Indirect stimulants such as almond, nuts, and broccoli should be part of regular diet for MS patients.

4.05.08 Cystic Fibrosis

Cystic fibrosis is an autosomal genetic disorder of lung, brain, and liver due to one gene inherited each from each parent. There are two mutations in mitochondrial DNA [605] causing an abnormal transport of chloride and sodium as thick viscous secretion. Transmembrane conductance regulator was identified in 1989 at 7q31.2 of chromosome # 7.

The disease of cystic fibrosis is tied to water chemistry and a dysfunctional redox system by way of poor voltage gated chloride [606] and poor acquaporin [607] water channel proteins. Organ functions change when water flow changes. At fault in this case is water-collagen network. Protons and hydronium ion flow with the help of light through the three layer prism of water to mitochondrial membrane, establish voltage, maintain magnetic moment. and improve redox.

604   https://suite.io/laura-owens/17v1266
605   http://www.ncbi.nlm.nih.gov/pubmed/12400067
606   http://www.ebi.ac.uk/interpro/entry/IPR001807
607   http://www.ks.uiuc.edu/Research/aquaporins/

The exclusion zone (EZ) of water in these three layers is the fourth living state of water. It is a few layers thick of water of thousands of H_3O^2 negatively charged liquid crystalline structures indifferent to charged solutes around hydrophilic protein surfaces [608]. We can call it living water as "solvent of life" capable of interacting with electromagnetic radiation and electromechanical properties. As such exclusion zone of water is a life supporting evolutionary design tthat facilitates protein dynamics, enzyme activity, cellular response, and mechanical signals in biology. Maintenance of its dense, viscous, and negatively charged alkanine state is essential to its critical functions [609], [610].

CFTR (cystic fibrosis transmembrane conductance regulator), a chloride ion channel protein in sweat glands, doesn't work. Chloride is trapped in the cell. If there is water channel there is array of magnetic particles (Orthogonal Array of Intermembrane Particles (OAPs) that contact collagen. OAPs assemble magnetic moment in cell membranes and creates voltage [611], [612]. There is problem of collagen crystallization and lack of aquaporin proteins. Actually, stress hormone cortisol destroys collagen by removing copper from its lysyl residues. There is no piezoelectric effect. Surprisingly the leptin receptor can sense this problem. We know that histamine as a cure rearranges OAPs. This is a good example of how critical is mitochondrial magnetism to health.

Simple exercise helps to amileorate cystic fibrosis and so do Yoga, breathing through skin, earthing and connecting to earth, walking on sandstone, and use of sense of touch. D shell electrons of transition metals can help due to their complicated electronic configuration of D shell electron and resultant magnetic field. Earth's current can conduct electricity through water-collagen network. Touch and message can change collagen. There is sufficient body of research suggesting that piezoelectric effects of pressure and electric and magnetic fields are propagated all over body including neocortex. Simple massage, therefore, is a good remedy for cystic fibrosis.

608   http://www.i-sis.org.uk/WFMEZ.php
609   http://www.wateriontechnologies.com/science.asp
610   http://www.ivoviz.hu/files/mr.pollack_005.pdf
611   http://www.ncbi.nlm.nih.gov/pmc/articles/PMC2784574/
612   http://jcs.biologists.org/content/108/9/2993.full.pdf

Diseases of Mitochondrial Gene defects

4.05.08 Lieber's Hereditary Optic Neuropathy (LHON)

When a photon hits our retina it puts 10,000 ions at work at our synapses. We are in trouble when we lose this power of mitochondria that controls perception of seeing.

LHON is characterized by painless bilateral sub-acute visual failure of one or both eyes beginning with ordinary blurring and then covering the entire central visual field. It is a single organ disease and the patient is declared legally blind [613]. *Actually, a single amino acid change in NADH: ubiquinine Oxidoreductase complex of the electron transport chain is the primary cause [614], [615].* This is the first complement of the chain encoded by the mitochondrial genome.

Vitamin E and coenzyme Q_{10} supplements may give some relief [616], [617].

4.05.09 Leigh Syndrome

Leigh syndrome is characterized by loss of energy production because of mitochondrial DNA mutation. The disease is characterized by increased lactate concentration in the blood. The symptoms show up between the age of three to twelve months. About 50% of affected patients die before their third birthday. Some 20-25% of patients are found to have this problem because of mitochondrial genome. Diagnosis is confirmed by genetic testing. The mutation is of course of maternal origin.

---

613   http://www.bec.ucla.edu/papers/Wallace_23.5.05_3.pdf
614   http://ghr.nlm.nih.gov/condition/leber-hereditary-optic-neuropathy
615   http://www.ncbi.nlm.nih.gov/pmc/articles/PMC3129042/
616   http://www.santhera.com/downloads/Sadun_2010_CurrOpinionReview.pdf
617   http://www.ncbi.nlm.nih.gov/pmc/articles/PMC3202309/

4.05.10 Retinitis Pigmentosa

Retinitis pigmentosa is also characterized by loss of energy production because of mitochondrial DNA mutation [618], [619]. Retina in the back of the eye is like the film in the camera. This is where the first stage of seeing begins. With loss of energy production both cone and rod type cells are affected and their millions of receptors fail to work.

Eyes receive and use the highest dose of glucose and oxygen from brain to be able to complete their job of seeing. The cone cells in our retina have twice as much large and packed mitochondria compared to the rod cells, all busy producing ATP energy for fast sequences of repolarization and depolarization for millions of photoreceptors. This is why they have high level of cytochrome C oxidase, complex IV of the electron transport system. *Low ATP supply thus means poor eye sight and the culprit is the mitochondrial gene.* Retinitis pigmentosa is primary retinal degenerations with autosomal, X-linked and mitochondrial modes of inheritance. A total of 40 genes have been identified to date that, when mutated, cause different forms of nonsyndromic retinitis pigmentosa [620].

4.05.11 Myoneurogenic Gastrointestinal Encephalopathy (MNGIE)

This is a disease that often occurs during the second and 5th decade in life. It can affect kidney, paralyse eyes, and affect drooping of eye lids. MNGIE gets worse with time. Luckily, only seventy people with this disorder have been reported globally [621].

MNGIE affects multiple body parts but mainly gastrointestinal tract and nervous system[622]. Caused by mutations in both copies of TYMP genes (autosomal recessive) that encodes enzyme thiamidine phosphorylase, MNGIE is characterized by dismotility of nerves and muscles of digestive system that cause early satiety, nausea, vomiting, mal-absorption, insufficient peristalsis, stomach rumbling, diarrhea, constipation, diverticulitis, and continuous weight loss. A build up of thiamidine causes not only the damage of mitochondrial

618   http://www.blindness.org/index.php?option=com_content&id=50&Itemid=67
619   http://www.ncbi.nlm.nih.gov/pubmedhealth/PMH0002024/
620   http://www.medscape.com/viewarticle/578594
621   http://ghr.nlm.nih.gov/condition/mitochondrial-neurogastrointestinal-encephalopathy-disease
622   http://ghr.nlm.nih.gov/condition/mitochondrial-neurogastrointestinal-encephalopathy-disease

DNA, but it interferes with DNA repair also. Another type of MNGIE (without leucoencephapathy) is caused by mutations in gene POLG.

Stem cell transplant seems to be a possible cure [623]. Another treatment is hemodialysis in order to remove circulating thiamidine [624].

4.05.12 Hearing Loss and Deafness

Mitochondrial hearing loss and deafness is characterized by mutations of genes that encode ribosomal and transfer RNA_s. Annual audiometric testing should be used to assess stability and progression. Hearing aids, speech therapy, culturally appropriate language training, and cochlear implantation are helpful. Aminoglycoside type antibiotics (streptomycin, gentamicin, kanamycin, tobramycin, and neomycin) must be avoided and so should be the foods with their residues [625], [626]. Biotin deficiency is also implicated in hearing loss and, therefore, a methylation diet with biotin rich weekly complements of berries, fruits, Swiss chord, carrot, almond, walnut, and eggs can be helpful.

4.05.13 Creatinine Deficiency Syndrome

Cerebral Creatinine Deficiency Syndrome(CCDS) occurs at the age of three months to three years [627]. Actually, there can be three deficiencies: guanidinoacetate methyltransferase, L-arginine glycine amidinotransferase, and that of creatine transporter. Mental disability, seizures, and autism like symptoms are common.

Diagnostic tests of urine ceatinine, creatin, and guadiniacetate are very helpful. Management of diseases includes dietary restriction on arginine and feeding of creatine rich beef, cod, and salmon. Vegetarian patients need to opt for supplements.

623 http://journals.lww.com/neurotodayonline/Fulltext/2008/07030/Stem_Cell_Transplant_Effective_for_Mngie.3.aspx http://www.neurology.org/content/67/8/1330.extract
624 http://www.neurology.org/content/67/8/1330.extract
625 http://www.farad.org/publications/digests/072005AminoglycosideResidues.pdf
626 http://www.livingnaturally.com/ns/DisplayMonograph.asp?StoreID=E32FA6C399AB-4C99897032581851D45D&DocID=condition-aminoglycosideinduceddeafness
627 http://www.ncbi.nlm.nih.gov/books/NBK3794/

4.05.14 Pyruvate Dehydrogenase Complex Deficiency (PDCD)

PDCD is a more common neurodegenerative disorder because of abnormal mitochondrial metabolism [628]. The disease is characterized by lactic acid build up and breakdown of citric acid cycle. Poor muscle tone, abnormal eye movement, and seizures are common and such symptoms can start at birth because of grey matter degeneration in the brain stem. Lactic acidosis is the most serious problem [629].

The disease is rare and affected individuals have right and left hemisphere disconnect. The inability to produce pyruvate dehydrogenase and associated enzyme for converting pyruvate to acetyl-CoA simply creates problems in partial and incomplete citric acid cycle.

4.05.15 Overuse of Antibiotics and Mitochondrial Dysfunction

Current research confirms that a majority of commonly prescribed antibiotics such as amionoglycocide, ampicillin, beta-lactams, ciprofloxan, kanamycin, macrolides, quinolones, streptomycin, and tetracycline cause mitochondrial damage [630]. This is found to more true of high dose prescription of antibiotics [631]. Certain antibiotics and drugs targeted to control bacterial infection may cause mitochondria to failure and dysfunction [632], [633]. **Drug induced mitochondrial toxicity seems to be a problem that health service providers have to contend with [634].** Antibiotics and drugs that kill bacteria by stopping protein synthesis can also stop protein synthesis and ATP production in mitochondria. Also, the very process of killing bacteria requires a surge of free radicals that cause collateral damage to mitochondria.

More serious is now often encountered food born poisoning by Lysteria, a bacteria that can get into our cytoplasm [635]. This is a very adaptable bacterium

628   http://emedicine.medscape.com/article/948360-overview
629   http://ghr.nlm.nih.gov/condition/pyruvate-dehydrogenase-deficiency
630   http://www.ncbi.nlm.nih.gov/pmc/articles/PMC3760005/
631   http://aac.asm.org/content/51/1/54.full
632   http://www.the-scientist.com/?articles.view/articleNo/36329/title/The-Downside-of-Antibiotics-/
633   http://stm.sciencemag.org/content/5/192/192ra85.editor-summary
634   http://www.mitoaction.org/blog/may-mito-meeting-drug-toxicity-mitochondria
635   http://www.nature.com/nsmb/journal/v12/n1/full/nsmb0105-1.html

capable of fooling our immune system. The practice of treating Lysteria infection by ampicillin poses collateral problem of damage to mitochondria [636].

Given the surge of free radical production by antibiotic administration to treat bacterial infection, it stands to reason that antioxidant N-Acetyl-L-Cysteine seems to prevent mitochondrial function. So should daily methylation diets rich in antioxidants, vitamins B-complex, A, C, E, and K. Mineral manganese is part of antioxidant enzyme super oxide dismutase and one needs to boost its intake by intake of nuts and seeds.

Diagnostic Methods and Procedures

4.06 Diagnostic Methods

Diagnosing mitochondrial diseases is difficult, diverse, and not well defined. Test results are not easy to interpret because diseases of diabetes, disorders of thyroid and parathyroid, and collagen vascular problems can have similar symptoms. All uncertainty notwithstanding, there are a number of approaches to diagnosis including testing for point mutation, biochemical examination of the muscle tissue, and visual examinations. Table 4.06.01 lists main methods of diagnosis.

Table 4.06.01 Diagnostic Methods for Mitochondrial Diseases	
Thor-Byrne-ier Method	**Secondary Evaluation**
> 2% Ragged Fiber in skeletal Muscle Biopsy.	Blood lactate and serum pyruvate
< 20% mean activity of Electron transport Complex (Polarography)	Lactate Pyruvate Ratio Amino acids in blood, urine, and cerebral fluid.
Abnormality of mitochondrial DNA	Organic acids in blood and cerebral fluid.
Lactate ^{31}P Magnetic Resonance Spectroscopy	Carnitine in blood, urine, and muscle biopsy specimen
Primary Evaluation	Ketones in blood and urine

636   http://www.ncbi.nlm.nih.gov/pubmed/10852095

Blood Pressure, routine EKG and echocardiogram	Urinary acylglycine as indicator of beta oxidation of fatty acids
Hemoglobin Ac Blood Counts Blood Lactate	Skin biopsy for mitochondrial structure by electron microscopy.
Serum Electrolyte	**Laboratory Evaluation**
Abnormal lactate, ketone, pyruvate, and 3-methylglutaconic acids in urine.	Repeat Testing
Point mutation of mitochondrial DNA	Repeat testing after fast or intravenous infusion of specific meals.
Assessment of retinitis pigmentosa	Point mutation confirmation as to specific mitochondrial phenotype.
	Southern Blot testing for a given mitochondrial phenotype.

Note: Mitochondrial phenotype refers to a patient with maternally inherited mitochondrial gene defects characterized by variations in complexes of electron transport chain [637].

Diabetic neuropathy and retinopathy are a common features of mitochondrial disease. Once a phenotype is determined clinically, mutational analysis on blood lymphocytes can offer further confirmations. Although Southern Blot detects large deletions and duplications, a dozen or so mutations can be assessed. The fact that mitochondrial structure is determined by nuclear DNA and that it can influence many mitochondrial diseases should not be overlooked. Unfortunately nuclear DNA effects remain unmapped. A stepwise diagnosis scheme of Table 4.06.01 is the only way to proceed. Muscle tissue is tested for electron transport chain activity and glycogen storage disease. Mitochondria from muscle and liver can be examined by polarographic method to assess the state of oxidative phosphorylation. In addition to not being definitive, the diagnoses based on electron microscopy, electron transport chain activity, enzyme analyses for fatty acid beta-oxidation, determinations of Coenzyme Q_{10}, carnitine, and acylcarnitine, and of oxidative phosphorylation are very expensive.

---

637   http://www.plosone.org/article/info%3Adoi%2F10.1371%2Fjournal.pone.0035160

Cure and Treatment of Mitochondrial Diseases

4.07 Treatments of Mitochondrial Diseases

Management of mitochondrial disease may include early diagnosis and treatment of diabetes mellitus, cardiac pacing, ptosis correction, and intraocular lens replacement for cataracts. Individuals with complex I and/or complex II deficiency may benefit from oral administration of riboflavin. There are very limited treatments for diseases due to genetic mutations are deletions. Our readers may like to review 34 citations that deal with mitochondrial diseases caused by mitochondrial DNA methylation, deletion, and /or mutations. Cases on diabetes and multiple sclerosis will no doubt receive critical scrutiny in near future. Too many challenges in fixing mitochondria gene mutations and deletions remain unattended [638]. A good methylation diet can be of definite value in prevention and even cure of mitochondrial diseases.

- A daily dose of vitamin B Complex is always good.

- Exercise and a restricted calorie methylation diet can reverse diabetic and cardiovascular problems.

- Resveratrol type phytoalexin and antioxidants PQQ and coenzyme Q_{10} may help even further by preventing damage to mitochondrial DNA.

Neurons don't turnover and we are to live with the ones we have as an infant and then adult. **There is always a possibility of 50 million mutations in one generation.** Such mutations can cause many unforeseen health problems. Zinc protein p53 and its gene on chromosome 17 are the guardian of genome [639], [640]. It is a tumor suppressor gene and if we get only one copy of this gene,

---

638   http://rarediseases.info.nih.gov/files/White_Paper_v3_8_FinalCGedits.pdf
639   http://www.ncbi.nlm.nih.gov/books/NBK22268/
640   http://ghr.nlm.nih.gov/gene/TP53

we are cursed to have cancer. Zinc deficiency per se can be carcinogenic [641]. Mother's gut bacteria affect fetus's brain via effective barrier [642], [643].

We can have our genome mapped for less than $1,000.00 and in less than 25 minutes for routine diagnostics. Old CRISPR (Clustered Regulatory Interspersed Short palindromic Receptors) mechanism that bacteria use to chop the DNA of their viruses uses a single nuclease protein Cas 9 is a "search and prune" enzyme. Potential values of CRISPR/Cas technology, literally a boon, are evolving in the areas of pathogen resistant crops, phage-free food fermentations, genome engineering, and treatment of single gene diseases of sickel-cell anemia and cystic fibrosis. We may soon be able to highjack and reprogram our cells by hand held sequencing machines capable of detecting malaria drug resistance, genetic variation as they relate to migraines, and relationship of gut bacteria with diabetes.

Sacropenia or loss of muscle mass as we age is a common problem. Muscle strength declines three times faster than the muscle mass as we age beyond the our 40th birth day because of multiple reasons: increased oxidative damage, increased uncoupling of proton motive force, decay of mitochondrial DNA, alterations of mitochondrial RNA and enzyme proteins, low energy production, decreased biogenesis of mitochondria, changes in mitochondrial fission and fusion, changes in mitochondrial turnover, and increased cell death [644]. Increased myostatin is the main cause of loss of muscle mass [645]. Strength-training exercise including simple lifting of weights or exercising with dumbbells or kettle bells helps reduce myostatin. A methylation diet, as a constant epigenetic switch, designed for a full complement of vitamins and minewrals can tone our muscles by supplying optimum energy. Vitamin D_3 supplement of 100 IU per day is known to reduce myostatin by 70% . We need to accept that cancer is a disease of aging because older cells are progressively more prone to development of tumors.

Included below is the list of major research institutions that our readers can consult for timely research on clinical and routine therapeutics against diseases due to mitochondrial gene defects. Nanobots are going to be the key answers to DNA (gene) editing and reprofiling of our mother's gene's in us for better health sooner than we can predict.

---

641   http://www.ncbi.nlm.nih.gov/pubmed/11077439
642   http://www.the-scientist.com/?articles.view/articleNo/41476/title/Mother-s-Microbes-Protect-Baby-s-Brain/
643   https://endgametime.wordpress.com/the-awakening-quantum-mechanics-of-the-human-brain-and-consciousness/

644   http://biomedgerontology.oxfordjournals.org/content/50A/Special_Issue/11.short
645   http://diabetes.diabetesjournals.org/content/58/1/30.full

Major research Institutions

Australian Mitochondrial Disease Foundation

Georgetown University, Medical Center

Foundation for Mitochondrial Medicine

Mitochondrial Research Guild

Mitochondria Research Society

North American Mitochondrial Disease Consortium

Wayne State University Mitochondrial Disease Program

University of Miami, Miller School of Medicine

University of Pennsylvania, Medical School

University of Rochester, Medical Center

United Mitochondrial Disease Foundation

University of Newcastle upon Tyne, Newcastle, UK, and Center for Brain

Research, Medical University of Vienna, Vienna, Austria.

5

Mitochondria may occupy almost fifth of the cell's volume and its matrix occupying 50% of total volume is a very powerful and yet crowded place. A human cell of miniscule 1000 cubic micron volume can have up to 5000 mitochondria in it with their 4 nanometer outer and inner membranes and 7 nanometer intermediate space. Most of electron carrying NADH and $FADH_2$ are created in Krebs Cycle for processing around 32-38 moles of electrons per day in the mitochondrial matrix. Our body is a self-organized processing center critically dependent on information flow, communication, and very tight regulation. It appears that quantum coherence is essential to portals of life energy and geometrically adept protein molecules, next in importance to DNA, make and shape our daily living.

Our 2000 Kcalories/day diet translates to 83.3 Kcalories/hr. Thus we are a small 310.56 BTU_s/hr or 90.99 Watts/hr nano-factory. It is the nano-scale operation that gives mitochondria the power to raise this power on demand to 400 Watts for a cyclist or much more for a heavy weight lifter. Our 7.5 trillion cells make 1.4×10^{21} ATP molecules per second by enzyme ATP synthase that revolves 47 times a second [646]. Every second, a single ATP synthase enzyme turning clockwise makes 100 ATP molecules by facilitating a flow of 300- 564 protons through its structure. We live by breathing protons and using their energy.

Fundamental to the grand process of power production is coupling of reduction-oxidation reaction. Our body in chemical terms is a REDOX system and we live by using free-energy and electrons and protons that make it possiblee. Behind 99.99 watts per hour power is the power of

---

646   http://www.bmb.leeds.ac.uk/illingworth/motors/calculat.pdf

nuclear genes, mitochondrial genes, the proteins that they make, and overall dynamics of immortal mitochondria. Cellular power derives from what we eat: antioxidants, essential minerals like iron, magnesium, copper, selenium, and zinc and vitamins A, D, E, K, and other isoprenoids and porphyrins heme proteins. Nutrients empower the molecular mechanics of protein molecules central to our life processes. Nutrients are are the key to tune up of our NAD^+ driven circadian clock. Llife is the spin of electrons and their game of track hurdle over enzyme proteins containg metallic conductors. Diets for good health, healthy mind, and longevity are embedded in our evolutionary startup from electrons and protons.

Chapter 5
SUMMATION

Our life processes are quantized and we live by the spins of electrons.

Triveni P. Shukla

Life and living is possible only by the power of mitochondria that act in our cells like magnetically sensitive **spintronic transistors**. If we were to travel through mitochondria, organ by organ, just for a day, week, or in some cases a month, we will find that these sausage like stiff and elongated cylinders in our cells are very mobile and versatie capable of changing their shapes better than a piece of play dough. We will see them fusing, separating, and changing their orientation. *We will see them living different lives in different cells of our organs.* They can take a fixed position to deliver ATP in case of heart muscles and can be wrapped around the flagellum in case of sperm. We will see how they kill our poorly performing cells and give birth to new vigorous ones for a longer life. Also, we will see them postpone our death If we were to travel long enough. Actually, if we started in the beginning of formation of a single cell from ovum and sperm, we will see why mitochondria from the mother's ovum gain dominance in providing initial energy. We will see virtually the power of ATP and the power of mitochondria in deciding the death and birth of our cells. We will see how mitochondria manage the spin of electrons. This travel will for sure constitute a knowledge in molecular biology of mitochondria which has yet to unfold in its entirety as a quantum phenomenon.

Biotechnology is progressing exponentially and It is possible that we will engineer a *picobot* **with nano-infrared camera** that will do the travel for us and reveal the life of mitochondria which, truth be told, is revealing our own life. Much greater social values will result if the picobot were to tell us as to how daily nutrients impact on the life of mitochondria as biobatteries that run our body functions and vital signs. We do know now that nutrition and life style choices are critical to mitochondrial functions as summarized below.

Maintaining Mitochondrial Health	
Close to 65% of all cancer is a matter of chance, a simple random error [647]. With the exception of basal cell carcinoma, liver cancer, and lung cancer, most other types of cancer including cancer of bone, ovarian cancer, and pancreatic and skin cancers are caused by errors by stem cells in copying DNA. Healthy mitochondria can be a boon in controlling cancer.	
Cellular Homeostasis	Homeostasis is direct result of calorie restricted methylation diet on time via a planned schedule. Good health is a physiological balance. osteoporosis and bone fracture are organizational failures.
Stable and Healthy mitochondria	Require complete methylation diet containing appropriate RDA of omega-3 fatty acids, magnesium, vitamin D, vitamin B complex, adaptogens, and antioxidants.
Stable DNA and RNA	Epigenetic control means control of exposure to X-rays, electric power grids, pesticides, herbicides, and antibiotics.
Our Stem Cells	We should never misuse our body during the first 40 years of life by smoking, drinking, and staying sedentary [648].
Healthy Cells	We must avoid overdose of refined carbohydrates and sugars. We need to ingest B_6 and magnesium for ATP production, breathe a lot for oxygen and increase blood flow for oxygen. Oxygen deficiency simply means death.

647   http://science.slashdot.org/story/15/01/01/2317246/65-of-cancers-caused-by-bad-luck-not-genetics-or-environment

648   http://wws.weizmann.ac.il/resdev/sites/weizmann.ac.il.resdev/files/stem%20cell%20update%20booklet%20160311.pdf

Maintaining Mitochondrial Health	
Healthy Mitochondria	The lysosome system in our cells should not be allowed to kill us. We need to consume a lot of polyphenolic antioxidants via colored fruits and vegetables and optimize production of free radicals.
Melatonin	Pineal gland is our soul as the regulator of endocrine system.Night hormone produced by pineal gland controls circadiam rhythm. We need to sleep at least 7 hours a day.
Preprogrammed Cell Death	Healthy mitochondria can manage death of our cells, prevent defective signaling and leptin resistance, and avoid obesity.
Master Gene p53	Unmutated tumor suppressor gene on chromosome 17 is critical to cancer free long-life. Loss of this gene means onset of cancer. The methylation diet must deliver zinc.
Leptin Sensitivity	Proper leptin level means good energy metabolism No leptin gene means obesity and osteoporosis. Leptin resistance precedes insulin resistance. Leptin tells **hypothalamus** via lateral hypothalamus receptors what all other cells in the body need in terms of hormonal balance, reproductive rate, cellular regeneration, and the very beginning of digestive process. Sunlight and leptin are tied by 50,000 hypocretin neurons. Leptin is also communicates with PPAR gamma, the Peroxysome proliferator activated receptor, in regulation of energy metabolism.
ROS Free Radicals	Reactive oxygen species are produced by mitochondria for signaling and fighting bacteria and viruses but too many of them are bad for our health and longevity.
MTOR	**Mammalian target of rapamycin** is responsible for nutrient signals, amino acid utilization, insulin production, and growth factors, and onset of cancer. Serine-threonine kinase necessary for cell proliferation and cell death, is inhibited by rapamycin.
SIRTUINS	These genes are guardians of our cell. They control NAD+/NADH ratio, DNA repair, stimulate antioxidant production, and work well in calorie restricted diets [649].

649   http://www.ncbi.nlm.nih.gov/pubmed/18419308

Maintaining Mitochondrial Health	
Heat Shock Proteins	Only 800 Daltons in size, **Ubiquitin** can also work as heat shock proteins. We can call them stress proteins that defend against inflammation and infection. We need them for staying healthy and ubiquination for autorepair during our sleep.
Inflammation	Methylation diets of chocolate, red wine, tea, herbs and spices, high protein, mushrooms, fruits and vegetables, omega-3 fatty acids, vitamin D, and whole grain products control inflammation.
Cortisol	Cortisol is the King of hormones in our evolution and flight-or-fight response in regard to stress is conserved in evolution. Exercise, yoga, and meditation keep it low.
Cold Thermo-genesis	Brown and beige fat cells produce more heat as infra-red radiation in place of ATP. Hormone leptin helps. CT is greatly therapeutic against weight gain and obesity [650].
Immune system	Consume probiotics, simple water, tea, cabbage, oats and barley, garlic, shell fish, chicken soup, sweet potato, and mushrooms. Take vitamin D supplements.
Exercise	Exercise leads to long telomere which in turn leads to longevity. We must consume antioxidants and exercise regularly.
High Sugar	High Sugar leads to glycation of Proteins and diabetes. We must keep refined sugar consumption below 20 grams a day and avoid consuming oxidized polyunsaturated fats via our daily diet.
Synergy of central nervous system and enteric brain	Digestive health is a barometer of good Health To ensure good enteric brain is to eat less, eat on time, eat variety, eat probiotics, avoid deficiency and overdose, and eat all essential fatty acids and amino acids, vitamins, and minerals present in a methylation diet.

This chapter includes many citations including antibacterial defense-1, calcium regulation-1, cell death and differentiation-3, cellular stress 2 and oxidative stress and cell death-6, epigenetic programming-5, gene

---

650   http://genesdev.cshlp.org/content/27/3/234.full

methylation-5, xenobiotic reactive oxygen species-2, glucose homeostasis by nutrient control-1, resveratrol-1, mitochondria and aging-1, mitochondria and various cancer-12, inflammatory response-1, mitochondrial biogenesis-4, mitophagy-7, mitochondrial diseases-2, mitochondria in glycolysis-1, mitochondrial dysfunction-3, respiration in cancer tissue-1, mitochondria and antioxidant dysfunction-1, mitochondrial genome instability-1, and thermogenic cofactors in mitochondria-1. These citations highlight the role of mitochondria as organelles that operate by quantum rules in using electrons, protons, and ions for running and controlling our life [651].

Power of Mitochondria

Let us now probe into cells in our body a bit deeper [652]. Our body has more than 10 trillion cells of 200 types. Some 7.5 trillion of them divide two trillion times a day [653]. There are estimates on number of cells in human body ranging from 10 to 30 trillions. Let us stay conservative at 10 trillion. The largest egg cells in ovarian follicles, the secretory cells in ovarian glands, cone cells in the eye, nerve cells in the brain, cells in our bone, and the smallest cell of sperm, all have the same DNA but perform different functions.

Nerve cells conduct impulses and electricity, muscle cells contract, and gland cells secrete. We grow by their specific function and their division. *The cells have their own life and chemistry with specific mix of proteins.* Two and a half trillion red blood cells are designed specifically for oxygen delivery and carbon dioxide removal. **Twenty billion of them die each day and are reborn**[654]. So do 400 billion plateletts and 10 billion white blood cells. They are reborn of stem cells in the bone marrow. Just to emphasize a total of two trillion of our cells die each day and then they are reborn [655]. **The rejuvenation of these cells is rigorously controlled**. When birth rate falls behind the death rate we begin to age. The cells are made of plasma membrane, a phospholipid bilayer comprised of polar heads on in and outside, of proteins embedded in the membrane for various tasks of transferring molecules, transporting ions, recognizing and communicating with cells by glycoproteins, receptor proteins, enzyme proteins, and junction

651   http://arxiv.org/ftp/arxiv/papers/1012/1012.3371.pdf
652   https://highered.mcgraw-hill.com/sites/dl/free/0072886161/323275/samplech04.pdf
653   http://www.newton.dep.anl.gov/askasci/mole00/mole00482.htm
654   http://www.biosbcc.net/doohan/sample/htm/Blood%20cells.htm
655   http://www.ncbi.nlm.nih.gov/pmc/articles/PMC1120576/

proteins. Inside the cell is membrane bound nucleus containing DNA, and various organelles including *double layered mitochondria* with its own genome of 37 genes capable of producing most of the enzyme proteins for the electron transport chain.

Mitochondria are known to have taken up residence in eukaryotic (including human) cells some 1.45 billion years ago. Their inner membrane is 800 nm long including 37 nm long cristae accommodating a 25 nanometer long electron transfer chain. *This permits about 320 chains with 60 electron careers capable of transferring electrons and translocating enough protons for producing 10^{21} ATP molecules per second.* An enzyme multiplicity in the matrix of mitochondria runs our life by running and controlling metabolism, producing proteins, killing and renewing the cell and the mitochondrion itself, and prolonging life by a cycle of daily birth and death of our cells. Water, hydrogen bonds between hydrogen and oxygen present in DNA and enzyme proteins, a bare hydrogen atom without its electron we call proton (H^+), unfolding and purposeful folding of enzyme proteins, and free radicals with their spins are the key to our evolution and the life today. We spin in action and thought just as the electrons spin in our mitochondria as each cell in our body uses around 3 X 10 $^{-10}$ Watts power [656]. In terms of ATP, a cell with a volume of 3000 mm^3 uses 10^9 molecules per day.

We exist in good health because our exclusively maternal mitochondria are endowed by our genetic makeup to efficiently and successfully process electrons and protons for energy production from foods we consume. We can succumb to many diseases of muscles, brain, nerves, kidneys, heart, liver, eyes, ears, pancreas, and other body systems when our mitochondria become inefficient and underproductive. High energy consuming organs like brain and muscles suffer the most because mitochondrial dysfunction simply means loss of energy and control of locomotive power.

Electrons can move at a speed that equals $1/137^{th}$ of the speed of light or 1,300 miles per second. In comparison sound travels at 1100 feet per second and light travels at 186,000 miles per second. The electrons spin 100 x faster than the speed of light or 1644 X 10^8 meters/second. That is 18.6 million miles per second. The spin angular momentum of an electron is 1/2 of the reduced Planck's constant. Free radicals also spin like electrons. Amazingly, magnetic memory of an electron spin is 1000 times that of a proton. It is amazing that human body has the wherewithall to interconvert and digitise speed of light we see, speed of sound we hear, and frequency of

---

656   http://book.bionumbers.org/what-is-the-power-consumption-of-a-cell/

vibration of an odorous molecule we smell. Even more amazing is the coding of these events in and on time by our DNA that helps make all the proteins and enzymes which in turn do actual works of metabolism including brain functions and consciousness.

5.01 Mitochondrial Evolution

Humans came from a single women, the mitochondrial Eve, some 200,000 years ago [657], [658], [659]. Y-chromosomal Adam lived only 190,000 years ago. This tracing is done by maternal mitochondrial genes. Simply follow mutations in your mitochondrial DNA and you will find who you are related to. A much more convincing understanding of human genetic variations can come when maternal mitochondrial DNA is studied side by side with paternal Y-chromosome [660], [661]. Of a very old endosymbiotic bacterial origin mitochondrial DNA of maternal inheritance has high copy numbers, suffers from greater mutations by substitutions and deletions, and doesn't recombine. [662],[663]. Take the example of a muscle cell with 1000 mitochondria each with 1000 copies of circular DNA. This gives the cell highly amplified 1 million DNA pool compared to only 2 copies in the nuclear DNA [664]. These 1 million genes are responsible for much of our daily metabolism, energy production, apoptosis or programmed cell death, birth of new cells, protein transformation, and polarization of membranes for ion movement. Being in the vicinity of electron transport chain, 16,500 base pairs of mitochondrial DNAs are prone to somatic mutation in our life time due to free radical damage. Thus the unstable and poorly regulated mitochondrial genes cause numerous health problems [665].

Metabolism by mitochondria and immunity tied to diet dependent gut bacteria seem to be related [666]. Neurological diseases like autism seem to have their origin in functions of our gut microbiome and mitochondria

657   http://www.nature.com/nature/journal/v325/n6099/abs/325031a0.html
658   http://evolution.berkeley.edu/evolibrary/news/071101_genealogy
659   https://www.eva.mpg.de/fileadmin/content_files/staff/paabo/pdf/Fu_Revised_CurrentBiology_2013.
       pdf
660   http://www.ncsu.edu/project/bio183de/Black/genetech1/genetech1_news/ingman.html
661   http://www.ncbi.nlm.nih.gov/pubmed/16124858
662   http://www.ruf.rice.edu/~bioslabs/studies/mitochondria/mitorigin.html
663   http://www.ncbi.nlm.nih.gov/pubmed/10690412
664   http://www.geneticorigins.org/mito/mitoframeset.htm
665   http://www.surrey.ac.uk/qe/O2.htm
666   http://www.ncbi.nlm.nih.gov/pubmed/24416709

[667]. Many chronic diseases have multiple origins in gut microbiome, mitochondria, and nuclear DNA [668]. Our default diet of low fiber and high refined sugar is known to cause colorectal cancer and inflammatory bowel syndrome [669]. Not known for sure but it is suggested by credible research that appropriate pre- and probiotic diets of restricted calories may have considerable health benefits. Mitochondria with oldest bacterial symbiotic DNA system dedicated to our evolution are the gate keeper of our life and cell's health [670, 671].

To repeat and to re-emphasize, mitochondrial dysfunction is known to be responsible for aging, neurological disorders, cardiac dysfunction, diabetes, and muscular problems. Biogenesis of new mitochondria is a dire daily need for our health and satisfactory vital signs and much of it depends on what, when, and how we eat. Also, in order to stay healthy in the long haul we need to avoid over use of antibiotics and intake of refined sugars and drugs in general because they ruin mitochondria.

Power of Hydrogen in Our Daily Foods

5.02 Conversion of Food into Electrons and Protons for Energy

The Quantum Conundrum

Mitochondria seem to function by the quantum play book. Looking keenly at what goes on in mitochondria in terms of electron tunneling or hopping in cytochrome C called electron transfer, we are witnessing meeting of quantum physics and biology in a little clearer terms [672]. *The molecules in retina change shape with just a few photons* and other biomolecules are known to be photon sensitive. *Magnetic resonance image depends on many*

---

667   http://www.psychology.uwo.ca/pdfs/autism/GAHMJ-Nov2013-MacFabe.pdf
668   http://www.discoverymedicine.com/Alain-Li-Wan-Po/2013/05/24/the-human-genome-its-modifica-
       tions-and-interactions-with-those-of-the-microbiome-and-the-practice-of-genomic-medicine/
669   http://www.sciencedaily.com/releases/2011/05/110503132658.htm
670   http://jgp.rupress.org/content/139/6/395.full
671   http://www.ohsu.edu/nod/documents/2012/05-03/Duchen2010.pdf
672   http://www.ncbi.nlm.nih.gov/pmc/articles/PMC2839811/

trillion simultaneous spins in a macroscopic biological sample. The spinning protons act like a mini-magnet. Actually, perception per se may be a matter of spin coherence[673],[674]. Furthermore, functions of protein complexes and enzyme reactions appear to have quantum dimensions. This may very well be true of nutrient conversion, modification, and extraction of energy by mitochondria directed to good health and disease control in each cell of our body [675]. The molecular machines of electron transport, ATP synthesis, and protein making as directed and commanded by DNA via ribosome seem to have quantum dimensions as well [676]. Quantum laws operate when we hear, touch, smell, taste, and see. They operate inside mitochondria where molecular motor ATP synthase and ATP hydrolase function and inside the nucleus where enzyme helicase separates two strands of our DNA by a molecular ratchet. Our perception and may be even consciousness, as is now suggested by large body of research, are quantum mechanical in nature.

Quantum physics and electrodynamics define all molecules including the molecules of life involved in molecular recognition and workings of proteins and DNA within our cells. *Orbitals of big and small molecules define and direct stability of matter no matter where and* quantum effects, it appears, do apply to nano-scale bioconversions, signaling, and enzyme functions in and outside mitochondria. Our daily metabolism, cellular communications, health and life, and even consciousness are seemingly governed by quantum effects because they deal with photons, electrons, photons, ions, and atoms. For example

- **Quantum coherence plays a big role in electron transport in mitochondria [677]. There is an electron tunneling effect in complex I (NADH-ubiquinone oxidoreductase) where electrons are transferred across 90 A from NADH to ubiquinone and protons are translocated across inner mitochondrial membrane to the intermediate space for eventual ATP production [678]. The enzyme translocates four protons simultaneously. Actually, Fe/S clusters of enzyme NADH-Ubiquinine oxidoreductase have tunneling pathways.**
- **ATP synthase works by quantum mechanical principle. It does so by way of a continuous change in its conformation and geometry.**
- **Proton tunneling is known for most enzyme reactions that break bonds and split molecules. Energy produced by breaking of ATP**

673   http://www.ncbi.nlm.nih.gov/pmc/articles/PMC3800149/
674   http://journal.frontiersin.org/Journal/10.3389/fpsyg.2014.00554/full
675   http://www.sciencedaily.com/releases/2013/06/130627142404.htm
676   http://www.sciencedaily.com/releases/2015/01/150107101405.htm
677   http://rsfs.royalsocietypublishing.org/content/2/4/522.full
678   http://www.pnas.org/content/107/45/19157.full

bond by a spoonful of enzyme ATPase can produce as much torque as an average car's engine. An arginase finger acts as spark plug for current conduction. We are beginning to understand that the nano-scale Brownian motors like ATPase that hydrolyses ATP for producing mechanical energy presents a quantum phenomenon [679], [680]

- Mitochondrial proteins in retinal ganglion and their special neurons with photoreceptors interact with light [681]. *The trick is in photon directed transition of cis to trans isomers by quantized energy.* Mitochondria emit light[682] and they interact with visible light. Actually, we emit a million more Infrared photons than we often receive visible light photons with open eyes.

- A simple amino acid of positive charge plays wonders in converting photons to electrons by protein rhodopsin. Research shows that our nerve cells guide photons and are capable of producing biophotons [683].

- High speed lasers have been used at University of California, Berkeley by Greg S. Englet to study cellular quantum processes, e.g., movement of light energy in bacterial cells [684], [685].

- We have evidence of electron tunneling and electron transport in DNA [686]. DNA is separated into two strands by a motor like enzyme helicase that scoots along DNA to do its job via a ratchet like two hand mechanism

- Spontaneous DNA mutations take place by quantum effects also [687].

- Smell , a dominant determinant of food flavor, presents a case of quantum tunneling involving vibrational energies [688], [689]. We choose to eat by smell and taste and therefore by indirect quantum effects.

- Quantized set of spectral lines used in biology routinely for fingerprinting molecules are much more common place example.

No doubt all this is abstruse, abstract, and often incomprehensible. But this spooky wonder of quantum mechanics may soon turn into a little more

679   http://www.ncbi.nlm.nih.gov/pubmed/23345777
680   http://www.cnr.berkeley.edu/~goster/pdfs/RSReview.pdf
681   http://en.wikipedia.org/wiki/Photoreceptor_cell
682   http://arxiv.org/ftp/arxiv/papers/1012/1012.3371.pdf
683   http://arxiv.org/ftp/arxiv/papers/1012/1012.3371.pdf
684   http://hplusmagazine.com/2009/06/01/spooky-world-quantum-biology/
685   http://www.solvayinstitutes.be/publications/Report2010.pdf
686   http://www.pnas.org/content/107/45/19157.full
687   file:///C:/Users/Owner/Downloads/mcfadden_and_al-khalili.pdf
688   http://www.safaribooksonline.com/library/view/quantum-effects-in/9781139949040/Text/chapter12.html
689   http://www.ncbi.nlm.nih.gov/pmc/articles/PMC2839811/

understandable *biological relativity*. Quantum mysteries may be akin to protein folding, gene mutations, brain as a quantum computer, and many critical neuronal processes. We need to know quantum effects in proteins, DNA. RNA, and other macromolecules of life with much more clarity than we know today. **One hundred fifty years ago Thomas Hennery Huxley said that soon humans will take evolution in their own hands.** *Let us keep in mind that life is a molecular process that operates by the quantum playbook and q*uantum biology is emerging as a new frontier in medicine, nutrition, and health sciences. We have not taken evolution in our hands yet but for sure we are expediting it fast by way of genetic engineering. Our cells *continuously emit ultraweak infrared electromagnetic radiation . In case of* nerve cells, the intensity of biophotons correlates with blood flow in the brain, neural activity, cerebral energy metabolism, oxidative processes, and alpha-wave production; they deal with electron, proton, and photon type quantum particles.

The big question is "how does a cell mange coherence by dampening noise?" How does it respond to toxins? How do cells adapt? How does DNA repair itself? Even bigger question is information coding by DNA for 26,000 proteins. *Are genes written in quantum letters involving hydrogen bond and information is coded quantum mechanically*? Does vision involve quantum computing and is the body-mind interaction and consciousness itself quantum effect? Too many questions remain unanswered. Answers to these questions may not unravel soon but they will soon once we understand the quantum behavior of mitochondria.

Erwin Schrödinger way back in 1944 rightfully began with question of what is life [690]. Research works during the last 10 to 15 years do demonstrate that quantum mechanics can describe nanoscale life processes [691]. **Life, no doubt, is about constant fighting for Gibb's free energy, call it negative entropy.** Lets leave the spooky physics aside and expand on what we know of nutrition that sustains life.

Electrons and Protons from Daily Food

By now we have established that mitochondria in our cells are electron and proton processing organelle for producing chemical energy ATP from

---

690   http://www.ncbi.nlm.nih.gov/pmc/articles/PMC2839811/#c80
691   http://www.ncbi.nlm.nih.gov/pmc/articles/PMC2839811/

the electronic energy in C-H bonds of glucose or other foods that we eat. As a matter of fact, electron transport chain is a molecular machine that facilitates transfer of electrons to oxygen for its reduction to water. Stepwise transfer of energy takes place as electrons travel the ladder of reduction potentioal. Concomitant translocation of protons also happens as a coupled process used for production of chemical energy (ATP) by the molecular rotary motor called ATP synthase. Five complexes of proteins of electron transport chain, including the one that makes energy molecule ATP, reassemble and reorganize themselves for energy extraction and coversion [692]. Our cells respire and harvest back the sun's energy via workings of the electron transport chain. One mole of electron delivers an energy value of of 216 KJ. Sun helps us day by day by letting plants harvest **photon power** and make energy molecule ATP, transfer and store it in glucose, amino acids, and fats. **Photosynthesis *process makes electron rich glucose molecule at the expense of 18 ATP molecules* [693], [694]**.

One KCal is 4.184 KJ. Dividing 2000 Kcal or 8368 KJ present in an average diet by 216 KJ/mole of electron yields *38.74 moles of electrons required to sustain* an average human body. We should note that each pair of electrons produces 10 protons which become energy molecule ATP for running our daily life.

Do we need 38.74 moles of electrons per day? For an average person of 70 kg, the answer is a probable no. He or she needs to restrict calories in daily diet a little and stay on the lower end of a range 32-38 moles of electrons per day.

Let us reexamine then a daily diet of 1,880 Kcal comprised of 30 gram fat (270 Kcal), 55 gram protein (220 Kcal), and 377.5 gram total carbohydrate composed of 30 gram dietary fiber and 347.5 gram complex carbohydrate (1,390 Kcal) . Of the latter, no more than 20 gram per day should be refined sugar. Our mitochondria can extract 34.86 moles of electrons from the restricted diet allowing themselves for a 10% relief from overwork.

Daily calories from glucose alone calculates to be 347.5 X 4.00 = 1,324 kilocalories per day. This assumes that we have no deficiency of electron carriers for ATP production due to poor functioning of glycolysis and Krebs cycle (Table 6.01.01). On an average bonds in glucose have 680 kilocalories and our cells get 613 kilocalories by burning glucose to carbon dioxide. This

692   http://stringentresponse.blogspot.com/2011/02/observer-effect-in-biology-schrodingers.html
693   http://www.mrothery.co.uk/photosynthesis/photosynth&respnotes1.htm
694   http://dwb.unl.edu/Teacher/NSF/C10/C10Links/mills.edu/RESEARCH/FUTURES/JOHNB/path-
        ways/806.html

is 613/680 = 90% efficiency. The burning or oxidation process produces 10 Moles of NADH and 2 Moles of $FADH_2$ accounting respectively for 100 and 12 Moles of electrons (Table 5.01.01). The total proton power thus is 112 Moles.

Note: Since glucose has molecular weight of 180 gram, the daily intake of 347.5 gram glucose is 1.93 Moles of glucose. Thus we have 11.62 X 1023 molecules of glucose supporting our body per day.

I calculate that a total of 112 moles of protons translocate across the inner mitochondrial membrane at the expense of 22.4 moles of high energy electrons from electron carrier molecules. The electron carriers recycle because at a given instant we have no more 2 gram or 18.06×10^{20} molecules of NAD in our body. The daily need of electron carriers (table 5.01.01) must be met by an intake of prerequisite amount of NAD^+ and, therefore, vitamin B_3 niacin becomes a key nutrient of methylation diet (table 5.01.02).

Table 5.01.01 ATP Production per Glucose Molecule		
Stages	**Molecules/Glucose Molecule**	**ATP Yield**
Glycolysis (cytoplasm)	2 ATP used in preparatory work	- 2
	Production of Triose Phosphate	4
	NADH Produced	6
Link Reaction	2 NADH produces i pyruvate	6
Krebs Cycle (Mitochondrial Matrix)	2 ATP per Acetyl CoA	6
	6 NADH /3 Acetyl CoA	18
	2 FADH per Acetyl CoA	4
Total		38
Note: 1: average yield is believed to be 32; Note 2: There is 2 gram NAD in our body at a given instant.; Note 3: 10 Protons translocate with each pair of electron.		

Since mitochondria on average produce 36 molecules of ATP/molecule of glucose, 1.93 Mole of glucose produces 61.76 Moles of ATP and uses 1.93 X 6.00 = 11.58 moles of oxygen. *Every liter of oxygen thus accounts for 11.58 Kcal.* It stands to good reason then that both glucose and oxygen have got to be controlled well for good health. Control of oxygen delivery by exercise, deep breathing, restriction of calories, and even oxygen restriction to the electron transfer system of mitochondria is very healthful and therapeutic [695], [696], [697].

Table 5.01.02 RDA of Electron Transfer Nutrients in Methylation Diet that Promote Electron transfer in Mitochondria by Electron Carriers		
Key Cofactor	Precursor	Niacin RDA
NAD/NADH[698]	Niacin (B_3), tryptophan, aspartic Acid	20 mg
FADH/FADH$_2$	Riboflavin (B_2)	1.7 mg
CoenzymeQ$_{10}$	A benzoquinone with 10 isoprenes, High concentration in heart and lung mitochondria	1200 mg
Note: Methylation diet is perfect for health of mitochondria.		

Tight Control of Daily Living Process:

Our daily living is by no means random and a tight control of glucose is a physiological necessity. Glucose enters our cells by an elaborate control mechanism involving a carrier protein gated by hormone insulin. Basal glucose level in the cell is 5 mMole or 0.9 gram per liter. Its entry in the cell is regulated by glucose transporter proteins[699], [700]. Our nerve cells use only glucose for energy and they need just-in-time supply because they can't store it [701]. The major activities of neurons including manufacture and transport of neurotransmitters and transmission of signals are energy intensive and, therefore, glucose intensive. I should relate a story of my childhood here.

All through grades 7 through 12, I never ate lunch and neither did other students in schools all over India in my region. That is the low calorie side of my diet. Also I am aware of the fat that whenever a guest was given a glass of water, some sweets, sugar, or high sugar snacks were a must accompaniment. This I now believe gave the guest a boost of glucose. I for

695   http://www.ncbi.nlm.nih.gov/pmc/articles/PMC390920/
696   http://www.ncbi.nlm.nih.gov/books/NBK54112/
697   http://www.pnas.org/content/82/24/8384.full.pdf
698   http://www.ncbi.nlm.nih.gov/pmc/articles/PMC2905054/
699   http://www.ncbi.nlm.nih.gov/pubmed/7926364
700   http://life.umd.edu/classroom/bsci426/glucosetransport.pdf
701   http://www.fi.edu/learn/brain/carbs.html

sure had a restricted calorie diet because I never consumed more than 1600 calories during my teen years. How did my mitochondria managed temporal and quantitative glucose control in this *calorie restriction case* and how did they manage when I succumbed to an altogether different dietary habit when I came to the United States in 1964 remains a burning question in my mind even today? Our body it appears makes a lot of needed adjustments in a wide range.

The Case of Brown and Beige Fat and Thermogenesis

Brown fat cells are loaded with iron containing mitochondria. They are thermogenic and can generate a lot of heat. Regulated by norepinephrine, a small 33,000 MW protein thermogenin found in inner mitochondrial membrane of brown fat cells can uncouple ATP production and help produce non-shivering heat[702]. These are anion carrier proteins that return proton H^+ back to inner mitochondrial membrane from the outer membrane making them unavailable for ATP production[703].

We need to get rid of ectopic fat, fat in places where it doesn't belong, at all cost by a combination of balanced diet, induced thermogenesis, exercise, and yoga. **Examples of ectotic fats are paracardial fat, intramuscular fat, and fatty liver that readily lead to inflammatory cytokine production, type II diabetes, insulin resistance, and osteoporosis.** What we want is more and more of brown fat. Shivering a little in house kept at 60 degrees F can be a great idea for themogenesis and weight control. Ectopic fat secretes less of hormone adipopectin that regulates glucose and fatty acid metabolism, energy balance, and insulin resistance [704], [705].

The question then is "Can we control weight gain by diets that induce thermogenesis by brown fat?" Does cooling help lose weight? Can we alter mitochondrial function to increase metabolic rate and diet induced thermogenesis? There is only 0.492 moles or 250 gram ATP in our body at a given time but it uses 100-150 moles ATP or 50-75 Kg per day by recycling just in time. Shouldn't we control this wide range? Can we control the recycle rate for ATP? Can dietary ingredients increase thermogenin production by stimulating mitochondria? *The answer is yes because caffeine, green tea,*

---

702   http://www.ncbi.nlm.nih.gov/pubmed/9597749
703   http://www.ncbi.nlm.nih.gov/gene/7350
704   http://care.diabetesjournals.org/content/26/8/2442.full
705   http://www.nature.com/nm/journal/v7/n8/full/nm0801_941.html

fucaxanthin, and resveratrol do so by stimulating UCP 1 (uncoupling protein 1) production [706]. Peptide hormone irisin (encoded by gene FNDC5 and named after a Greek Goddess) increases when we do aerobic exercise and it can slim us down by converting white fat into thermogenin UCP 1 producing beige fat [707]. The Irisin in beige fat seems to have different yet unidentified genetic pathways including that of longevity[708].

Major thermogenic nutrients in our diet are short chain fatty acids of cheeses, caffeine, EGCG (eggalocatechin gallate), bitter orange, capsicum, ginger, guar gum, and pyruvate are dietary thermogenics. Catecholamine like norepinephrine and leptin can modify thermogenesis for weight reduction. To get maximum benefit, we must reduce alcohol and fat consumption in view of 13 ATP molecules produced per molecule of alcohol and 324 molecules of ATP from an average fat molecule (see note below) and increase consumption of methylation diet that includes avocado, coconut oil, egg , oatmeal, olive oil, quinova, sweet potato, tomato, nuts and seeds for low calories and low fat but rich in vitamins and minerals.

The best way to slow rate of ATP production is to do high rate intermittent exercise, intermittent calorie restriction and fasting two days a week like in Norway, and intermittent oxygen restriction. Routine cardio exercise program should incorporate chin up, sqauting, and squat thurts. Doing cortisol reducibg and stress reducing yoga should be part of the exercise program.

Add to this a whole grain and lentil based balanced dish topped with well ripened cheddar cheese and flavored with hot pepper with coffee or green tea as a beverage should make a great methylation diet for uncoupling oxidative phosphorylation and inducing weight loss by thermogenesis. Our daily diet can be a good mitochondrial medicine (Table 5.01.02). Vitamin B$_3$ or Niacin for balanced NAD/NADH ratio and an adequate coenzyme Q$_{10}$ RDA should be part of daily diet for people of advanced age.

A dietary warning is to avoid sugar, eat antioxidants and fatty acids as thermogenics, restrict calories, and exercise regularly.

---

706   http://web4.biotivia.com/bioshapeweightloss/ingredients.html
707   http://www.thepeachfactor.com/smoother-firmer-slimmer/irisin-the-new-hormone-that-makes-your-fat-cells-burn-fat.html
708

> Note: An electron rich fat molecule with 3 fatty acids of 18 carbons generates (3 X 18)/2 = 27 acetyl CoA molecules capable of making 27 X 12 = 324 ATP molecules. We need to always control our total fat intake to 25% of total calories and avoid trans fat. Twenty five percent of an 1,800 Calories diet is 450 Calories from 50 gram fat from eggs, butter, and all other sources of plant oils, seeds, and nuts.

The Health of Mitochondria

5.03 Mitochondrial Health

Mitochondrial health is all about daily diet and lifestyle. Self-regulating and self-auditing mitochondria are a system of enzyme structures and cofactor molecules. Their health is our health and longevity. Optimum assembly of Complex I subunits determines aging by keeping production of reactive oxygen specis to a minimum. Mitochondria enhance longevity by regulating sress response and apoptosis or death of cells. Behind it all is body wide signaling and communication[709]. A restricted calories methylation diet and holding breath for restricted oxygen supply does seem to enhance longevity.

A turtle can live 150-193 years with a small 16.787 kilobyte genome. Do changes in structure per se account for this difference [710]? Why do bowhead whales live 200 years? Flatworms and lobsters are almost immortals and jellyfish (Turritopsis nutricula) is truly an immortal. Does the secret lie in their ability to repair and control quality of DNA? or is it the ability of mitochondria to manage its proteins selectively and more precisely [711]. From what we know today in the human case, we can live longer in good health by preventing free radical damage to mitochondrial DNA and by restricting total daily calorie intake. Exercise and calorie restriction are great complementary therapies [712]. Although behind Japan and UK, US has already attained a male life expectancy of 79 years. The problem in US is incidence of chronic cardiovascular and neurological diseases, cancer, and diabetes.

---

709   http://www.sciencedirect.com/science/article/pii/S0014579301021998
710   http://www.pnas.org/content/95/24/14226.long
711   http://www.the-scientist.com/?articles.view/articleNo/35673/title/Inhibit-Mitochondria-to-Live-Longer-/
712   http://www.ncbi.nlm.nih.gov/pmc/articles/PMC2801852/

5.03.01 Exercise, Yoga, Meditation, and Mindfulness

Exercise, yoga, meditation, and mindfulness have similar effects on our daily health because everyone of these lifestyle choices tune our metabolism up by dealing with mitochondria and its electron and proton managing system. They have direct effect on the rate of oxygen supply. Oxygen transport to our cells is critical and our current understanding of the mechanism of transport and its delivery is a bit poor [713]. The question is "how do our cells optimize oxygen delivery under a condition of very low partial pressure of 0.0053 KPa (0.0000398 mm of mercury) ? Oxygen concentration in our cells is far less than in the blood. How does intermittent oxygen restriction prolong longevity and mitochondrial health [714]? What controls rate of consumption of oxygen by cytochrome oxidase, the fourth complex of the electron transport chain. Does oxygen itself modifies the rate [715].

There is no doubt that exercise increases health span [716]. Exercise delays age-associated frailty and it can increase mitochondrial function and cortical BDNF (brain derived neurotrophic factor) [717]. Over expression of genes that encode antioxidant enzymes glutathione peroxidase and manganese superoxide dismutase increases life span [718],[719]. *But as we age, number of mitochondria decreases and grip strength and neuromuscular coordination declines because of lack of antioxidant enzymes. A simple standing up, longer than we spend time sitting, can help lose 500-1000 calories per day* [720], [721], [722] *and yet make more* new mitochondria for strength and vigor [723].

The real remedy lies in self-examination and introspection. I should call it relaxation response taught today in 60% of medical schools. A Harvard study shows that yoga affects genes for mitochondrial energy production [724], [725] and yoga can be used as a cure for PTSD [726]. Mindfulness or my practice of age old *Akaagrata, that I can personally testify, to* can reduce

---

713   http://jeb.biologists.org/content/210/12/i.2
714   http://www.ncbi.nlm.nih.gov/pubmed/16770005
715   http://www.jbc.org/content/271/31/18672.full
716   http://www.longevityandhealthspan.com/content/2/1/14
717   http://circ.ahajournals.org/content/130/Suppl_2/A12182.abstract
718   http://www.ncbi.nlm.nih.gov/pubmed/7824577
719   http://www.agrigenic.com/enzymes.htm
720   http://www.precisionnutrition.com/sitting-standing-walking-work
721   http://www.bbc.com/news/magazine-24532996
722   hthttp://fitstar.com/high-intensity-exercise/tp://www.mayoclinic.org/healthy-living/adult-health/expert-answers/sitting/faq-20058005
723   http://fitstar.com/high-intensity-exercise/
724   http://www.mdmbac.com/meditation-yoga/harvard-study-shows-meditation-immediately-alters-gene-expression/
725   http://hms.harvard.edu/news/harvard-yoga-scientists-find-proof-meditation-benefit-11-21-13
726   http://commonhealth.wbur.org/2010/12/harvard-brigham-medical-study-yoga-veterans-ptsd

chronic pain [727]. Relaxation response secured by transcendental meditation, Zen Yoga, or practice of mindfulness reduces stress which is the mother of all inflammatory chronic diseases [728]. Positive health benefits, it is believed, come from making new mitochondria and preventing mutation of their genes.

5.03.02 Calorie and Oxygen Restriction

Calorie restriction diet and its effect on overall health, longevity, weight control and mitochondrial function is a very hot and productive research area today [729], [730], [731],[732],[733]. *It accounts for reduced electron flow, reduced proton leak, and reduced production of Reactive Oxygen Species (ROS) or free radicals.* Furthermore, it relates to hormone homeostasis, insulin sensitivity, inflammation, death of cells, antioxidant response, redox system of the plasma membrane, and protein turn over. **Calorie restriction is the best non-genetic intervention for longevity because it eliminates mitochondrial dysfunction, prevents diabetes and obesity, reduces blood pressure and arteriosclerosis, and combats neurological diseases of Parkinson's Alzheimer's, and even multiple sclerosis by proper fatty acid transport, and lipid composition shift.** It can reduce DNA mutation and help manage diseases of eyes, kidney, and liver. This is too much to claim but it seems to be true because restricted calorie intake influences

- Bioenergetic sensors NADH and free radicals.

- Master integrators AMP kinase, SIRT 1, SIRT 2, and SIRT 3.

- Antioxidant Response elements (ARE) and Nnuclear transcription Factors Nrf1 and Nrf2 for enzyme antioxidant production in response to stress due to environmental chemicals[734]. DNA does respond to electrophilic chemical toxins, produces ARE that works by binding with transcription factors. There are 84 genes involved including those for glutathione peroxidase, peroxiredoxin, and superoxidedismutase [735].

727   http://www.prohealth.com/me-cfs/library/showarticle.cfm?libid=17870
728   http://www.plosone.org/article/info%3Adoi%2F10.1371%2Fjournal.pone.0062817
729   http://www.ncbi.nlm.nih.gov/pubmed/24387308
730   http://ajcn.nutrition.org/content/78/3/361.long
731   http://www.biomedcentral.com/1471-2458/14/886
732   http://www.theskepticsguide.org/meta-analysis-all-diets-essentially-equal
733   http://www.nature.com/nrd/journal/v13/n10/full/nrd4391.html
734   http://www.ncbi.nlm.nih.gov/pubmed/15110384
735   http://www.sabiosciences.com/rt_pcr_product/HTML/PAHS-065A.html

- Mitochondrial biogenesis.

- Activities of PGC-1α and NRF2

Note: PGC-1α , a transcription coactivator, is a key regulator of energy metabolism as Peroxisome proliferator-activated receptor-γ coactivator and NRF2 is a powerful protein that binds with DNA at the site of antioxidant repair action. SIRTs are proteins that act as silent information regulators implicated in gene transcription, expression , cell death, and aging.

The key is in NAD$^+$ dependent regulation and reprogramming by SIRT2 and SIRT 3 of mitochondrial proteins including cytochrome C oxidase.

Intermittent calorie restriction (ICR) by fasting once or twice during the week and intermittent oxygen restriction (IOR) by simple holding of breath leads to longevity of mitochondria and cancer resistance [736]. Thus exercise mitigates many deleterious effects of aging [737]. Like the yoga practice in India in olden days and today, intermittent hypoxic training may be a valuable therapy in prolonging life and postponing death. **IOR and ICR help bioengineer selective suicide of poor mitochondria under heavy Reactive Oxygen Species Overload [738].** We know that preventing oxidative damage of mitochondrial DNA by high antioxidant diet can prolong life [739]. Calorie restriction helps by making more efficient mitochondria [740], [741]. My high school physical education teacher in India during late fiftees used to take students through a "Hold Your Breath" routine as an exercise in IOR.

Mitochondria, Chronic Diseases and Longevity

5.04 Obesity and Mitochondria

Mitochondria are tied to energy production. Since mitochondria control ATP production, energy expenditure, energy balance, disposal of reactive oxygen species or free radicals, and lipid and glucose metabolism, they

---

736   http://www.ncbi.nlm.nih.gov/pubmed/18072884
737   http://www.ncbi.nlm.nih.gov/pubmed/23217257
738   http://www.researchgate.net/publication/5775329_Theoretical_paper_exploring_overlooked_natu-ral_mitochondria-r
739   http://www.fasebj.org/content/14/2/312.long
740   http://www.pnas.org/content/103/6/1768.abstract
741   http://www.ncbi.nlm.nih.gov/pubmed/23217257tp://www.plosone.org/article/info%3A-doi%2F10.1371%2Fjournal.pone.0074644

literally control routine functions of all cells including fat cells. [742]. The "diabetes protein system" devoted to energy metabolism is a set of key mitochondrial proteins[743], [744]. Mitochondria may be able to reinvigorate insulin production in beta cells of pancreas even in case of Type I diabetics [745],[746]. **Nutritional intervention by methylation diet and selective practices of calorie and oxygen restriction play a big role in controlling and managing diabetes.** Increased uncoupling of electron transport chain and decreased capacity of ATP production influence energetics of heart function among diabetics [747]. Mitochondria, it appears, can spur and stop obesity[748].

Almost twenty six percent of Americans are obese and 430,000 of them are on hemodialysis. Those on three times a week regimen of hemodialysis lose their water soluble vitamins C and B complex that they need to compensate by appropriate vitamin supplementation [749]. These are key nutrients for mitochondria.

Since we eat intermittently we need hormones insulin and glucagon to regulate glucose homeostasis. Insulin gene on chromosome 11 and glucagon gene on chromosome 2 do just that. We also have hunger hormone ghrelin controlled by its gene on chromosome 6 and appetite control hormone leptin controlled by its gene on chromosome 7. There is also a critical need to control 60% of water in our body by a only 9 amino acid long **arginine vasopressin** which is controlled by a gene on chromosome 20. Why are these genes scattered all over the genome? Why do ghrelin and leptin receptors work by same brain cell [750]? Why does every fat cell secrete its own leptin and create a situation of exponential increase in leptin [751]? It is true that all energy and homeostasis hormones critical to mitochondrial function must be in balance. We don't have an answer today but cells must be signaling and coordinating food intake and energy expenditure day by day.

5.05 Mitochondria and Human age

---

742 http://www.ncbi.nlm.nih.gov/pubmed/23217257Actually mitochondria are involved in routine functioning of fat cells.
743 http://www.sciencedirect.com/science/article/pii/S221296341300003X
744 http://www.proteomesci.com/content/8/1/4
745 http://diabetes.diabetesjournals.org/content/54/suppl_2/S108.full
746 http://www.cell.com/trends/endocrinology-metabolism/pdf/S1043-2760(12)00094-X.pdf
747 https://circ.ahajournals.org/content/112/17/2686.abstract
748 http://scitechdaily.com/mitochondria-can-either-spur-stop-obesity/
749 http://www.kidneycarepartners.org/chronic_kidney_disease.html
750 http://www.ncbi.nlm.nih.gov/pubmed/21674492
751 http://www.cs.stedwards.edu/chem/Chemistry/CHEM43/CHEM43/Leptin/REGCNTRL.HTML

To explore our age and longevity is to explore longevity and bogenesis of our mitochondria and to explore mitochondria is to explore glucose (meaning calories) and oxygen supply that determine the fate and flow of electrons. A good diet for mitochondria is good for a relatively disease free healthful long life [752], [753]. We need to understand the mysteries behind mitochondria of turtle and whales that sometimes live well over 200 hundred years.

Methylation food with electron managing antioxidants, oxygen, and good supply of water is critical to mitochondrial function and methylation diet and exercise can add extra years to our life [754], [755]. Nagano in Japanese Alps is a winner in maximizing longevity for women to 87.2 years and for men to 80.9 years by good diet, physical activity, and even working beyond retirement at 65. *Miso soup three times a day has become an elixir for long life for Nagoans.* One should make a life extending "probiotic Soup-Salad" every alternate day by adding sour kraut, kale leaves, ginger, and garlic to Miso Soup. *Other life extending foods are mushrooms, pumpkin, and bitter gourd and vegetables.* Nagoans eat a lot of vegetables. Twenty five percent of these work beyond age 65. Jeanne Calment, the famous French women who died in 1997, lived for 122 years. Her long life, in addition to her genes from mom and dad, is often attributed to consumption of olive oil, 2.5 lb chocolate every week, and Port wine augmented by routine exercise by riding bicycle wherever she went. A long life by good diet and good physically activity is possible.

Power of Mitochondrial Genes

5.06 Mitochondrial Genes

Let us recollect that each cell in our body on an average has 500 to 1000 of mitochondria and each of them have 1000 or more copies of a circular DNA with 37 genes: 13 of them for making enzyme systems of electron transport chain, 22 for making transfer RNA, and 1 for making ribosomal RNA. All of them were fully sequenced in terms of their nucleotide base pairs in 1981, some 10 years ahead of the initiation of human genome project. These genes,

---

752   http://www.clinicalepigeneticsjournal.com/content/4/1/19
753   http://www.plosone.org/article/info%3Adoi%2F10.1371%2Fjournal.pone.0063855
754   https://matthew2262.wordpress.com/tag/genetic/
755   http://newsfeed.time.com/2013/05/23/happy-114th-birthday-to-jeralean-talley-the-oldest-living-american/

although no more than 37/2500 = 1.48% of all human genes, determine our daily health much more directly because they define (1) energy production from foods we eat and allocation thereof (2) death and birth of our cells, and (3) even production of cholesterol and hemoglobin. The problem is that all of them are prone to damage and mutation by free radicals produced by the mitochondria themselves. Although not inheritable, such somatic mutations do cause health havocs in our own life time in a single generation [756], [757], [758], [759]. This can be avoided by an active life supported by a calorie restricted methylation diet [760], [761], [762].

Somatic mutation of mitochondrial DNA are known to be the cause of a number of diseases including cancers of breast, colon, stomach, liver, and kidney, diabetes and deafness, leukemia and lymphoma. Uncontrolled cell division and tumor growth, too many free radicals, autoimmune disorders including those of digestive system, deficiency of cytochrome c or Complex IV of the electron transport chain, weak eye muscles in case of Kearns Sayre syndrome, Leber optic Neuropathy, and delayed development of complex V (Leigh Syndrome) are other diseases due to mitochondrial DNA mutations [763]. Many mitochondrial dysfunctions are caused also by nuclear DNA (gene)[764]. The following is a list of mitochondrial genes responsible for various diseases [765].

To this list we can add MT-CYB that controls deficiency of complex III (cytochrome b), **LRRK2**, PARK2, PARK7, PINK1, or **SNCA** gene for Parkinson's disease [766],[767]. and APOE ε 4 allele □□□ □□□□ 2 □□□ 3 □□□□□ □□□ Alzheimer's disease [768].

756 http://www.ncbi.nlm.nih.gov/pubmed/23154810
757 http://www.ncbi.nlm.nih.gov/pubmed/9806551
758 http://www.pnas.org/content/109/35/14087
759 http://www.uam.es/personal_pdi/ciencias/genhum/biblioparte2/SEMIN1.pdf
760 http://theprogressivepatient.com/decoding-methylation-and-23andme/
761 http://www.dramyyasko.com/resources/autism-pathways-to-recovery/chapter-2/
762 http://www.whfoods.com/genpage.php?dbid=19&tname=faq
763 http://www.nature.com/nrg/journal/v13/n12/full/nrg3275.html
764 http://www.springer.com/biomed/human+genetics/book/978-1-4614-3721-5
765 licy%2Femed%2FGenetic+Testing_Mitochondrial+Disorders.html&keywords=<!123-321!>&-source=emed&page=id=169&me=index.p
766 http://www.ncbi.nlm.nih.gov/pubmed/1904141
767 http://www.ncbi.nlm.nih.gov/pubmed/22718549
768 file:///C:/Users/Owner/Downloads/00463521ef97ae2cde000000.pdf

List of Diseases Specific Mitochondrial Genes		
Syndrome	Main clinical manifestations	Major genes involved
MELAS	Stroke-like episodes at age <40 Seizures and/or dementia Pigmentary retinopathy Lactic acidosis	MT-TL1, MT-ND5 (>95%) MT-TF, MT-TH, MT-TK, MT-TQ, MT-TS1, MT-TS2, MT-ND1, MT-ND6 (rare)
MERFF	Myoclonus Seizures Cerebellar ataxia Myopathy	MT-TK (>80%) MT-TF, MT-TP (rare)
CPEO	External ophthalmoplegia Bilateral ptosis	Various deletions of MT-DNA
KSS	External ophthalmoplegia <20yo Pigmentary retinopathy Cerebellar ataxia Heart block	Various deletions of MT-DNA
LS	Sub acute relapsing encephalopathy Infantile onset Cerebellar/brain stem dysfunction	*MT-ATP6, MT-TL1, MT-TK, MT-TW, MT-TV, MT-ND1, MT-ND2, MT-ND3, MT-ND4, MT-ND5, MT-ND6, MT-CO3* MT-DNA deletions (rare)
LHON	Painless bilateral visual failure Male predominance Dystonia Cardiac pre-excitation syndromes	*MT-ND1, MT-ND4, MT-ND6*

List of Diseases Specific Mitochondrial Genes		
NARP	Peripheral neuropathy	*MT-ATP6*
	Ataxia	
	Pigmentary retinopathy	

Bacteria have been our friends for a long time helping us make probiotic foods like kimchi, sour kraut, and yogurt and medicine like antibiotic penicillin. Just in the last two years they have been found to come to our aid in a big way. CRISPR technology is advancing fast and it may soon become a standard genetic therapy, a means of editing defective disease causing genes. We need to learn how bacteria use CRISPR (Clustered Regularly Interspersed Short Paliondronic repeat) RNA to defend themselves against viruses. An endonucleage enzyme that has genetic memory, that can question and search, and then cleave like a scissor. The enzyme can be used for genome editing very much like the find and replace function of Microsoft Word processor. **For simplicity let us call this bacterial gift RNA Guided DNA Cleaving enzyme.** It permits much more accurate genome editing and gene manipulation than Zinc Finger Nucleases (targets for unique sequences) and TALEN (transcription activator like effector nuclease). Technology is being used to treat muscular distrophy, liver diseases, eye diseases, and blood disease of beta-thalassaemia. Cancer treatment has now become highly successful with Chemeric Antigen Receptor T cells (CAR T), a protein that knows how to find tumor cells. We may soon have treatments for neurological disorders. Monsanto and AstrZeneca are using the technology to create nutritious foods (grains, fruits, and vegetables) at higher production rates and yield. Hopefully, we will have better foods and better health via genetic engineering and gene therapy by CRISPR.

No doubt, dietary factors can enhance mitochondrial heath and thus our daily health and well being [769]. *Nutrient therapies in order to prevent and stabilize mitochondrial DNA include proper intake of folic acid, acetyl-L-carnitine, lutein, vitamin C, vitamin E, lipoic acid, Zeaxanthine, and vitamin K_3 as electron acceptors, all a kind of antioxidant available in a well designed methylation diet.*

Fruits, vegetables, and nuts can supply most critical nutrients says Cleveland Clinic. Although not approved by Food and drug Administration, Table 5.16.02 and 5.16.03 later present suggested daily intake of major

---

769   http://www.clinicalepigeneticsjournal.com/content/4/1/19

nutrients [770],[771]. Personalized medicine including dietary prescription and exercise plans shall become routine for us once we understand genetically critical nutritional pathways.

5.07 Production of Reactive Oxygen Species

Too many uncontrolled free radicals, in excess of 3% of total oxygen uptake by mitochondria, are bad for health. Ironically free radicals are also good because they help making of mitochondria, making of our immune system, and controlling death and birth of cells. **The key word is control.** There is a rather low production of reactive oxygen species when there is maximum ATP (chemical energy) production. The flux of superoxide (SO_2) production in mitochondrial matrix depends on concentration of electron donors, coenzyme Q_{10} level, $NADH/NAD^+$ ratio, and local oxygen concentration [772]. A good methylation diet should deliver an optimum of these nutrients.

5.08 Mortal and Immortal Cells

Unlike the multicellular jellyfish, humans are mortals. Biological aging can't be prevented because shortening of telomere (the cap of DNA) at each cell division is unavoidable. We know that enzyme telomerase helps cancer cells divide infinitely and thus they render our tissues and organs completely dysfunctional. Poor protection of telomere is an epigenetic effect [773]. As a genomic scribe, telomeres react and record nutritional and environmental stress factors over of life time. A methylation diet can optimize production of enzyme telomerase for longevity [774]. We also know that stem cells are relatively immortal. *That the two strands of DNA in human cell do not uncoil equally gives us another clue.* This is why research on telomerase and its role in cancer biology and longevity is now an area of active research[775].

Our stem cells containing a single helix of DNA are a kind of immortal cells and so should the mitochondria in our undifferentiated stem cells that

---

770   http://www.marksdailyapple.com/managing-your-mitochondria-nutrients-and-supplements/#ax-zz369h0rXwR
771   http://nutritionreview.org/2013/09/mitochondrial-dysfunction/
772   http://www.ncbi.nlm.nih.gov/pmc/articles/PMC2605959/
773   http://www.ncbi.nlm.nih.gov/pubmed/23850488
774   http://naturalmedicinejournal.com/journal/2013-06/optimal-longevity-hinges-telomeres
775   http://www.ncbi.nlm.nih.gov/pmc/articles/PMC3258147/

can devide and produce more cells indefinitely [776], [777]. Cancer is mutation in stem cells caused by high rate of division and random error in preserving the DNA. How do we keep the immortal DNA strand forever [778]? is the big question. Cancer cells on the other hand enjoy telomerase protection and become immortal like bacteria [779], [780]. *Loss of telomere , it appears, can be prevented by extra telomerase and therein lies a clue to biological immortality or at least extension of the life of human cells, the brain cells in particular*. **A physically active lifestyle can increase telomerase [781] and so can a methylation diet containing astaxanthin, curcumin from turmeric, folate from asparagus, magnesium from okra, polyphenols from whole grains, probiotics from sour kraut and yogurt, ubiquinol, vitamins A, D, K$_2$, and B$_{12}$.** "What foods or elixirs can we design against cell senescence?" is the big question of the day. The easy and practical answer is a *restricted calorie methylation diet and a lifestyle that incorporates d*aily practice of exercise, yoga, proper sleep, and a scheme of as interactive living as possible.

5.09 The Mitochondrial Human Proteome Initiative

Italian Proteomics Association has started a study on mitochondrial proteome and protein interactions encoded by mitochondrial DNA that control metabolism [782]. Mitochondria, as described earlier, control Krebs cycle functions, operation of electron transport chain and production of ATP, and metabolism of glucose, amino acids, and free fatty acids [783], [784]. Receptor proteins are capable of signaling and thus controlling gene expression and metabolic activities and associated signal transduction, transmission, and modulation (sending and receiving). They are also involved in tumor cell growth and cancer development [785].

Notch signaling in particular deals with identity and behavior of a cell including its death. It all depends on how well and how controlled is

---

776   http://www.ncbi.nlm.nih.gov/pubmed/23970416
777   http://www.fasebj.org/content/21/14/3773.full
778   http://www.ncbi.nlm.nih.gov/pmc/articles/PMC3918731/
779   http://www.hiccc.columbia.edu/news/what-makes-cancer-cell-immortal
780   http://www.ncbi.nlm.nih.gov/pubmed/23326372
781   http://www.ucsf.edu/news/2013/09/108886/lifestyle-changes-may-lengthen-telomeres-measure-cell-aging
782   http://scitechdaily.com/mitochondria-can-either-spur-stop-obesity/
783   hthttp://www.gibsonproteomics.org/research-focus/mitochondrial-proteomicstp://accelerating-science.com/proteomics/the-mitochondrial-human-proteome-initiative/
784   http://www.gibsonproteomics.org/research-focus/mitochondrial-proteomics
785   http://www.ncbi.nlm.nih.gov/pubmed/12496471

localization and transport of protein molecules, molecules that run our life [786]. *The hard fact of life is that proteins and messenger RNA are the basis of cellular polarity and plasticity [787].* Notch (a binding site or indentation on the surface) signaling is an evolutionarily conserved pathway in all multicellular organisms including humans. It regulates fate of cells and tissue homeostasis. A few proteins (Notch1, Notch2, Notch3, and Notch4) spanning in and out of the width of cell do a lot of communicating. Ligand -receptor cross-talks mediate justacrine or contact dependent cellular signaling. This includes signals for cardiac, immune, neuronal, and endocrine systems.

Signaling pathways are connected to metabolism. *Notch 1 signaling alters close to 8 proteins affecting glutamine metabolism, Krebs cycle functions, and production of ATP, NADH, and NADPH [788].* **We know that mitochondrial protein expression is tied to heart failure** [789], a process of involving 39 proteins responsible for its routine function [790]. Faulty Notch signaling is implicated in diseases like multiple sclerosis and T cell leukemia. It is central to neuronal function and cardiac valve homeostasis. Receptors are single pass transmission proteins and transmembrane receptor proteins span cell membranes from in to outside [791].

Various proteins are now known to be involved in cancer, aging, and many neurological diseases. An understanding of structure and functions of proteins (proteomics) may lead to diet based therapeutics at the cellular level. We still need to understand, however, the expression of mitochondrial genes for controlling aging and age-related diseases. Although proteome research began 15 years ago, exact knowledge of protein types and their functions has yet to be fully mapped out. Proteins run the life of mitochondria and our cells die when mitochondria die. Without mitochondria we cease to be a biological being. We must know of and about the geometry, notches, and spatial projections on these key proteins in greater detail than we do at the present.

786   h http://www.nasonline.org/programs/sackler-colloquia/completed_colloquia/molecular-kine-sis-in-cellular-functi http://www.nasonline.org/programs/sackler-colloquia/completed_colloquia/molecular-kinesis-in-cellular-function-and-plasticity.html on-and-plasticity.html ttp://www.pnas.org/content/98/13/6997.full.pdf
787   http://www.nasonline.org/programs/sackler-colloquia/completed_colloquia/molecular-kine-sis-in-cellular-function-and-plasticity.html
788   http://www.jbc.org/content/early/2014/01/28/jbc.M113.519405
789   http://www.ncbi.nlm.nih.gov/pubmed/24548633
790   http://www.ncbi.nlm.nih.gov/pubmed/19834913
791   http://www.cellsignal.com/contents/science-pathway-research-stem-cell-markers/notch-signal-ing-pathway/pathways-notch

5.10 Mitochondria and Quantum mechanics of Our Daily Life

Research in quantum biology is advancing fast and much more about it should be pointed out than described in section 5.02 of this chapter under quantum conundrum. Quantum mechanics, if Einstein holds, must apply to ionization, bond vibrations, and chemical bonding in metabolic reactions in all living creatures. Actually, it applies to very shape and topology of protein and DNA molecules. Metabolic reactions involve movement of electrons and protons within living cells and our biology seems to be a special case of **quantum** operations in biological electromagnetics [792]. As a matter of fact quantum mechanics dominates Iron/sulfur clusters of cytochromes of electron transport chain in quantized mitochondria [793]. Acting as solid-state electronics, mitochondria use electromagnetic field masterfully. Also, ATP produced right in the inner membrane of mitochondria helps unfold (or uncondense) protein polymers so water can bind in order to power quantum information and energy. Protons are pushed out off cytochromes at various steps and cytochrome c oxidase combines electron and proton to produce water. ***Three protons are delivered by proton tunneling every second.*** Very little ATP is made during deep sleep (REM, Rapid Eye Movement) when our brain is in a coherent quantum state. **It appears that electrons and protons are made quantum coherent during sleep.** The free radicals with two electrons spinning in the same direction play a very important role in memory and communication. Since mitochondria have both magnetic and electric fields, they can manage spin of electrons well for signaling.

Infrared radiation produced by "electromagnetic compass" of enzyme complexes of electron transport chain is very important for coherence of free radicals. Entangled proteins and their quaternary structures during folding and unfolding decide the free energy landscape.

Also it appears that the hydrogen bonds in protein and DNA molecules play a quantum role. Protons roam and move freely in these bonds and they help transfer energy and information. They act as quantum measuring device for a pair of electrons. Water is ionic and interaction of light with liquid water generates quantum coherent domains in which water molecules oscillate between ground and excited states close to ionization potential of water, a phenomenon that we don't fully understand [794]. An excited water

---

792   http://www.nature.com/news/2011/110615/full/474272a.html
793   http://jackkruse.com/tensegrity-9-magnetic-mitochondria-memory-creates-coherence/
794   file:///C:/Users/Owner/Downloads/entropy-16-04874.pdf

molecule is the source of superconducting protons necessary for rapid communication by transfer of energy and information[795]. Coherent domains trap electromagnetic frequencies for biochemical reaction and regulatory gene functions.

As pointed out in section 5.02, a *mutation may involve a shift of a single proton (hydrogen atom) from one side to adjacent one in a genome which appears to be a **coherent linear superposition** that can be maintained on biological time scale and DNA, held by quantum entanglement, may persist unmutated.* This phenomenon is describable by a single wave function no matter how far apart. Forms of nucleotide bond in DNA oscillate in different directions and account for superposition and stability. ***Phonons, quantum energy of vibrations of a crystal lattice , have same wavelength as the size of DNA.*** Enzyme reactions and mutations involve **proton and electron tunneling**. We could visualize it as movement and hopping of electrons through and around protein molecules of the electron transport system in the inner mitochondrial membrane within *1.4 X 10^{-9} meters. ATP production is now being considered as a case of nano-scale (1.4 X 10^{-9} meters) quantum tunneling[796], [797],[798].* This is a rather ultra-fast phenomenon and it appears that ordered structures in biology are created for retention of quantum coherence because decoherence wipes out the quantum phenomenon.

When the genome becomes correlated or entangled with the environment, it decoheres and accelerated decoherence causes mutation involving quantum jump events such as tautomeric shifts (position of electrons and protons) in a single proton in DNA bases. ***Thus coupling of quantum state represents the mutational state.***

Our ability to smell, to absorb light of specific frequencies by our retina, and DNA mutation are special cases of quantum mechanics[799]. So is the ATPase (hydrolase) which functions like a Brownian motors in living organisms [800]. ***Pigments and packed chromophores in our organs are a good example of quantum coherence also where waves of electrons extend over multiple molecular complexes.*** *The system works like an one way rectifier.* Nano-crystals make quantum dots[801] and spin up and spin down of electrons can

---

795   http://jackkruse.com/tensegrity-6-hydrogen-bonding-networks-water/
796   http://www.ks.uiuc.edu/Research/quantum_biology/
797   http://www.pbs.org/wgbh/nova/blogs/physics/2014/03/quantum-life/
798   http://qubit-ulm.com/quantum-effects-in-biology/
799   http://www.ncbi.nlm.nih.gov/pubmed/8111728
800   http://users.df.uba.ar/marcos/309.pdf
801   http://www.marketwatch.com/story/quantum-materials-acquires-bayer-technology-services-quan-tum-dot-manufacturing-and-quantum-dot-solar-cell-patents-201

serve as quantum bits in information processing by our brain [802]. *Magnetic resonance imaging, we know, is a result of zillions of spins in a macroscopic human tissues.*

In enzyme catalyzed reactions, protons move from one molecule to another by tunneling and thus bypassing an energy barrier. Smell in olfactory system may have its origin in molecular vibrations[803] and electronic tunneling[804]. Electrons in this case travel at less than 2200 kilometers per second which is only 1% of speed of light but it is fast enough to make complete round of earth in only 18 seconds . Action potentials by our neurons can travel up to 100 meters per second. It appears that quantum mechanics pervades all cellular functions. *Our health then is sum total of many ultra-fast quantum events but how do mitochondria manage olfaction in our nose and the view of the world in our eyes where a single photon can cause 1,000 ions to get to action are still huge mysteries [805].* Neural response is also a quantum phenomenon[806] just as the functions of myriads of functional enzyme proteins [807], [808]. The genes that code these proteins mutate by quantum effect. Genes mutate and go bad, they make inefficient proteins or don't make them at all. We lose signaling and perception. We die. Let us examine a few chronic problems that we have come to know of during a short period of only past five decades.

- **Somatic mitochondrial DNA (mtDNA) mutations have been increasingly observed in human cancers. As each cell contains many mitochondria with multiple copies of mtDNA, It is possible that wild-type and mutant mtDNA can co-exist in a state called heteroplasmy. During cell division, mitochondria are randomly distributed to daughter cells [809]. Over time, the proportion of the mutant mtDNA within the cell can vary and may drift toward predominantly mutant or wild type to achieve homoplasmy (identical copies of mitochondrial DNA). Thus, the biological impact of a given mutation may vary, depending on the proportion of mutant mtDNAs carried by the cell. This effect contributes to various phenotypes observed among family members carrying the same pathogenic mtDNA mutation. Most mutations occur in the coding sequences but few result**

802   http://arstechnica.com/science/2012/09/reading-and-writing-quantum-bits-on-a-single-electron-spin/
803   http://www.bbc.com/news/science-environment-21150046
804   http://phys.org/news89542035.html
805   http://www.nemenmanlab.org/~ilya/images/4/43/Rieke-baylor-98.pdf
806   http://www.informationphilosopher.com/presentations/Milan/papers/QB_Salzburg_jedlicka.pdf
807   http://endgametime.wordpress.com/the-awakening-quantum-mechanics-of-the-human-brain-and-consciousness/
808   http://www.livescience.com/37807-brain-is-not-quantum-computer.html
809   http://www.nature.com/onc/journal/v25/n34/abs/1209604a.html

in substantial amino acid changes raising questions as to their biological consequence. Numerous studies have revealed that mtDNA play a crucial role in the development of cancer but further work is required to establish the functional significance of specific mitochondrial mutations in cancer and disease progression. Origin of these mutations, their functional consequences in cancer development, and possible therapeutic implications are active areas of research today. The daily diet plays a huge role.

• Planned degradation of mitochondria (mytophagy) is an autophagic quality control mechanism that removes dysfunctional mitochondria. This is a very selective process. The drivers are the enzyme proteins and genes behind them. In this process, PINK1 (PTEN-induced putative kinase protein 1) recruits the cytosolic E3 enzyme ubiquitin ligase parkin to damaged mitochondria, which causes their engulfment by autophagosomes before lysosomal degradation. PINK1 and parkin mediate a mitochondrion. PTEN is a gene for phosphatase and tensin. It is an enzyme proteins of critical biological value including carcinogenesis.

• Mitochondria are primarily responsible for providing the contracting cardiac myocyte with a continuous supply of ATP. However, mitochondria can rapidly change into death-promoting organelles. In response to changes in the intracellular environment, mitochondria become producers of excessive reactive oxygen species and release prodeath proteins, resulting in disrupted ATP synthesis and activation of cell death pathways. Interestingly, cells have developed a defense mechanism against aberrant mitochondria that can cause harm to the cell. This mechanism involves selective sequestration and subsequent degradation of the dysfunctional mitochondrion before it causes activation of cell death. Induction of mitochondrial autophagy called mitophagy, results in selective clearance of damaged mitochondria in cells. In response to stress such as ischemia or reperfusion, prosurvival and prodeath pathways are concomitantly activated in cardiac muscle cells. Thus, there is a delicate balance between life and death in our cells during stress. The final outcome depends on effective communication or cross-talk between various pathways. In case of heart, mitophagy functions as an early cardioprotective response, favoring adaptation to stress by removing damaged mitochondria. In contrast, increased oxidative stress and enzymes of death (apoptotic proteases) can inactivate mitophagy, allowing for the execution of cell death [810].

---

810   http://circres.ahajournals.org/content/111/9/1208.abstract

- As to routine health maintenance, mitochondria of brown and white adipose fat cells have different activities [811], [812]. Brown fat cells have many mitochondria because their function is thermogenesis. On the contrary white adipose fat cells have very few because they need just enough ATP for fat storage. High level of mitochondrial biogenesis in brown adipose fat is indicative of high metabolism. Also, brown adipose fat cell utilizes uncoupling proteins (UCPs) to uncouple oxidative phosphorylation in the mitochondrial Electron Transfer Chain reaction, thereby reducing ATP production. Thus there is efficiency in dissipating energy as heat [813]. Brown adipose fat cells are organized to have distinct lobules, rich supply of blood, and communication with central nervous system[814]. They produce heat during shivering.

- Genes of mitochondria are still being worked out. Mutations in these genes cause breast, colon, kidney, leukemia, liver, lymphoma, prostate, stomach cancers. Parkinson's disease is a great example of mitochondrial DNA dysfunction. The big question is how to control it by gene therapy and food supplements. Even bigger question is connection between mitochondrial and nuclear DNA_s for proper functioning of cells and their life span [815]. Free radicals generated during respiration do have an impact on type 2 diabetes in particular [816]. <u>Even in case of type 1 diabetes, electron transport complex IV is at risk because of mutations in mitochondrial DNA [817], [818].</u> Mitochondrial dysfunction leads to glucose insulin imbalance and eventually to death of beta cells of the pancreas [819]. Mitochondria integrate and generate metabolic signals, thereby connect glucose recognition to insulin secretion [820],[821].

- UK government is leaning towards permitting mitochondrial replacement [822] [823]. The technique involves fertilizing a healthy egg in- vitro with sperm and egg of a candidate couple, a kind of mitochondrial transplant. A study of European population reveals that there can be unidentical and different mitochondrial DNA types

811   http://hyperphysics.phy-astr.gsu.edu/hbase/biology/mitochondria.html
812   https://uk.answers.yahoo.com/question/index?qid=20130710105215AAdCjIO
813   http://www.imb.sinica.edu.tw/~leeyinghue/mitobiogenesis.htm
814   http://www.biochemj.org/csb/frame.htm
815   http://www.the-scientist.com/?articles.view/articleNo/34398/title/Mitochondria-Versus-Nucleus/
816   http://www.ncbi.nlm.nih.gov/pubmed/19650713
817   http://www.fasebj.org/cgi/content/meeting_abstract/26/1_MeetingAbstracts/lb748
818   file:///C:/Users/Owner/Downloads/12052520495246.pdf
819   http://www.cell.com/trends/endocrinology-metabolism/abstract/S1043-2760(12)00094-X
820   http://www.hindawi.com/journals/omcl/2012/740849/
821   mitochondria integrate and generate metabolic signals, thereby connecting glucose recognition to insulin exocytosis.
822   http://www.hfea.gov.uk/6896.html
823   http://news.sciencemag.org/health/2013/06/u.k.-government-plans-allow-mitochondrial-replacement

in the same individual [824] and the extent of heterogeneity may be up to 61%. This is not necessarily a negative with respect to health because there seems to be a self-correcting mechanism. Even more dramatic breakthrough is that a mutant DNA can be eliminated. It can be kept below 80%, a threshold necessary for onset of diseases [825]. This DNA elimination technique may cure Lieber's hereditary optic neuropathy and other brain and muscle diseases.

- An impressive research is about gene SIRT1 of sirtuin family of genes that make deacylase enzymes. This gene is activated by resveratrol and it helps maintain HIF1 level in order to maintain communication between nuclear and mitochondrial DNA[826] [827]. HIF1 is factor that helps transcribe or decode DNA into proteins. This communication and interaction between the nuclear and mitochondrial genes is necessary for the health of our cells and our longevity. To keep it going we must have enough NAD in our diet or vitamin B_3 supplement. Resveratrol from grapes and wine has been implicated in glucose control[828], longevity[829], [830] and blood pressure maintenance[831]. Decline in NAD^+ induces loss of communication when HIF-1α accumulates and creates havoc. It has been shown to accelerate by deleting SIRT1 gene in mouse. *NAD^+ levels regulate mitochondrial homeostasis and deficiency of niacin or vitamin B_3 should not be allowed to persist.* This is why niacin fortification of wheat flour began way back in 1938. Niacin derived NAD^+ acts like the SIRT1 gene.

Current research indicates that mitochondria are the key to gene therapy against cancer and a population of healthy mitochondria is essential to our disease free long life. *No doubt our daily nutrition is an epigenetic switch for good gene expression and health maintenance. There is ample science behind the concept that physical movement, exercise, and mindfulness amplify the beneficial effects of nutrition.* Already we can methylate cytosine for silencing expression and post-replication DNA repair [832]. Like wise we can hydroxymethylate for activating a gene very much like an

824   http://www.sciencedaily.com/releases/2013/10/131003093043.htm
825   http://med.miami.edu/news/breakthrough-dna-study-opens-door-to-potential-treatments-for-mito-chondrial
826   https://thinksteroids.com/community/threads/declining-nad-induces-a-pseudohypoxic-state-dis-rupting-nuclear-mitochondrial-communi.134348338/
827   http://hms.harvard.edu/news/genetics/new-reversible-cause-aging-12-19-13
828   http://ajcn.nutrition.org/content/early/2014/04/02/ajcn.113.082024.abstract
829   http://www.ncbi.nlm.nih.gov/pubmed/22718956
830   https://www.fightaging.org/archives/2012/06/a-resveratrol-meta-analysis.php
831   http://www.clinicalnutritionjournal.com/article/S0261-5614(14)00084-3/abstract
832   http://www.ncbi.nlm.nih.gov/pubmed/16570853

on-off switch. It has been shown that hydroxymethylations enhances the pluripotency of the stem cells [833]. The big question is "Can quantum biology of our being be regulated and moderated by foods we eat and beverages we drink and can it be punctuated by life style?" The answers seem to be yes.

5.11 Probing into Neuron Firing

Neuron firing is a great example of quantum effects in bionics and bioelectronics. Neurons fire and deliver motor messages to the rest of the body. Artificial devices can digitize these messages. For instance brain signals can be sent to a computer. Computer programs can be used for improving brain fitness and performance. We can buy an EPOC **(Effective Practice and Organisation of Care)** neuroheadset from Emotive of Australia for routine processing of our neurosignals [834]. The sensors of the headset tune into signals from the brain, detect our thoughts and feelings, and convert them wirelessly to computers in our lap. So we are now headed to understanding our EEG, understanding how brain works in real time, and managing our brain's fitness and performance. Inter Axon of Toronto, Canada offers similar seven sensor EEG headset system by the name of MUSE [835].

New science will soon fine tune mitochondrial bionics into specific signs of our health, fitness, and well being. Our brain, the most enigmatic quantum bit biocomputor, interprets every action of mitochondria. Can it interpret day to day health implications of our vital signs from vital organs and can such interpretations be digitized and logged in our physical laptop or even better in our smart phone? The answer seems to be yes.

5.12 Life from Artificial DNA

Can our mitochondria be modified to stay healthy and active longer than just a century? Can it fight oxidative stress day in and day out? The modified cytosine and guanidine, it appears, have opened new avenues for life in general and our day-to-day health in particular by supression or activation of genes[836]. Even gut bacteria can be brought to our rescue. Although it has a

---

833   http://www.ks.uiuc.edu/Research/methylation/
834   http://www.emotiv.com/store/hardware/epoc-bci/epoc-neuroheadset/
835   http://www.interaxon.ca/contact.html
836   http://www.scripps.edu/news/press/2014/20140507romesberg.html

long way to go, the work at Scripps research Institute in La Jolla, CA under Dr. Romesberg's direction has a very practical use of artificial bacteria. Artificial bacterial therapy may become a common practice for disease control and health management [837].

Also, life from artificial DNA is possible now [838], [839]. Two new hydrophobic base pairs in addition to existing four (A, T, G, C) can have the possibility of making proteins from 176 amino acids as opposed to only 22. This kind of synthetic life can be used for new vaccines, drugs toxic to cancer cells, antibiotics, nano-materials, and new RNAs. But can mutated mitochondrial DNA, short of mitochondrial transplant, be rendered normal by artificial bacteria and artificial DNA? Only future will tell.

5.13 Antioxidants and Quantum Power of Hydrogen transfer

Our cells maintain a reducing environment and antioxidants are present in them by design. Mechanisms of antioxidative actions involve sequential electron and proton transfer. The mechanism of sequential electron and proton transfer, a quantum process, is the key to quenching of the outer sphere of excited electron of a free radical. A majority of these are Oxygen Free Radicals called Reactive Oxygen Species (ROS) such as superoxide O_2, singlet oxygen $^1O_2$, H_2O_2, and OH^-. Let us keep in mind that oxygen is a diatomic molecule. Free radicals form when two electrons are missing in one of oxygen atoms making it positive and the other atom becomes negative. Following definitions are added for clarity for this subatomic phenomenon.

- **Molecular oxygen exists in a stable triplet state with an unusual electronic configuration. This is an exception because most other molecules exist in singlet stage. Addition of one electron to triplet oxygen makes superoxide radical. Addition of two electrons produces peroxide. These are toxic reduction products of oxygen with extra electrons.**
- **Oxy radicals are any group of compounds containing reactive oxygen radicals such as super oxide and singlet oxygen. Super oxide can give rise to hydrogen per oxide which in turn can produce hydroxyl radical.**

837   http://www.ncbi.nlm.nih.gov/pmc/articles/PMC1138267/
838   http://www.huffingtonpost.com/2014/05/07/living-organism-artificial-dna_n_5283095.html
839   http://www.nature.com/nature/journal/vaop/ncurrent/full/nature13314.html

- Fortunately only tiny amount of these radicals is produced by mitochondria.
- Addition of one single electron renders the diatomic oxygen anionic with charge of -1. This is the most common free radical in nature called superoxide.
- The singlet oxygen, with degenerate orbital and different spin, is an excited oxygen molecule capable of room temperature stability for no more than an hour. *The energy difference is 94.3 KJ/mole. It is very reactive and can kill even cancer cells.* It oxidizes LDL cholesterol and causes cardiovascular problems. Polyphenolic and carotenoid antioxidants quench it well.
- Hydroxyl radical are produced from hydroperoxides produced during oxidation of fats. They can also be the product of our immune system.
- Free radicals have unpaired *excited* electron, are short lived but very reactive.
- Free radicals are produced in different pathways localized in the cell. Complex I, ubiquinone, and complex III generate most of the superoxide O_2^+ radicals. Two electrons are used at the end of electron transport chain to reduce oxygen into water. When only one electron is donated, oxygen becomes a reactive free radical.

By their electronic structure, free radicals with one unpaired spin are paramagnetic in that their magnetic behavior is in the direction of applied magnetic field [840]. Consider an electron as a spinning ball of charge and its spin equaling to its intrinsic angular momentum- the impetus gained by a moving electron [841]. All moving charges produce magnetic field and electron spin represents a tiny magnetic field. They **order** the electron in atomic structure and determines all attractions and reactivities. This is unlike diamagnetic materials used to trap their spin in order to quantitatively measure free radicals by Electron Paramagnetic Resonance or Electron Spin Resonance techniques.

Free radicals are the agents of aging, cancer, cataracts, diabetes, emphysema, heart disease, osteoporosis, rheumatoid arthritis, senility, and strokes. The cure to these problems are antioxidants. This is precisely the reason for a detailed description of antioxidants in sections 5.13 and 5.14.

Free radicals are produced by our white blood cells, cytokines, and 40-75 % neucleophiles- special white blood cells that get ready to fight within

---

840   http://chemistry.about.com/od/chemistryglossary/g/paramagnetism-definition.htm
841   http://www.scientificamerican.com/article/what-exactly-is-the-spin/

minutes of injury and infection. ***Neutrophiles produce the dangerous superoxide free radical to kill the invading bacteria or virus.*** The leftover free radical damage our DNA, proteins, and lipids like LDL cholesterol often by oxidizing or abstracting a hydrogen. ***They influence gene expression and even death of a cell.*** The superoxide O_2 radical has two unpaired electrons that have same spin quantum number. It accepts electrons one at a time and damages the cell.

The remedial antioxidants donate electrons for quenching free radicals with unpaired valence electrons. Their activity as described earlier is governed by quantum effects. They are reduced compounds and get oxidized when they quench a free radical. As a matter of fact, antioxidants become a weak free radical by undergoing oxidation by a potent free radical but their large molecular size dilutes their oxidative power. Transfer of an electron or hydrogen in oxidation processes is tantamount to transfer of a discrete package of energy characterized by quantum yield. We now know that hydrogen or proton transfer is rather fast via tunneling effect in case of catechin[842], [843]. [844]. Galloylated catechin antioxidants are more potent antioxidants where the π-bond electrons in allyl and benzene rings offer the structural basis for potency. Vitamin E exhibits similar proton tunneling and charge transfer effects as an antioxidant [845], [846]. So is the case of vitamin E like fat soluble ubiquinol [847]. Quantum chemical approach to understanding and quantifying antioxidants is possible in case of ferulic and sinapic acids [848]. Quercetin from apple, onion, grape fruit, beans, and vegetables exhibits similarwell known quantum chemistry of hydrogen transfer[849], [850].

Human cells have many antioxidants in order to fight or quench free radicals. The list below classifies them by functional categories.

Carotenoids   Beta-carotene, lycopene, and lutein

Vitamins   α-tocopherol, vitamin C, vitamin K

Lipid solubles   Ubiquinone, N-acetyl cysteine, lipoic acid

Thiols   Glutathione

842   http://www.nobleharbor.com/tea/health/QuantumMechanicsExplainsTea.htm
843   http://www.rsc.org/chemistryworld/News/2007/April/23040702.asp
844   http://www.researchgate.net/publication/225765091_Antioxidant_effects_of_green_tea_polyphe-nols
845   http://pubs.acs.org/doi/abs/10.1021/j100185a065
846   http://pubs.acs.org/doi/abs/10.1021/j100185a065
847   http://www.ncbi.nlm.nih.gov/pubmed/24367903
848   http://bioinfo.swu.bg/velkov.pdf
849   http://pubs.rsc.org/en/content/articlelanding/2010/cp/b924521a#!divAbstract
850   http://worldwidescience.org/topicpages/q/quantum+pharmacology+held.html

Phenolics planning)	Quircetin and catechins (very important in diet
Saponins	Cortisone, estradiol, estriol
Minerals	Copper, selenium, zinc
Enzymes	Super oxide dismutase, catalase, and glutathione peroxidase.
Hormones	Melatonin, estrogens
Others	Resveratrol, lipoicacid, bioflavonoid rutin,

The redox potentials depend on structure, donor -acceptor groups, and polarizability and the antioxidant power is evaluated in terms of hydrogen ion transfer and/or oxygen radical absorbance capacity (ORAC) [851].

We now know that flexibility and stability in biology is maintained by conjugated (conjugated linoleic acid, omega-3 fatty acids, riboflavin) and isoprenoid (vitamin A, Carotene vitamin E, and coenzyme Q_{10}) biomplecules permitting tunneling of electrons via hydrogen bonds in DNA and protons in proteins. These are the molecules that offer environment for electron mobility. Redox potential and concentration of various antioxidants is listed below.

Although chapter 2 has a detailed listing of cofactors, vitamins, adaptogens, and antioxidants as special nutrients, we should examine here again in detail essential structures that seem to be the key to running our electronic life. Table 5.13.01 summarizes such structures for visual comparison of chemical analogy. Their planar configuration extends electronic delocalization between adjacent rings. As a matter fact, structure, geometry, and planarity are key to electron density, delocalization, and antioxidant effects.

---

851   http://www.scientificamerican.com/article/what-are-orac-values/

Redox Potential and Concentration [852],[853],[854],[855]

	Redox Potential (MilliVolts)	Concentration (microMoles/Kg)
Glutathione	+920	6,400
Beta-carotene	+695	5
Zeaxanthin	+537	
Gallic Acid	+532	
Vitamin E	+480	50
Vitamin C	+486	260
Caffeic Acid	+450	
Ascorbic acid	+282	
Rutin	+230	
Quercetin	+110	
Ubiquinol	+ 45	200

A five carbon unit structure, isoprene, seems to have multiple roles in our life as vitamins A, D, E, K, ubiquinone coenzyme Q_{10}, and menaquinone electron carriers. Phylloquinone known as vitamin K is also found in mitochondria. Other examples include lycopene, anthocyanidins, cinnamaldehyde, and conjugated linoleic acid. *Known for their conjugated system of alternating single and double bonds with π-orbitals and delocalized electrons, such structures are electrically conductive permitting electron mobility.*

Quinones in particular are known to have semiconductor property [856]. Biology at large is based on electron transfers and such structures are ubiquitous as special proteins containing porphyrins, cofactors for enzymes, coenzyme Q_{10} like oxidation-reduction carriers, and dietary antioxidants in general. Isoprenoid or terpenoid molecules make essential foods for mitochondria as presented in Tables 2.04.02 and 2.06.02. Routine chemistry

852   http://www.mdpi.org/molecules/papers/12102327.pdf
853   http://www.ncbi.nlm.nih.gov/pubmed/17660583
854   http://en.wikipedia.org/wiki/Antioxidant
855   http://siba.unipv.it/farmacia/art/Marrubini/ANTIOXIDANTS%20&%20REDOX%20SIGNALING.pdf
856   http://www.ncbi.nlm.nih.gov/pubmed/22483224

tells us that benzene like compounds are electron accepting, triterpinoid structures have sensing ability capable of warding off oxidative stress induced inflammation, and π-electrons are delocalized by conjugated cinnamaldehyde from cinnamon [857]. We know that vitamin E and D are potent fat soluble antioxidants [858] and that vitamin K fights oxidative stress [859].

Electron mobile structures seem to be central to human electrophysiology and listed below are structures of vitamins, antioxidants, and dietary nutrients that are central to our metabolism and physiology. The purpose here is to offer a visual view of molecules that control our life processes as electron transfer semiconductor systems. Noteworthy is the structural ananoly of various bioflavonoids included in in figures 33-53.

Quercetin or quircetol, a flavonol antioxidants, has special role in mitochondrial function, metabolism, nerve function, allergies, immune modulation, and fighting pain. *It promotes mitochondrial biogenesis[860] , cognition [861], and it has been tried in fighting pelvic and chronic prostatic pain syndrome with success [862], [863].* As a powerful flavonol antioxidant quercetin protects fats and cholesterol by donating electron and in the process becoming a less harmful radical. *Available from capers, green and black tea, onion, and apple it is no doubt a major nutrient for routine health.* A cup of afternoon tea has a big value in improving mitochondrial function. *An apple as snack, green and black tea as beverage, and capers as savory spice designed into our daily foods can easily deliver more than 100 mg of quircetin per day.* Actually, six servings of fruits and vegetables may deliver up to 500 mg/day. Consuming pine apple for enzyme bromelain increases the bioavailability of quircetin. Flavonoid rutin found in apples, asparagus, buckwheat, and citrus fruits is also a powerful antioxidant.

For centuries, both quircetin and rutin have been used in many countries as alternative medicine for antibacterial and antioxidant effects in treatment of diseases of heart and lung[864] . An extensive list of life supporting molecules is included in Table 5.13.01.

857   http://www2.chemistry.msu.edu/faculty/reusch/VirtTxtJml/react3.htm
858   http://www.ncbi.nlm.nih.gov/pubmed/8325381
859   http://www.jneurosci.org/content/23/13/5816.full.pdf
860   http://www.hindawi.com/journals/omcl/2013/154279/
861   http://www.ncbi.nlm.nih.gov/pubmed/24893798
862   http://www.chiro.org/nutrition/FULL/Quercetin_Is_Promising.shtml
863   http://umm.edu/health/medical/altmed/condition/prostatitis
864   http://www.sciencedirect.com/science/article/pii/S0039914011009386

Table 5.13.01 List of Conjugated and Isoprenoid Molecules That Sustain Life

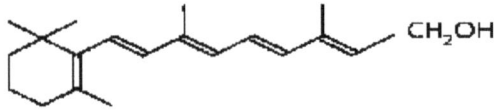

Vitamin A alcohol

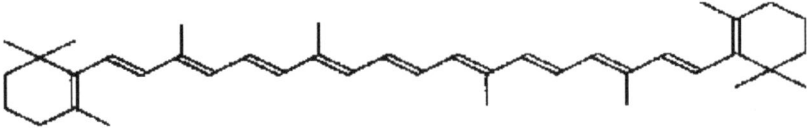

β-Carotene

Fig. 1: Vitamin A and β-Carotene

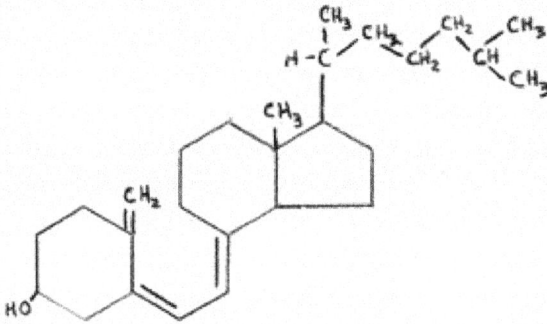

Fig. 2: Vitamin D

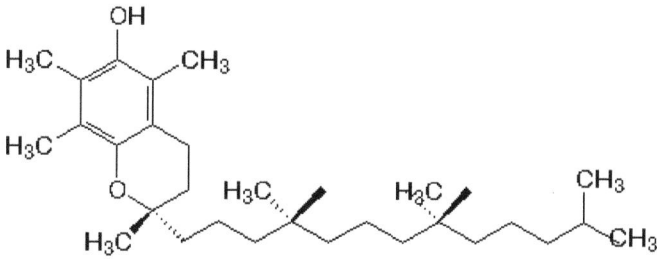

Vitamin E (α-tocopherol)

Fig.3 Vitamin E

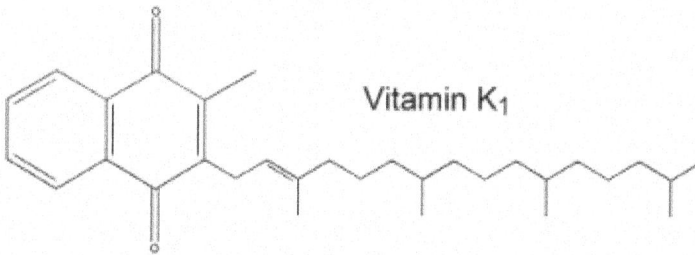

Vitamin K₁

Fig.4 Vitamin K₁

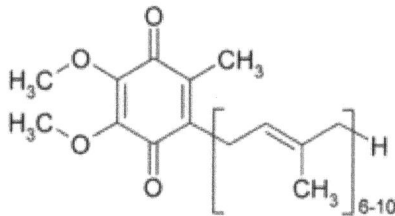

Fig. 5: Coenzyme Q₁₀

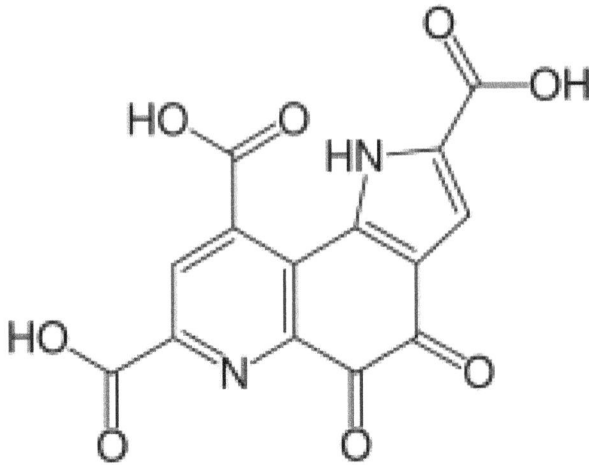
Fig. 6: PQQ (Pyrolloquinone quinoline)

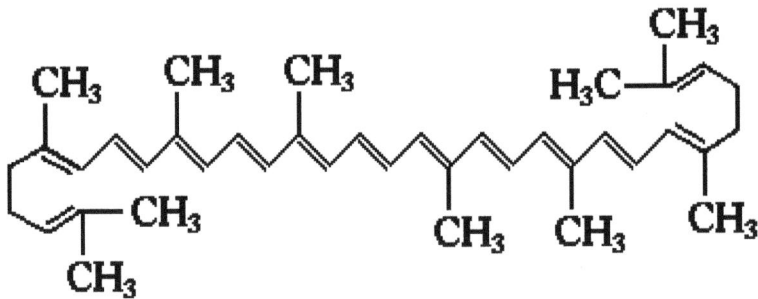
Fig. 7: Lycopene

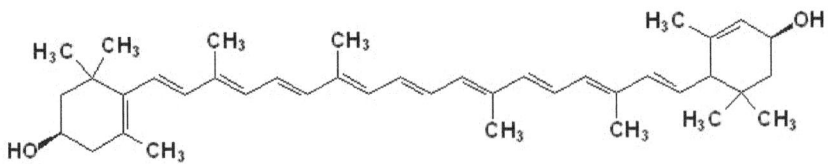
Fig. 8: Lutein

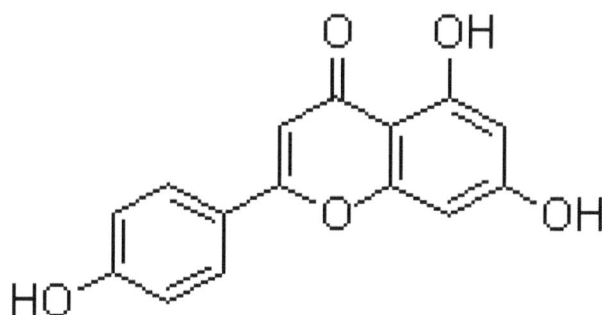

Fig. 9: apigenin

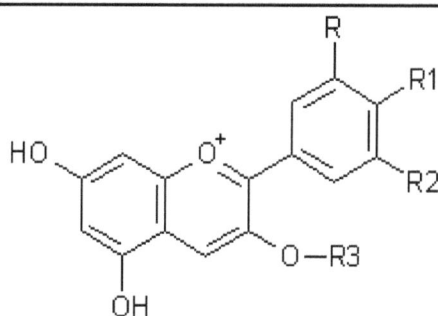

Fig. 10: Anthocyanins

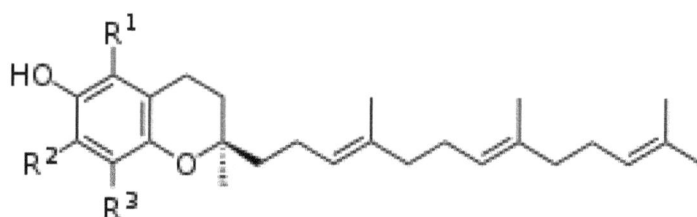

Fig. 11: Trocotrienol

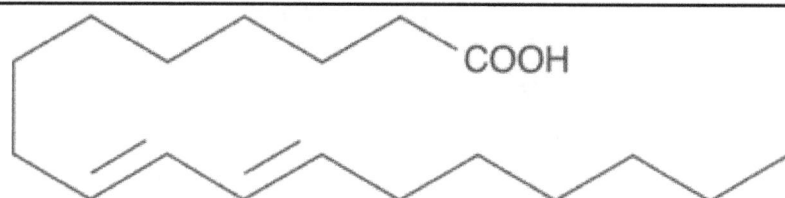

Fig. 12: Conjugated Linoleic Acid

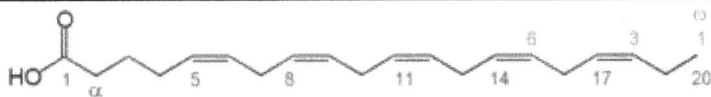

Eicosapentanoic Acid (EPA)

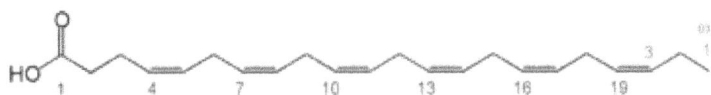

Docosahesanoic Acid (DHA)

Fig.13 : Omega-3 Fatty Acids

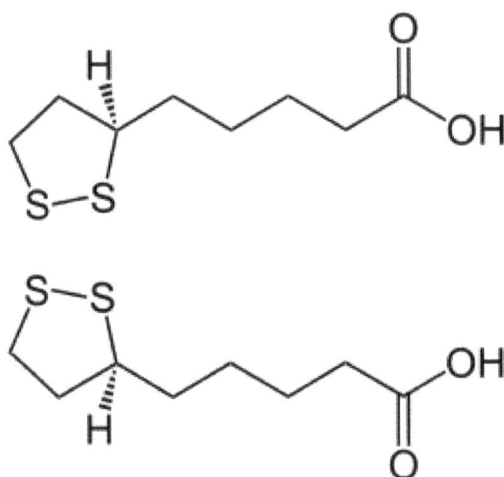

Fig. 14: α-Lipoic Acid

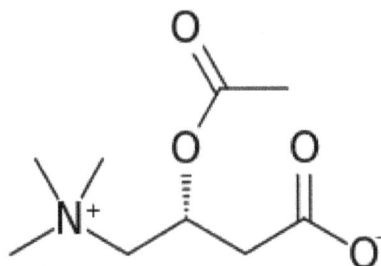

Fig. 15: Acetyl-L-carnitine

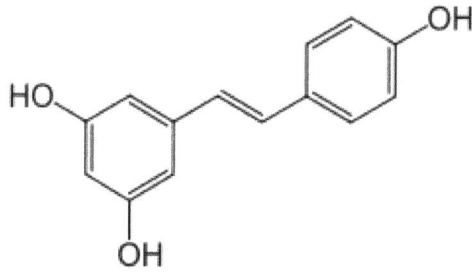

Fig 16: Resveratrol, a stilbenoid molecule

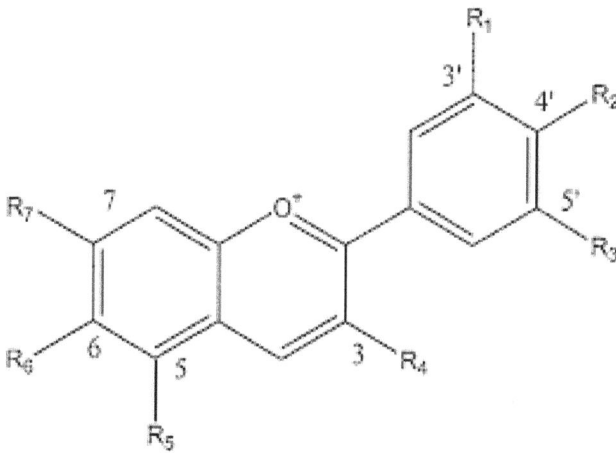

Fig. 17: Anthocyanidin

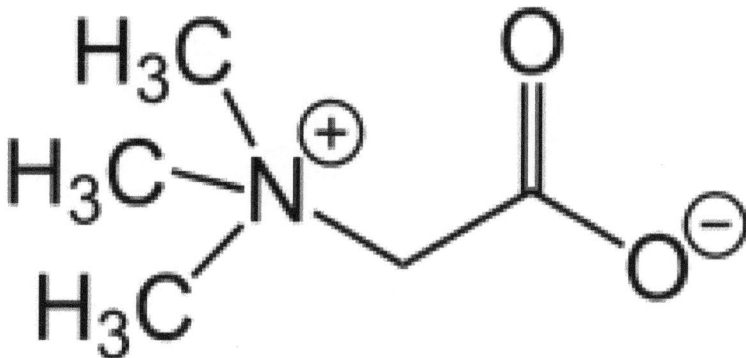

Fig. 18: Betaine

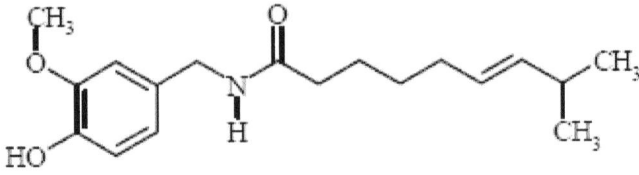

Fig. 19: Capsaicin from Chili Pepper

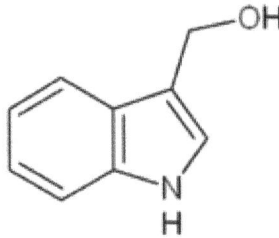

Fig. 20: Indol-3-Carbinol

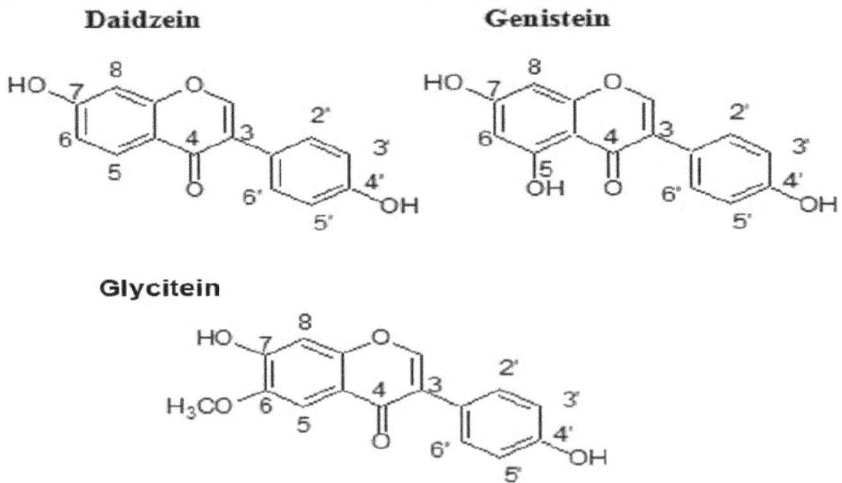

Fig. 21: Soybean isoflavones

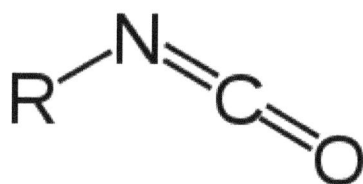

Fig. 22: Isocyanate

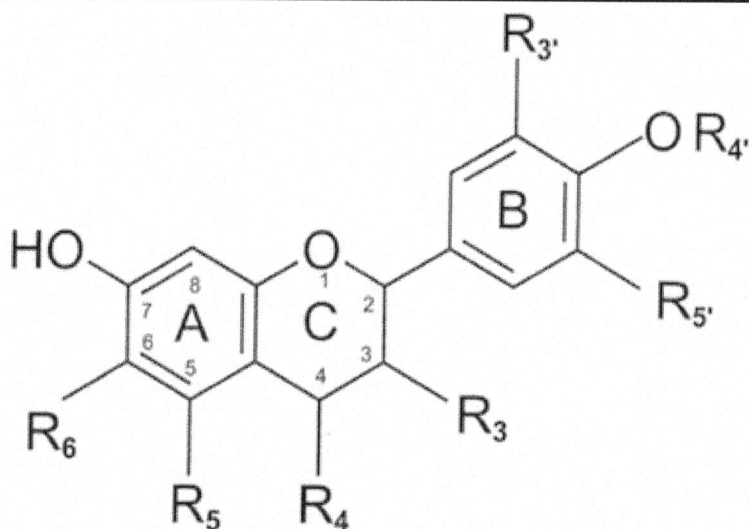

Fig. 23: Flavonoid Structures

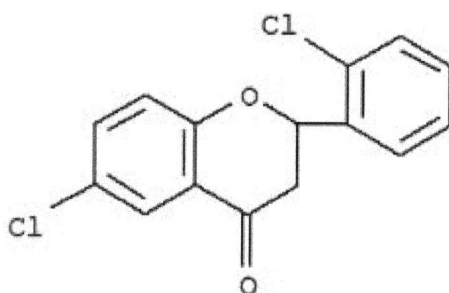

Fig. 24: Flavonone Structure

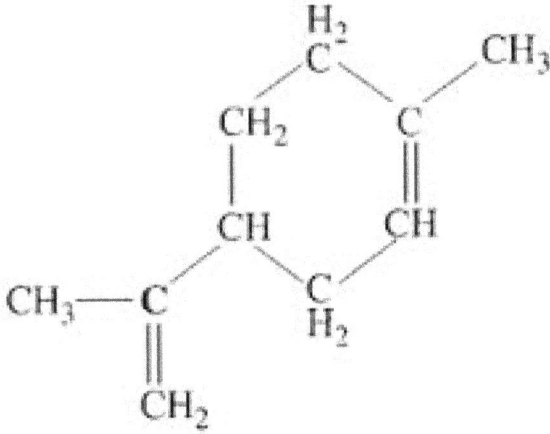

Fig. 25: A monoterpine

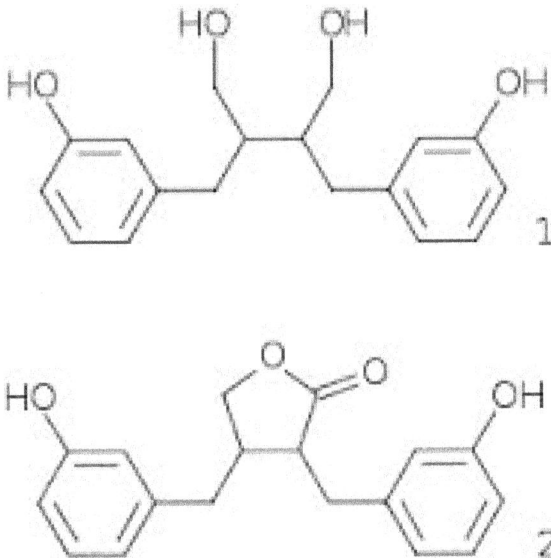

Fig. 26: Lignans from Flax seed

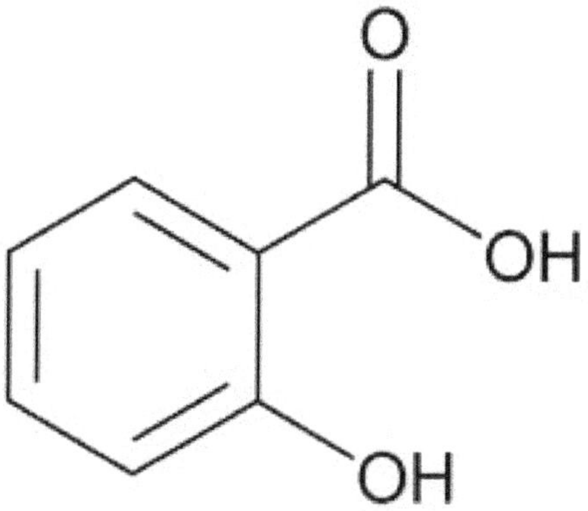

Fig. 27: Salicylic Acid

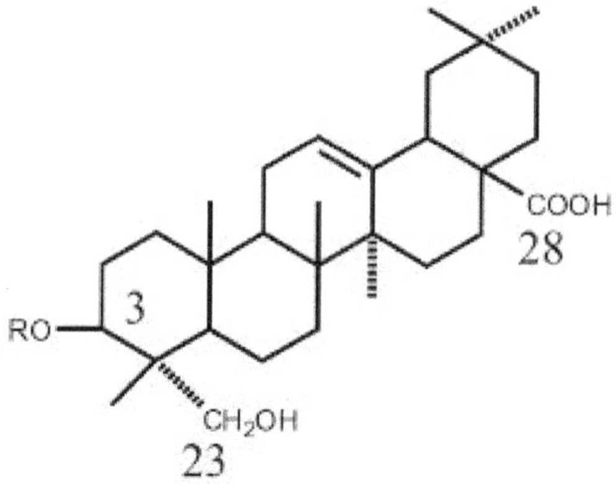

Fig. 28: Triterpinoid Saponin

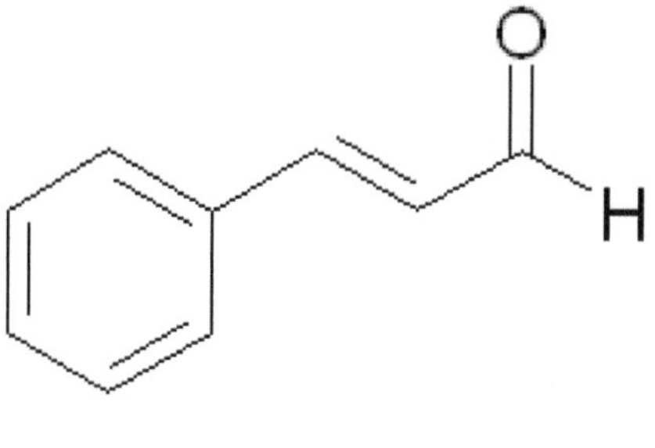

Fig.29: Cinnamaldehyde

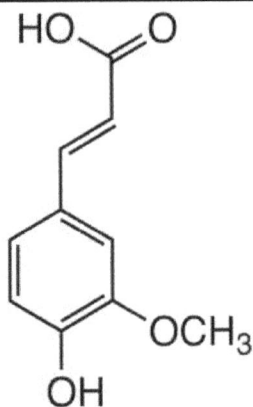

Figure 30 Ferulic Acid

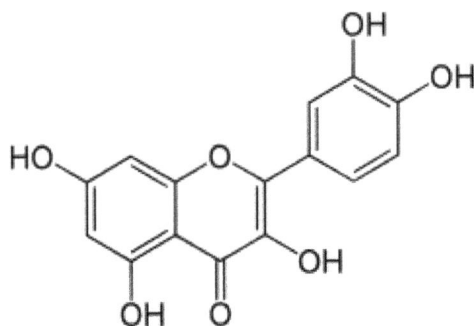

Figure 31 Quircetin

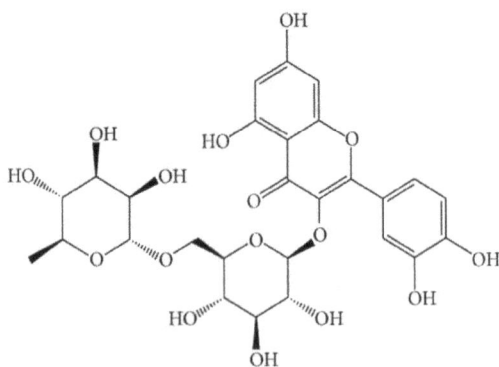

Figure 32 Rutin

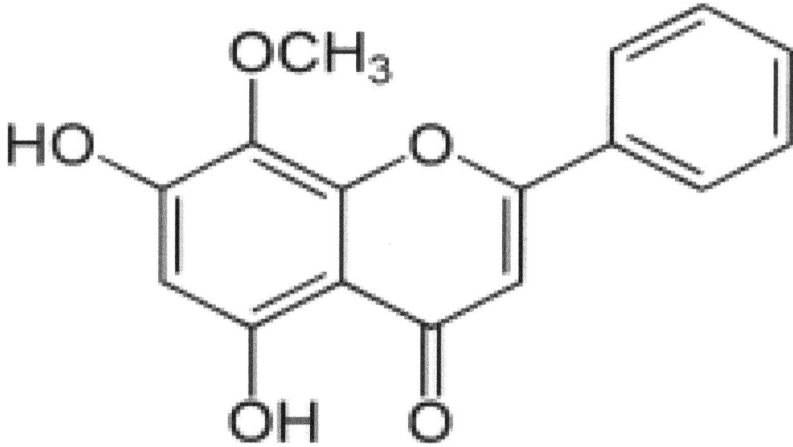

Figure 33. A Omethyl flavone, Wogonin, from Scutellaria herbs of Chinese and Japanese medicine causes death of cancer cells.

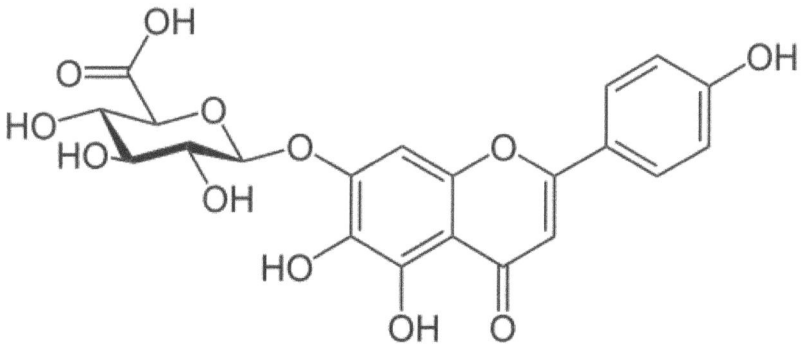

Figure 34. Scutellain, a phenolic flavone, causes death of breast and ovarian cancer cells.

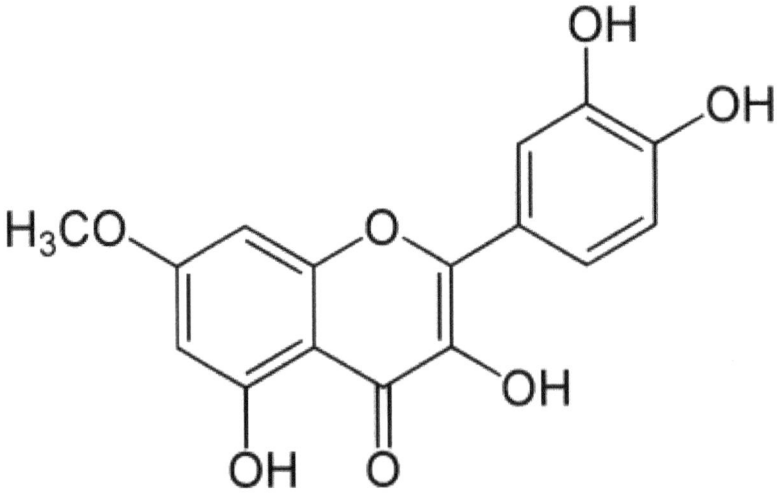

Figure 35. Rhamnetin, an O-methylated flavonol from clove, is an antiinflammatory antioxidant.

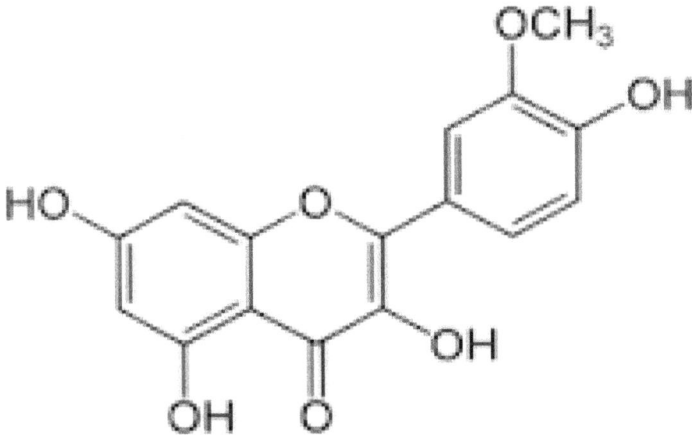

Figure 36. Isorhamnetin, as a 0-methylated flavonol from mustard green and red turnip, is an ontioxidant anticarcinogen.

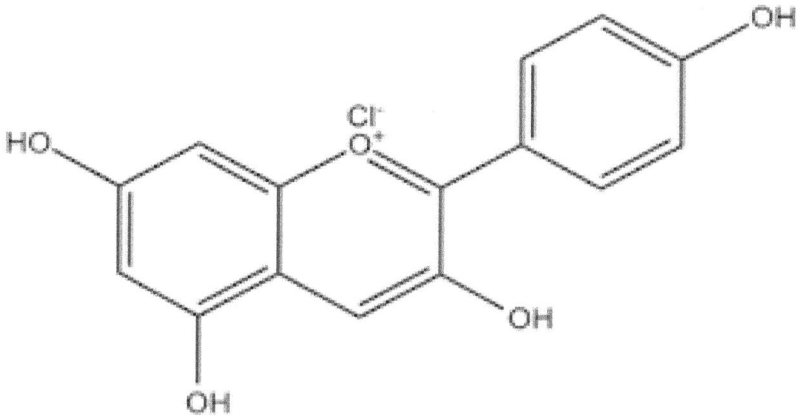

Figure 37. Pelargonidin, an antioxidant flavonoid, quenches Hydrogen peroxide.

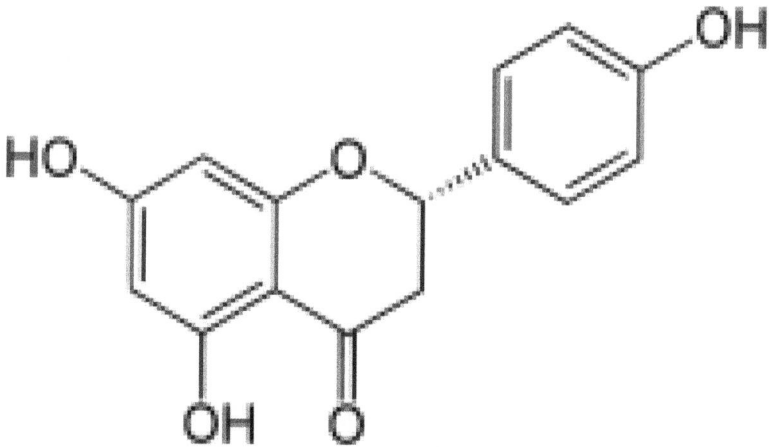

Figure 38. Antiinflammatory naringenin from grapefruit, orange, and tomato juices is known to modulate immune system and promote carbohydrate metabolism.

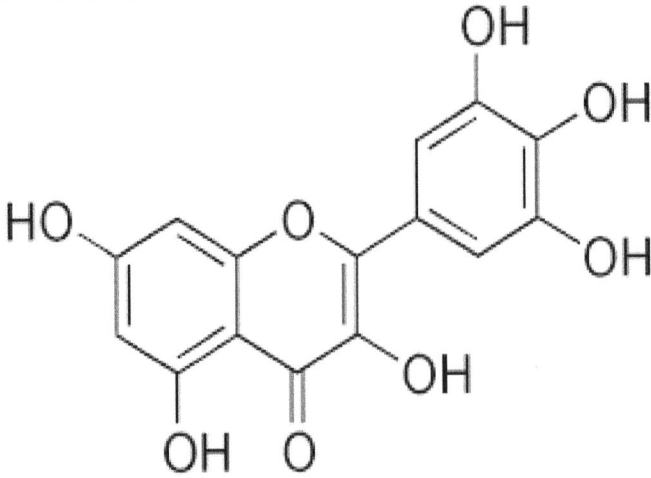

Figure 39. Myricetin, a fusetin and luteolin like flavonoid antioxidant, is found to be anticarcinogenic also. Consumers in Netherland get 23 mg/day from fruits, vegetables, and berries.

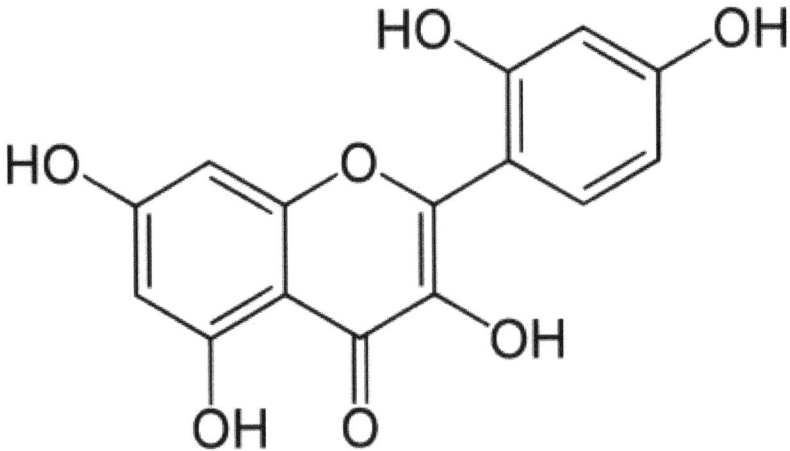

Figure 40. Morin, as an antioxidant flavonol from orange and gvava protects against free radical damage.

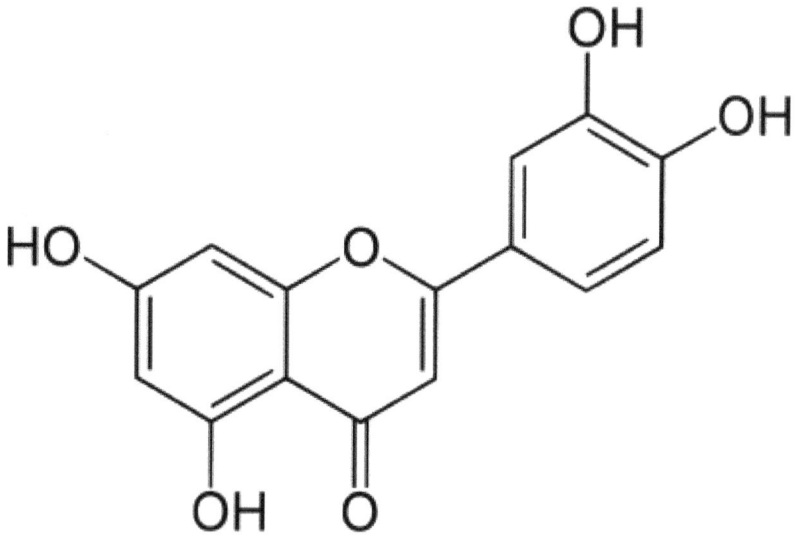

Figure 41. Luteolin, a flavoinoid antioxidant from broccoli, celery, grren pepper, and parsley, is an antiinflammatory anticarcinogen.

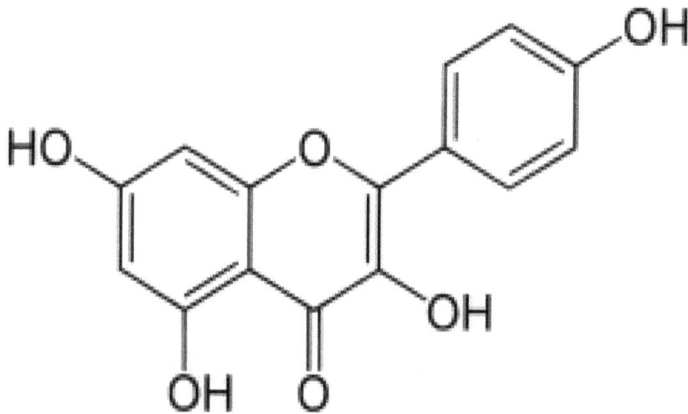

Figure 42. Kaempferol, a flavonol antioxidant from common fruits and vegetables, has effects reducing oxidative stress and preventing cancer.

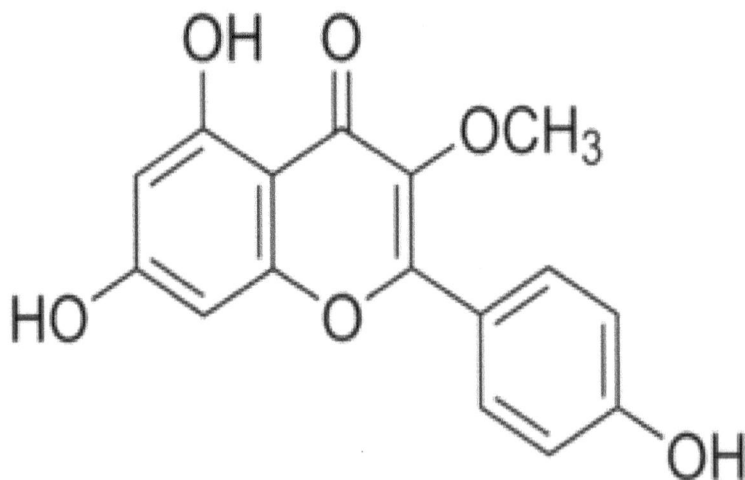

Figure 43. Isolaempferide or 3-methoxyapigenin is an antiinflammatory antioxidant with smooth muscle relaxant properties.

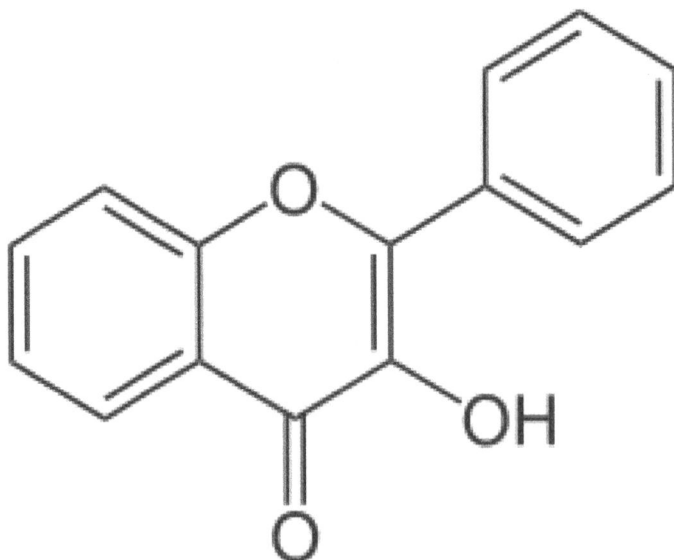

Figure 44. 3-Hydroxyflavone (or 6 or 7 hydroxy analogues) are antioxidants from caper, cocoa, chocolate, and tea. 3-Hydroxy is the flavone skeleton.

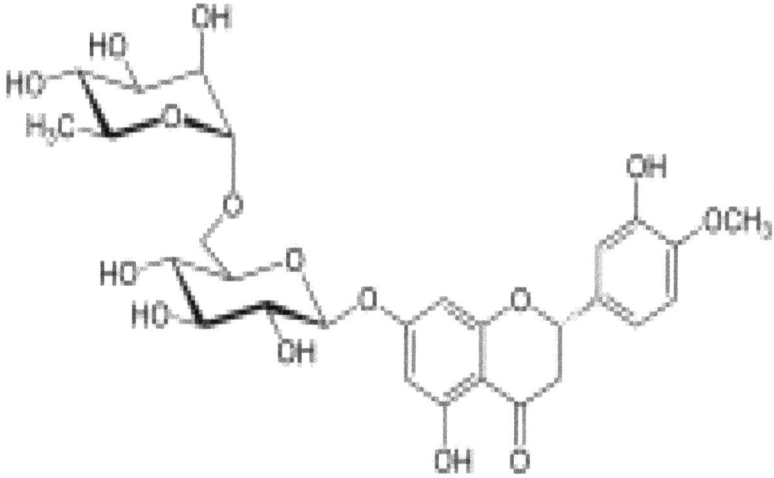

Figure 45. Hesperidinis a glycoside from citrus fruits. It is anticarcinogenic and is effective in preventing postmenopausal osteoporosis. Hesperetin is the aglycone (structure w/o sugar).

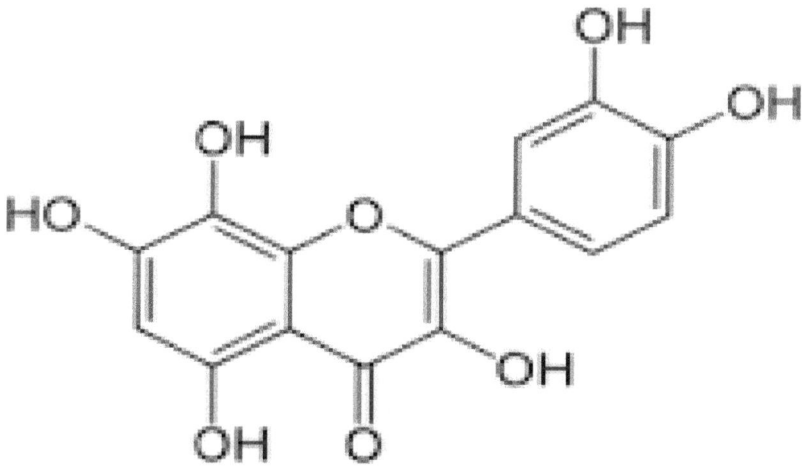

Figure 46. Gossypetin is hydroxylated quircetin with antiatherosclerotic effects. Apple, onion, and tea are good sources.

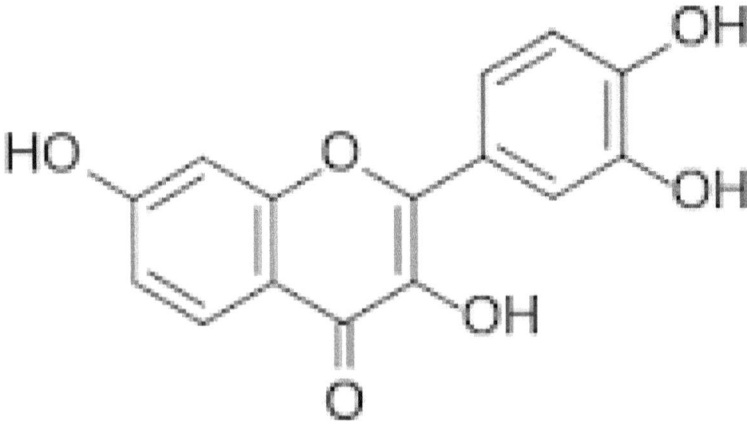

Figure 47. Fisetin, a flavonol from strawberry and onion marketed as memory enhancer, is an anticarcinogen that may protect nerve cells.

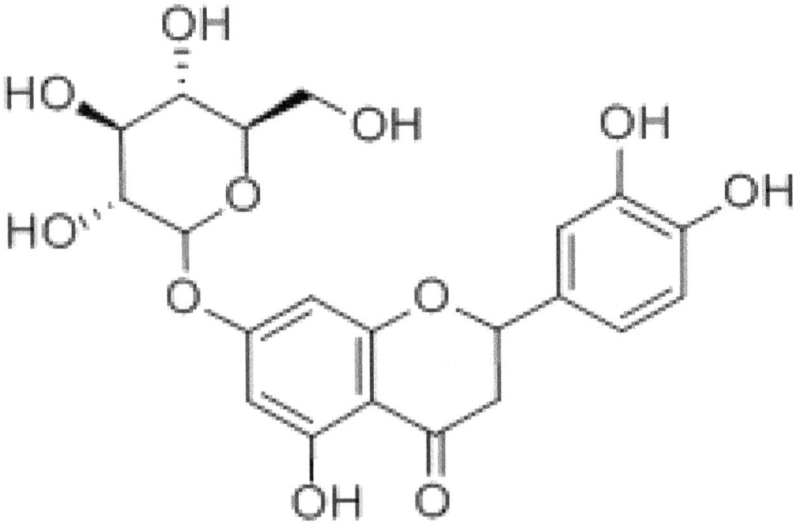

Figure 48. Eriodictyol glycoside, a common bioflavonoid from lemon peal can be a daily complement for B vitamins, vitamin C, and the flavonoid antioxidant.

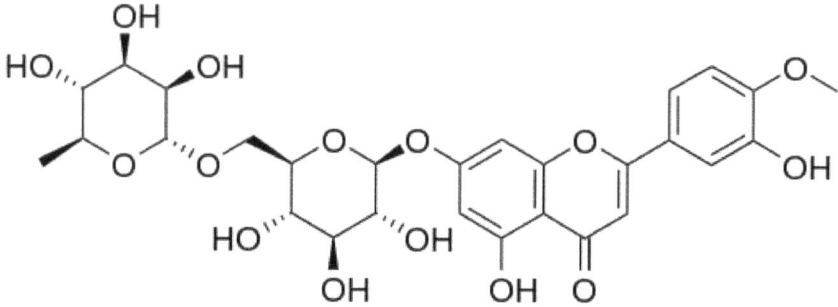

Figure 49. Diosmin is a modified synthetic hesperidin used to treat chronic venous insufficiency.

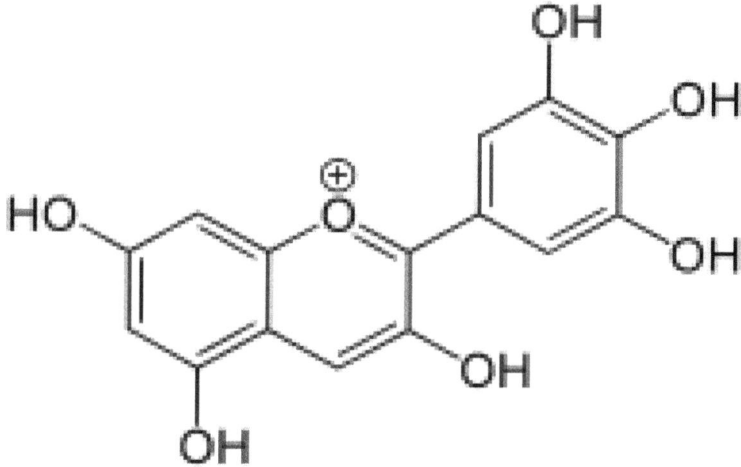

Figure 50. Delphinidin, an anthocyanidin antioxidant from wine, can kill colon cancer cells. It is a potent antioxidant and angiogenic against cancer cell from cranberry, grapes, and pomegranate.

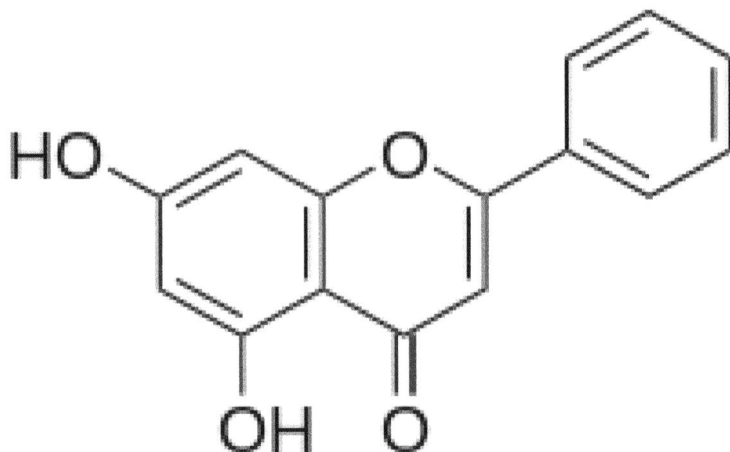

Figure 51. Chrysin, the flavonoid of passion flower, is testosteron boosting flavone.

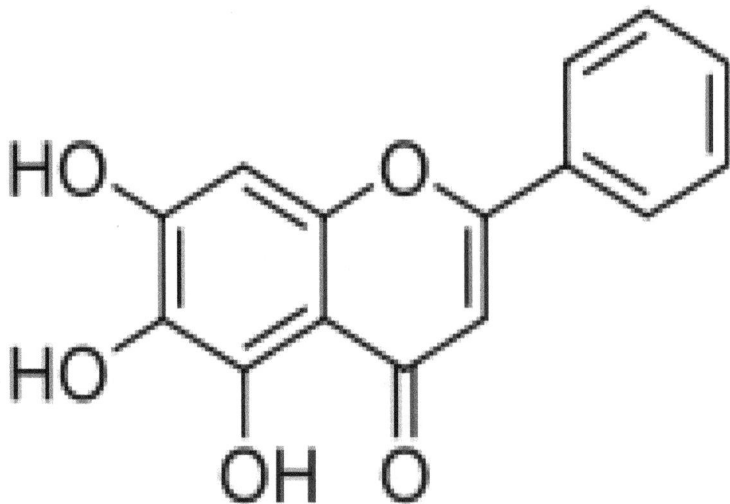

Figure 52. Biaclalein, a trihydroxyflavone, from roots of skullcap (Scutellaria baicalensis) is used against infection and cancer in Chinese medicine.

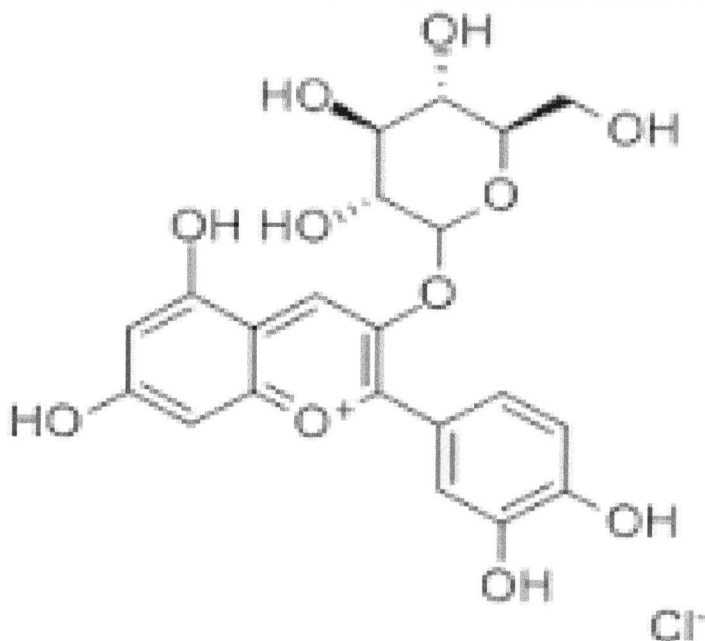

Figure 53. Cyanidin 3 glucoside, anthocyanin chrysenthamin, is used to treat hyperglycemia and insulin sensitivity.

Descriptions of Isoprenoid pigments, vitamins, quinones, and precursors of sex hormones are abundant in literature [865], [866]. Isoprenoids affect cytotoxic power of human natural Killer cells of our immune system [867]. These molecules are critical to living systems and have been conserved in plant and animal life. They play huge roles in respiration and membrane fluidity in case of humans[868]. Without these functional molecules and those listed in Table 2.07.02, there shall be no life for us. No wonder why antioxidants like flax lignans and soy isoflavones as main phytoestrogens have received maximum attention in clinical research [869].

PPQ, resveratrol, CoQ_{10}, Vitamins A, E, D, and K, isoflavones and flavonoids, glutathiones, and quercetin are readdresses in this section for the simple reason of their relevance to our daily methylation diet.

865   http://www.chem.qmul.ac.uk/iupac/misc/quinone.html
866   http://www.britannica.com/EBchecked/topic/296490/isoprenoid
867   http://www.ncbi.nlm.nih.gov/pubmed/23847096
868   https://www.rpi.edu/dept/bcbp/molbiochem/MBWeb/mb1/part2/lipid.htm
869   http://www.ncbi.nlm.nih.gov/pubmed/10082786

5.13.01 Pyroloquinoline Quinone (PQQ) for heart and the Nerve Cells

PQQ (Pyroloquinoline Quinone) is a polyphenolic antioxidants critical to mitochondrial performance in all living system[870] . PQQ is food for mitochondria and research on PPQ containing foods is extensive. *PQQ acts as an enzyme cofactor and a oxidation-reduction signaling vital to our daily living. It is a true longevity nutrient* [871] **vital to expression of 25% critical genes (238 out of 1000 tested) and thus a master molecule for making new mitochondria.**

Four major enzyme proteins depend on PQQ for their function: serine-methionine-protein kinase, Flavin reductase, Acetyl-coA synthase, and dopamine β-hydroxylase [872]. Mitochondrial DNA mutations cause not only aging but a majority of cancers . It is becoming clear now that mitochondria evolved cooperatively in our cells to manage electrons and protons, to balance good and bad free radicals, and to monitor death and rebirth of cells. We can maintain healthy mitochondria and proper balance of death and rebirth of our cells by consuming diets containing PQQ.

Furthermore PQQ has definite roles in protecting existing neurons and making new ones. It helps making of nerve growth factors vital to birth of new nerve cells [873] and strengthens heart muscles almost like beta-blockers like Metaprolol in protecting heart after serious attack and stroke. As to specific benefits it balances blood glucose by reducing insulin resistance [874], helps our cells function better by helping the key proteins that run our life processes, prevents aggregation of α-synnuclein, a protein associated with Parkinson's disease [875]. Also, it is involved in sulfur oxidation of cell signaling protein DJ-1, an important event for Parkinson's patients [876].

PQQ, call it the first new vitamin, discovered in last 55 years as a break-through anti-aging nutrient [877], that improves cognition, memory, and learning. It protects brain cells from beta-amyloid proteins linked to Alzheimer's disease, kills leukemia cancer cells [878], and modulates methyl

---

870   http://www.aorhealth.com/assets/Research/pdf/Advances_9_April_2006_Pyrroloquinoline_Qui-none_PQQ.pdf
871   https://www.facebook.com/organicherbalsolutions/posts/439368709433706
872   http://www.ncbi.nlm.nih.gov/pubmed/15689995
873   hthttp http://www.prohealth.com/library/showarticle.cfm?libid=16896://www.prohealth.com/library/showarticle.cfm?libid=16896tp://www.ncbi.nlm.nih.gov/pubmed/22843070
874   http://en.wikipedia.org/wiki/Pyrroloquinoline_quinone
875   http://www.ncbi.nlm.nih.gov/pubmed/16962995
876   http://www.pureencapsulations.com/education-research/newscaps/newscap-03-01-10
877   http://www.ncbi.nlm.nih.gov/pubmed/8403896
878   http://naturallysavvy.com/care/pyrroloquinoline-quinone-and-memory

D-aspartate (NMDA) receptor and as such helps control seizures [879]. PQQ promotes the master regulator PCG-1α (Peroxisome Proliferator Activator Receptor gamma cofactor 1α) [880]. To summarize, PQQ

- Affect genes involved in energy production

- Quenches free radicals with 500X efficiency

- Improves cognition, memory, and brain health

- Interacts with brain neurotransmitters

- Prevents cell death

- Cures ischemia reperfusion injury in case of heart patients

- Prevents Parkinson's disease by inhibiting α-synuclein

This powerful antioxidant pretty much can help run our daily life along with other antioxidants that protect our cell's membranes. Our daily diet can easily deliver about 30 nanogram per gram of PQQ foods. Heat stable and water soluble PQQ can last several thousand cycles before being all used up . Its biogenesis is well understood [881]. As an antioxidant PQQ works with glutathione for reactivation, protects mitochondria from oxidative stress, and promotes generation of new mitochondria. It has an anti-inflammatory role [882]. There is no official RDA yet.

Daily intake of PQQ is a necessity for freedom from neurological disorders and chronic diseases of heart, diabetes, and metabolic syndromes. For sure PQQ along with other antioxidants (hydroxytyrisol from olive oil, resveratrol from vine, quercetin from apple and onion, and catechins from tea) can prolong our life and enhance our daily health. Consuming copious servings of fruits and vegetable should be our daily priority. We must include papaya, and kiwi, broad beans, edamami, green soy bean, fermented soy Natto, parsley, and cruciferacea family vegetables such as cabbage and cauliflower in our methylation diet. *The power of spinach in effect is power of PQQ [883].* Using spinach as salad and drinking green tea for beverage can improve mitochondrial health and delay aging.

879   http://www.ncbi.nlm.nih.gov/pubmed/10704515
880   http://www.jbc.org/content/285/1/142.long
881   http://www.pnas.org/content/101/21/7913.full.pdf
882   http://informahealthcare.com/doi/abs/10.3109/03008209309014242?journalCode=cts
883   http://www.naturalnews.com/031236_mitochondria_cellular_energy.html

5.13.02 Resveratrol

The role of resveratrol, a stilbenoid phenolic antioxidant and phytoalexin , was briefly described in section 5.10. Mitochondrial impairment, a primary cause of fatigue, seems to be mitigated by resveratrol [884], [885]. A daily dose of 250 mg per day is often recommended for mitochondrial protection [886], [887], [888] because it is repeatedly shown to boost mitochondrial function, to improve longevity, and to act as an antiinflammatory and antiviral agents [889],[890]. Harvard medical school, NIH, University of New South Wales, Sydney, Mayo Clinic, Memorial Sloan Kettering cancer Center, Linus Pauling Institute of Oregon State University, and University of Southern CA have been working in this area with great intensity. However, FDA has not approved resveratrol because of considerable controversy on its therapeutic value[891],[892]. On the other hand research does suggest that it improves mitochondrial function by increasing superoxide dismutase activity, activating SIRT 1 gene that in association with NAD maintains mitochondrial connection with nuclear DNA, inhibiting enzyme topoisomerase, and having therapeutic values against Alzheimer's disease, cancer, dementia, and heart diseases. The overall effect is supported by many meta-analyses on glucose control [893], aging[894], longevity[895], blood pressure control[896], and diabetes[897]. *Mitochondrial function and post resveratrol consumption response can be measured electrochemically in terms of electron transfer to complex IV.*

Natural sources of resveratrol are red wine (0.001%), pomegranates, Japanese knotwood, berries, peanut (0.5%), and cocoa powder (0.3%). FDA considers it GRAS or Generally Recognized as safe but has not approved it for disease control [898].

---

884   http://www.sciencedirect.com/science/article/pii/S221464741400004X
885   http://www.ncbi.nlm.nih.gov/pmc/articles/PMC2680051/
886   http://www.medscape.com/viewarticle/745451
887   http://www.sciencedirect.com/science/article/pii/S0092867406014280
888   http://www.immunityageing.com/content/10/1/28
889   http://www.bloomberg.com/news/2013-03-07/red-wine-compound-activates-gene-needed-for-healthy-cells.html
890   hhttp://www.fda.gov/ucm/groups/fdagov-public/@fdagov-foods-gen/documents/document/ucm264051.pdfhttp://www.anh-usa.org/new-study-touts-big-health-benefits-of-resveratrol/
891   http://www.alzforum.org/news/research-news/dietary-resveratrol-makes-little-difference-health
892   http://www.the-scientist.com/?articles.view/articleNo/32208/title/Resveratrol-May-Not-Extend-Life/
893   jcn.nutrition.org/content/early/2014/04/02/ajcn.113.082024.abstract
894   http://www.impactaging.com/papers/v5/n7/full/100579.html
895   http://www.researchgate.net/publication/227710963_The_effect_of_resveratrol_on_longevity_across_species_a_meta-analysis
896   http://www.clinicalnutritionjournal.com/article/S0261-5614(14)00084-3/abstract
897   http://newhope360.com/breaking-news/resveratrol-does-indeed-help-diabetics
898   http://www.fda.gov/ucm/groups/fdagov-public/@fdagov-foods-gen/documents/document/

5.13.03 Coenzyme Q$_{10}$

Coenzyme q$_{10}$ is present in every cell of our body with high concentration in organs that need high energy on demand (heart, liver, kidney). Known as ubiquinone, Q in its name refers to quinone and 10 refers to electron mobile 10 isoprenoid side chain structure. Soluble in the lipid bilayer of inner mitochondrial membrane, it can exist in three oxidation-reduction states: fully oxidized ubiquinone, ubisemiquinone, and reduced ubiquinol. Its isoprenoid chain has a length similar to the width of inner mitochondrial membrane.

No other food molecule can perform functions of Coenzyme Q$_{10}$ which often coperforms with vitamin K$_2$. **Coenzyme Q$_{10}$ is a product of 12 genes.** Mutation of any one of these genes create deficiency of Q$_{10}$. Mutations of mitochondrial genes ETFDH, APTX, and BRAF make the situation even worse. Statins and beta blocker medicines inhibit synthesis of coenzyme Q$_{10}$ and we should decide on their daily dose only after careful consultation with our physicians.

As described in Chapter 1, Coenzyme Q$_{10}$ plays a huge role in electron transfer in inner mitochondrial membrane via Q-Cycle. Electrons from NADH and succinate pass through coenzymeQ$_{10}$, then to complex II and III and finally to oxygen via cytochrome oxidase. Simultaneous to electron transfer, translocation of protons from the mitochondrial matrix to intermediate space between outer and inner membrane facilitates production of ATP by ATP synthase, an enzyme that literally breathes protons.

Coenzyme q$_{10}$ is an antioxidant capable of inhibiting lipid peroxidation and production of lipid peroxy radicals. It prevents oxidation of DNA bases and generates vitamin E as an antioxidant. Deficiency of coenzyme Q$_{10}$ cause cancer, heart failure, high blood pressure, infertility, migraine headache, and Parkin's disease. Good food sources for coenzyme Q$_{10}$ are dark green vegetables, avocado, almond, peanuts, pistachio, grape seed, soybean, meats, and fish. Many common Coenzyme Q$_{10}$ containing foods for methylation diet are included in chapter 2.

5.13.04 Vitamins A, E, D, and K

Vitamins A, E, and K are necessary mitochondrial foods described in chapter 2. Methylation diets provide for sufficient daily dose of these vitamins even at reduced calorie diets as long as the variety of ingredients is willfully maintained by way of carrots and sweet potato for vitamin A, almond and nuts, and plant oils for vitamin E, and vegetables like brussels sprout, broccoli, kale, mustard green, scallion, spinach, and spices like basil.

5.13.05 Isoflavones and Flavonoids

Fruits and vegetables, soy bean, edamami, chocolate, tea, coffee, and various nuts are great sources of isoflavones and flavonoids. Chapter 2 has an extensive coverage. Again a good methylation diet should deliver recommended daily allowance.

5.13.06 Glutathione

Glutathione is a tripeptide (gamma linked cysteine with glutamic acid which in turn has a regular linkage with glycine) antioxidant involved in quenching free radicals, regulating nitric oxide cycle, DNA synthesis, and iron metabolism [899] [900]. *Our cells synthesize it in presence of zinc.* Its concentration increases by supplements of vitamin D_3, whey protein, S-adenosylmethionine, and N-Acetylcysteine. *This powerful natural antioxidant comes from fruits and vegetables, milk and eggs, turmeric, and whey protein.* It is very effective in reducing disulfide bonds of proteins in the cytosol [901]. Our methylation diet must deliver sufficient zinc by way of oyesters and lobster for high doisage and nuts and simple vegetables for routine diets.

---

899   http://www.medicinenet.com/script/main/art.asp?articlekey=50746
900   http://www.immunehealthscience.com/glutathione.html
901   http://www.rheumatoid-arthritis-decisions.com/Foods-that-boost-glutathione.html

5.13.07 Quercetin, a Potent Antiinflammatory Bioflavonoid

Quercetin, also known as sophretin and meletin like coloring pigment in plant kingdom, is a cousin of more commonly known antioxidant **rutin**. It is a great cure as an antioxidant for lowering C-reactive proteins, inhibiting inflammatory cyclooxygenase(COX) enzymes, and preventing cytokines (NF kappa β)[902],[903] . Quercetin is an antidiabetic and anti-aging bioflavonoid, proclaims Dr. Stephen C. Bischoff of Germany [904]. *We can get enough of quercetin from our daily wine, apples, onion, hot peppers, okra, grape and other citrus fruit, beans, sprouts, blackberries, cappers, and vegetables. Black and green tea leaves are the best source, around 250 mg/100 g. A cup of tea provides more quercetin than a medium size apple.* Bromelain, the enzyme from pineapple improves the bioavailability of practically water insoluble quercetin. Water soluble quercetin chalcones are also available.

Quircetin boosts endurance exercise capacity [905], [906], [907] . Sugar bound glycosylated quercetin as pentahydroxy flavone is more common in nature. Along with tannic acid it seem to prolong aging [908] by quenching free radicals. It donates electrons and delocalizes unpaired electrons by resonance. With powers of antihistamine and antiinflammatory agent [909], [910] this plant pigment fights cancer, congestion, other respiratory problems, rheumatoid arthritis, heart disease, and hypertension and lovers LDL cholesterol. It is an excellent stress reducing bioflavonoid.

5.13.08 Conjugated Linoleic Acid and Omega-3 Fatty Acids

Lets take a tally of common cis double bond containing electron rich (isoprenoid) molecules which support our health and well being. This group of molecules includes essential oils, pigments, cancer causing isoprenoid mutated RAS (reticular activating system) proteins, fragrances, vitamins, cofactors, and sex hormones. Three nutrients we hear often in this group

902   http://www.supplementfacts.com/BioflavonoidBookS3.htm
903   http://www.ncbi.nlm.nih.gov/pubmed/15053821
904   http://www.readcube.com/articles/10.1097/MCO.0b013e32831394b8
905   http://www.ncbi.nlm.nih.gov/pubmed/21606866
906   http://www.quercetinscience.com/Quercetin-Performance-MetaAnalysis-MSSE-D-10-00878.pdf
907   file:///C:/Users/Owner/Downloads/Kressler_2011.pdf
908   http://journal.frontiersin.org/Journal/10.3389/fgene.2012.00048/abstract
909   http://umm.edu/health/medical/altmed/supplement/quercetin
910   http://www.rxlist.com/quercetin/supplements.htm

are omega-3 fatty acids, conjugated linoleic acid (CLA), and coenzyme Q_{10}. These molecules are central to biology. DHA, a 22 carbon long Omega-3 fatty acid has a very long evolutionary history and then there are others known to common folks.

- Coenzyme Q_{10} like electron carriers and plastoquinones
- Polyphenols as antioxidants
- Vitamin K, a Phylloquinone critical to blood clotting
- Fat Soluble Vitamin as an Antioxidant.
- Vitamin D as a Cholesterol derivative necessary for Calcium and Phosphorus metabolism
- Vitamin A, β-carotene , and other pigments for vision and photoreception

Isoprene structure, $CH_2=C(CH_3)CH=CH_2$, is common to almost all molecular categories listed above. DHA (docosahexanoic acid, 22: 6 n-3)) and EPA (Eicosapentanoic acid, 20:n 5-3) are curved chemical structures because of all cis-configuration of 6 and 5 double bonds in 22 carbon and 20 carbon fatty acids respectively. *These electron rich omega-3 fatty acids and conjugated linoleic acid must be part our daily methylation diet.* These phenomena are linked to cell's ability to talk to each other about nutrient status and regulate communication with the brain. They are absolutely necessary for mitochondrial health in terms of maintaining and balancing endocytosis (energy intensive protein transport) and gene expression [911]. In SN_2 state, where C-2 position of glycerol is esterified, DHA acts like oxygen . Its π-electrons permit high electric and magnetic field. Electroencephalographs will simply not be possible without DHA. DHA tied to circadian rhythm turns sunlight to electric signal via water-collagen complex and it helps produce IR radiation in mitochondria [912]. Melatonin drops if there is less DHA in brain cells. Lack of DHA in SCN (Suprachiasmatic nucleus) of brain is responsible for destruction of leptin. Blue light (wavelength of 450-490 nm) destroys melatonin because human brain doesn't differentiate between blue light and sunlight.

DHA is tied to our evolution and low DHA simply means sick brain. Actually, the brain cells die under DHA deficiency [913]. Less oxygen in mitochondria means less DHA no matter what and how much omega-3 fatty acid we eat. **Loss of DHA destroys leptin receptor necessary for**

911   http://www.ncbi.nlm.nih.gov/pmc/articles/PMC3809566/
912   http://www.ncbi.nlm.nih.gov/pubmed/25144192
913   http://www.febsletters.org/article/S0014-5793(09)01059-X/abstract

neuronal development. DHA is necessary for cognition, photoreception, and intelligence [914]. A reasonable daily intake should be 120 mg/day.

Mitochondria must have paramagnetic DHA and oxygen for their normal power. As an electron rich molecule in our lipid membranes, DHA attracts oxygen. Its structure allows quantum transfer and π-electron communication. **DHA is involved in expression of more than 100 genes produced in our brain [915], [916].** Whereas EPA reduces inflammation, DHA, the most abundant type of fatty acid in our brain, produces electricity and acts in neuron signaling because of its spatial property [917]. It serves as the best electron and proton catching device.

No wonder 48% of all circuits in our body are dedicated to light. These fatty acids prevent neurodegenerative diseases[918], [919]. Conjugated linoleic acid in particular prevents mitochondrial oxidation [920], improves lipid metabolism, and prevents heart disease [921]. Let us remember that as a conserved acyl component of photoreceptor synapses for nerve cell signaling DHA is tied to evolution of our brain. It protects mood and memory, protects light receptors, reduces inflammation, and most importantly helps photoreceptors convert photons into electrons.

Our daily methylation diet should contain good fat *with DHA like fatty acids* for electron supply. Moderate inclusion of butter for conjugated linoleic acid, therefore, in our daily recipes is good. Trans and saturated fats destroy the membrane charge[922].

To emphasize again, DHA converts light energy into electricity as part of signaling mechanism in the brain and this is a 600 million year old evolutionary mechanism. **The flexible configuration of DHA molecule transitions within picoseconds and entire molecule becomes an electron wave [923].** What matters here is its π-electron system permitting flipping bond polarity by quantized sunlight as it absorbs light. Actually, the π-electrons on either side of CH_2 bond communicate.

Eating habits including proper RDA of vitamin D and DHA omega-3 and personal environment control mitochondrial function. Their deficiency is known to lower electric and magnetic fields in mitochondria. This also

914   http://www.ars.usda.gov/SP2UserFiles/person/4986/set4/Final%20DHA%202012.pdf
915   http://ajcn.nutrition.org/content/83/6/S1520.long
916   http://www.plosone.org/article/info%3Adoi%2F10.1371%2Fjournal.pone.0035425
917   http://www.terrapub.co.jp/onlineproceedings/fs/wfc2008/pdf/wfcbk_057.pdf
918   http://www.sciencedirect.com/science/article/pii/S0952327812000737
919   http://www.ncbi.nlm.nih.gov/pubmed/22727983
920   http://ajcn.nutrition.org/content/79/6/1169S.full
921   http://www.jlr.org/content/43/12/2112.full.pdf
922   http://www.indiana.edu/~oso/Fat/SolidNLiquid.html
923   http://www.ars.usda.gov/SP2UserFiles/person/4986/set4/Final%20DHA%202012.pdf

causes low production of IR light. Resolvins from EPA and protectins from DHA are neuroprotective proteins [924]. *Unique spatial property include a curved structure and an all cis-configuration for this very flexible molecule that can configure itself in picoseconds.* The π-electron system absorbs light. Alternating double bonds are like a hole- a positively charged electron deficient hole. Quantized sunlight flips the direction of bond polarity. Thus the structure has a great electron and proton catch system: captures electric current and acts as an e-wave.

DHA helps make vital copper, iodine, and selenium proteins. Our nerves contain DHA at exited membranes and synaptic junctions. Retina has it and photoreceptors and sperm cells have it. DHA is an excellent antiinflammatory nutrient. We must exercise in order to exploit full benefits of DHA in our cell membranes and mitochondria. A good deal of technical detail is discussed here just to unequivocally highlight the importance of omega-3 fatty acids in our day-to-day nutrition.

5.14 Porphyrins and Metallo-proteins for Life

Porphyrins and metallo-proteins, ubiquitous and vital in human body, are very rarely talked about by nutritionists and food scientists. Just as nucleotides are important for structures of DNA, RNA, and high energy electron carriers like NADH and $FADH_2$ and just as amino acids are important for structures of antibodies, enzymes, receptors, and neuro transmitters, **conjugated isoprenoids** are important for structures of antioxidants, vitamins, and hormones.. Conjugated porphyrin metal protein complexes are involved in routine gas and ligand transport, electron transport, and detoxification of xenebiotic substances in the liver. Fullerene biomolecules are the strongest antioxidants and their full life enhancing potential has yet to be realized [925], [926].

Heme protein cytochrome 450 enzymes of close to 1000 types are present in liver and intestine [927]. They are there to dispose of harmful substances simply by adding a OH radical or extra conjugation. These heme proteins determine drug actions and interaction [928], [929]. Of 50 of these

924   http://lipidlibrary.aocs.org/Lipids/eicresol/file.pdf
925   http://www.owndoc.com/pdf/fullerenes-help-familial-als.pdf
926   http://www.hindawi.com/journals/bmri/2013/821498/
927   http://www.ebi.ac.uk/interpro/potm/2006_10/Page1.htm
928   http://www.ncbi.nlm.nih.gov/pmc/articles/PMC1312247/
929   http://www.nutritionandmetabolism.com/content/5/1/27

enzymes, six metabolize most of routinely used drugs [930]. Nutritional status and iron deficiency can affect the function of cytochrome 450 enzymes causing abnormal liver functions [931].

It is well known that vitamin B$_{12}$ is a porphyrins structure dedicated to formation of red blood cells, building proteins, and functions of nervous system. Actually, it is a brain vitamin. Oxygen, carbon dioxide, and nitric oxide carrying hemoglobin and heme b myoglobin are other critical biomolecules of life. Gas transport in body is rather exclusive work of conjugated porphyrin heme proteins characterized by π-electron orbital systems. As pointed out earlier, the alternating single and double C-C bonds and delocalization of electrons support life as we know it today.

Hemoglobin and myoglobin contain heme b proteins for oxygen, carbon dioxide, and nitric oxide exchange. Up to 0.5 liter oxygen is carried per minute by these iron proteins from lung to heart and finally to every cell in the body via capillaries [932]. A low oxygen level in case of lung disease or anemia tells the stem cells in bone marrow to make more red blood cells. Nutrients iron, folic acid, and vitamin B$_{12}$ are necessary to maintain up to 400,000 red blood cells per micro liter blood, at least 600 red blood cells for each white blood cell and at least 40 for each platelet.

Even more important iron containing heme proteins in regard to mitochondrial function are cytochrome C and Cytochrome C oxidase, a cousin of heme b called heme a proteins. Cytochrome C transfers electrons from complex III (CoEnzQ-cytochrome C reductase) to complex IV or cytochrome C oxidase. It is a small 12,000 Dalton heme-protein. On the other hand, Cytochrome C oxidase is a large transmembrane protein. It receives one electron each from cytochrome C family of enzyme proteins. They do have the structural novelty of π-π overlapping orbital complex and symmetry for electron affinity. Their properties of diverse functions depend on the environment. *The key point to note is that binding of gases by hemoglobin's heme b is an electron phenomenon and heme a of cytochromes in electron transport chain is also involved in letting electrons hop around. Conjugated cis structures are critical to a whole host of biological function. Important nutrients in regard to functions of cytochrome c and related structures are iron, sulfur, folate, and vitamin B$_{12}$.*

---

930   http://www.aafp.org/afp/2007/0801/p391.html
931   ht http://www.ncbi.nlm.nih.gov/pubmed/24379667
932   http://medical-dictionary.thefreedictionary.com/oxygen+consumption

5.15 The Power of Sleep

Chronic sleep deprivation ages our brain by stress, causes failure of repair our bones, prevents proper sugar digestion and pancreatic function, prevents making of growth factor for good skin, prevents muscle repair, and shrinks neurons by arresting timely removal of debris at the end of the day [933]. Our body takes care of itself during sleep by calibrating and defraging our brain [934], [935]. Naturally we must right size our sleep for 8 hours a day and optimize our chronobiology and circadian rhythm.

We are beginning to understand that circadian clock of NAD$^+$ cycle drives mitochondrial oxidative metabolism in mice [936] and sleep deprivation endangers mitochondria [937], [938]. Actually, sleep apnea is due to mitochondrial dysfunction [939].

High melatonin foods such as tart cherries, lettuce, cheese, ginger root, and walnut help us sleep naturally by creating in vivo the best drug that there is in the namr of melatonin. Also, we can induce sleep by warm bath, eating of a favorite chocolate food before going to bed, and a simple daily commitment to exercise and yoga.

5.16 Optimization of Mitochondrial Function for health and Longevity

The fact that mighty mitochondria are behind our vigor, energy, and well being is least talked about by the health and fitness gurus. Expanding waistline, weakening muscles, and frequent trauma are sure signs of mitochondrial dysfunction and loss of mitochondrial count and efficiency. Their dysfunction causes 40 different diseases and 160 other body ailments. *High empty calories without proper nutrient intake is the biggest problem for mitochondrial healt and our daily health and longevity.*

Why do we age? How does cancer develop? What is the connection between heart disease and Alzheimer's? What is the cause of infertility? What is the cause of hearing loss? We don't have answers to these questions

---

933   http://jonlieffmd.com/blog/the-five-secrets-of-brain-health
934   http://ieeexplore.ieee.org/xpl/articleDetails.jsp?reload=true&arnumber=6294346
935   http://sleepbetter.org/sleep-calibrates-your-memories/2147483647/
936   file:///C:/Users/Owner/Downloads/Science-2013-Peek-.pdf
937   http://www.ncbi.nlm.nih.gov/pubmed/20176368
938   http://www.health-inspiration.com/html/protecting_the_mitochondria.html
939   http://www.cpmedical.net/newsletter/mitochondria-resuscitation-the-key-to-healing-every-disease

in detail but behind it all is the biology of mitochondria. Antioxidants are molecules that can prevent problems of autism, cancer, heart failure, type 2 diabetes, and neurological disorders such as Alzheimer's , Huntington's, and Parkinson's diseases. Healthy mitochondria are essential for our brain and vigor of stem cells. What we need for optimal mitochondrial function is a well designed methylation diet. A careful study of chapter 2 should help select foods for such diets based on varieties of fruits, vegetables, nuts, and seeds.

Avoiding inflammation, keeping immune system balanced, maintaining gut and digestive health with pro-biotics, staying away from toxins, and consuming twice the RDA of antioxidants as we go beyond our sixtieth birthday are great guidelines for health maintenance. Table 5.15.01 is further detailed beyond Table 5.06 with respect to additional nutrients and choices of restricted calorie consumption, exercise, and even mindfulness. For mitochondria to be free of mutation and deletions withous free radical damage and for keeping Krebs cycle operation to an optimum we must cosume methylation nutrients for the best of their efficiency. The methylation diet must deliver Vitamins A, B_1, B_2, B_3, C, D, E, K, Coenz Q10, PPQ, carnitine, carnosine, lipoic acid, taurine, idequinone, omega-3 fatty acids, and minerals copper, iron, magnesium, manganese, selenium, sulfur by way of high sulfer proteins, and zinc [940].

Table 5.16.01 Mitochondrial Nutrients[941] Compared with RDA by Cleveland Clinic (Table 2.07.01).

Nutrient	RDA by Cleveland Clinic, Table 2.07.01	Mg Per Day (80 Kg Person)
Alpha Lipoic Acid	400	649
Acetyl-L-carnitine	3.75	1297
Biotin, B_7		1
Nicotinamide, B_3	350	195
Riboflavin, B_2	400	78
Pyridoxin, B_6		78
Folate, B_9 mcg	2,000	

---

940   http://nutritionreview.org/2013/09/mitochondrial-dysfunction/
941   https://www.google.com/search?q=food+and+nutrients+for+mitochondria&tbm=isch&tbo=u&-source=univ&sa=X&ei=ho2xU5GZKM6XqAb6woIg&ved=0CF4Q7Ak&biw=973&bih=706

Creatine		649
Coenzyme Q$_{10}$	750	65
Vitamin E, (IU)	750	
Resveratrol		65
Selenium, mcg	50	
Taurine		1257

5.17 Mitochondrial Control of Fatty Acid Oxidation

Although energy production in our body is local and specific to the needs of organs; extra load of glucose or fatty acids is bad for mitochondria. β-oxidation of long chain fatty acids is under genetic control both in terms of making of DNA code to RNA code and further translating the RNA code to a new protein sequence[942]. Is a simple ratio of carbohydrate to fat in our daily diet a good enough control of energy production? Or does the ratio activate certain nuclear or mitochondrial genes? We don't have answers to these questions. For the time being the best approach is to keep the ratio constant through a planned pattern of restricted calorie consumption of a methylation diet in right amount at right time.

Table 5.16.02 Foods for Healthy Mitochondria		
Nutrients	**Functions**	**Mg/Day**
Coenzyme Q$_{10}$		300.00
PPQ		20.00
Carnosine	Human body makes this amino acid	400-500
Carnitine		No Official RDA
Alpha-Lipoic Acid		Unofficial, 100.00
Resveratrol		Unofficial, 200.00
Shilajit	Supports defense system	250.00
Vitamin B$_3$	Most retail foods are fortified	14.00

---

942   http://lipidlibrary.aocs.org/animbio/fa-oxid/index.htm

D-ribose	Core of DNA and RNA mole-cules	3.00
Carotenoid Fucaxan-thin		150.00
Omega-3 Fatty Acid	Brain Food	500.00
Aerobic exercise	Creates new mitochondria	
Calorie Restricted Diet	Creates new mitochondria	
Note: Balance your hormones		

5.18 Human Body and Brain: Ions and Low energy Hydrogen Bonds

Our body fluid is like seawater, the largest depository of salt where life began. Our living will simply not be possible without salt or what scientists call sodium chloride. This salt and others of calcium and potassium exist as ions surrounded by water. **Human body has the largest amount of sodium which is necessary for nerve impulses and signal transduction in the brain. Common positive ions like sodium, potassium, and calcium matter to molecular mechanics of life.** We know of problems of hypertension corresponding to daily salt consumption of more than 3.5 gram compared to the ideal of below 1.5 gram. Excess salt creates problems in mitochondrial function [943],[944].

Key biomolecules like DNA, RNA, and proteins construct and shape by hydrogen bonds. As pointed out earlier protons can tunnel through the hydrogen bonds in DNA. The base pairs in DNA exemplify hydrogen bonds, critical for the stability of the double helix [945].

Although weak (*a dipole-dipole interaction of 4.73 to 28.41 BTU$_s$*), these are the bonds that hold most soft matter and condensed phases of water together. They are known to exhibit quantum effects of tunneling over energy barriers and are essential to life on earth [946], [947]. Electrons always behave as electrons. They behave the same way whether in hydrogen bonds of water and those of DNA or protein.

943   http://pubs.rsc.org/en/Content/ArticleLanding/2014/CC/c3cc48709a#!divAbstract
944   http://www.cell.com/biophysj/pdf/S0006-3495(13)04144-1.pdf
945   file:///C:/Users/Owner/Downloads/0fcfd5053027a98e66000000.pdf
946   http://www.pnas.org/content/108/16/6369.full
947   http://www.sciencedaily.com/releases/1999/01/990121074852.htm

We do know now that mitochondria, as molecular machines, do have electromagnetic fields [948]. ATP synthase is a proton powered turbine[949], cytochrome C oxidase is powered by electrons and it captures and pumps protons across inner mitochondrial membrane[950], iron-sulfur structures in mitochondrial complexes are wired [951], ATP hydrolysis involves proton diffusion and tunneling [952], and quantum coherence seems to be essential to portals of life energy [953]. Although quantum biology of mitochondria is not the main theme of this book, it seems central to life of our cells and good health comes from good cellular function.

The Power of the Molecular Motor of Life

5.19 A. Structures of respiratory Enzyme Complexes I through IV

No doubt our biological being depends on electrons, protons and ions. Moving and jumping around of electrons from one orbital to another is almost universal in respiration in our mitochondria, mitochondria of other animals, photosynthesis, and nitrogen fixation. The energy in bonds of food molecules is deposited in NADH and $FADH_2$ during glycolysis, pyruvate decarboxylation, and operation of Krebs cycle in the human case. It then is transferred in small steps through four special enzyme complexes in order to make life energy ATP. Electrically connected enzyme complexes I, III, and IV are designed to pump 4, 4, and 2 protons respectively across the inner mitochondrial membrane from matrix to the intermediate space. The protons are in a sense pumped through the enzyme ATP synthase in order to produce energ molecule ATP. This is a biomechanical enigma conserved in biology ever since the evolution of living organisma. Bacterium and human beings are alike in this respect. The key is proton gradient.

One glucose molecule delivers its bond energies to 10 NADH electron carriers that receive electron as a hydride ion. The electrons move in steps

---

948   http://pubs.rsc.org/en/content/articlehtml/2013/ib/c3ib40166a
949   http://www.atpsynthase.info/FAQ.html
950   http://www.ncbi.nlm.nih.gov/pubmed/21545285
951   https://www.rpi.edu/dept/bcbp/molbiochem/MBWeb/mb1/part2/redox.htm
952   http://www.cell.com/biophysj/abstract/S0006-3495(11)03349-2
953   http://www.sciencedaily.com/releases/2014/01/140116085105.htm

from one carrier to another (from a lower to higher reduction potential) and finally to the highest potential of oxygen which gets reduced to water. **Each NADH expediting pumping of 10 protons accounts for moving a total of 100 protons from matrix to the intermediate space and each electron passing through the electron transport chain in theory can produce three ATP.** The transfer happens through metalloproteins containing Iron-Sulfur clusters of different oxidation states. **These cluster are involved in facilitating redox reactions, donating sulfur for making lipoic acid, making free radicals, and regulating gene expression.** We can say that iron-sulfur proteins have a big role in origin of life and we live by electrical currents typified by electrocardiogram and EEG or electroencephalogram.

Please read carefully and digest the details below with a belief that supply of electrons (from good foods) is necessary for a good health and just as necessary is supply of antioxidants (vitamins C, D, E, K, Q_{10}, glutathione, melatonin, and minerals) for our life which has evolved in the presence of oxygen. The critical players beyond oxygen and antioxidants are omega-3 fatty acids, conjugated isoprenoids phytochemicals, heme proteins, cytochrome proteins, and other enzyme metalloproteins containing zinc, copper, and selenium including enzyme glutathione peroxidase. Let us review the enzyme complexes of the electron transport system once more.

NADH: Ubiquinone Oxidoreductase or Complex I is one of the largest membrane bound enzyme structures that acts like a proton pump [954]. Three dimensional structure of L-shaped (ankle and foot like) complex I made of 45 subunits is not yet determined and neither are the electron and proton pathways [955]. It is a combination of flavoprotein and an iron protein capable of generating four protons. The subunits of structure are encoded both by nuclear and mitochondrial DNA[956], [957] and the enzyme with its iron-sulfur clusters is central to electron transfer from NADH. While we don't know how it works, we do know that its malfunction by way of inefficiency and mitochondrial genome mutation causes many disorders [958]. Major unknowns to date are mechanisms of ubiquinone reduction and proton translocation. Also, complex I produces reactive oxygen species and superoxide free radical that cause Parkinson's disease. A single nucleotide change in the

---

954   http://www.scripps.edu/yagi/ci/overview.html
955   http://www.life.illinois.edu/crofts/bioph354/complex_i.html
956   http://www.nature.com/nature/journal/v515/n7525/full/nature13686.html
957   http://www.ncbi.nlm.nih.gov/pubmed/20552642
958   http://www.mrc-mbu.cam.ac.uk/research/mitochondrial-complex-i

mitochondrial DNA causes Leber's hereditary optic neuropathy (LHON) because of mutated complex I[959].

Succinate dehydrogenase: ubiquinone Oxidoreductase or **Complex II** is an integral inner mitochondrial membrane protein used both in Krebs cycle and Electron transport chain [960]. **Encoded by nuclear genome**, it is located on the matrix side of the inner mitochondrial membrane. It oxidizes succinate to fumerate in Krebs cycle and reduces ubiquinone in the electron transport chain. Complex II is made up of two hydrophilic subunits (a FAD containing flavoprotein and a three iron-Sulfur cluster containing $F_e S$ Protein) and two hydrophobic transmembrane subunits (a cytochrome b560 and a small cytochrome, embedded in the membrane). $FADH_2$, iron-sulfur centers, heme b, and ubiquinone are electron carriers. Succinate oxidizes via FAD producing electrons that tunnel along the $F_e S$ relay until they reach 3 X $F_e S$ cluster. Subsequently electrons are transferred to a ubiquinone. Together complexes I and II transfer electrons from NADH or $FADH_2$ to ubiquinone which can freely diffuse through inner mitochondrial membrane [961]. This enzyme complex pumps four protons out through mitochondrial membrane to the intermediate space for each NADH or oxygen when transporting electrons. Reduction of quinone, we should note, needs 2 electrons and 2 protons. Complex II is known to produce reactive oxygen species of superoxide and H_2O_2[962],[963].

Leigh Syndrome, late onset of neurodegenerative disorders, and reduced tumor suppression are common problems associated with complex II.

Ubiquinol: Cytochrome c reductase or Cytochrome bc1 Complex III The catalytic subunit cytochrome b of complex III is encoded by mitochondrial DNA (mtDNA). All other subunits are encoded by nuclear DNA, made in the cytosol, and translocated into the organelle for assembly at the inner membrane. The core protein is **ubiquinone: cytochrome C reductase** with 1 mitochondrial and 10 nuclear subunits.

It is the third enzyme within the mitochondrial inner membrane, the large protein complex of approximately 250,000 MW made up of 11 different subunits. It forms a dimer in the mitochondrial inner membrane and catalyses pumping of protons across the inner membrane and transfer of electrons from ubiquinol to cytochrome c by a mechanism known as the Q

959   file:///C:/Users/Owner/Desktop/Mitochondrial%20complex%20I%20-2014.htm
960   http://www.cell.com/cell/abstract/S0092-8674(05)00504-0
961   http://www.jbc.org/content/282/1/1.full.pdf
962   ww.ncbi.nlm.nih.gov/pubmed/22689576
963   http://www.sciencedirect.com/science/article/pii/S000527281300008X

cycle in which ubiquinol (Q) the electron carrier exists as a reduced, partially reduced or oxidized form.

Complex III can exist as a supercomplex of I, II, and IV where II and IV may be stabilized by cardiolipin. Also redox complexes I, III, and IV are reported to make supramolecular complexes [964].

Three dimensional structure and electron path is known to some extent but not the proton pumping path. There are three REDOX centers: cytochrome b, cytochrome c, and Rieke FeS protein. Cytochrome b binds to ubiquinone and the core protein is ubiquinol: cytochrome C reductase. Electron transfer takes place from ubiquinol to cytochrome C and the transfer process is coupled with electron transfer in the inner mitochondrial membrane [965].

Complex III oxidizes ubiquinol in the inner membrane phase, reduces cytochrome c in the intermediate space, and then uses thus generated free energy to transport two protons across the membrane (matrix to intermediate space). Finally it releases two more protons in the intermediate space. Please examine the quinone cycle below.

NOTE: Coenzyme q_{10} is a fat soluble (inner membrane soluble) ubiquinone rather ubiquitous in biological systems. In case of humans, there are 10 isoprenoid repeats in the tail of the molecule. The functional group is a 1,4- benzoquinone which can accept and donate electrons and exist in three oxidation states: fully reduced ubiquinol QH_2, radical semiquinone QH, and fully oxidized Q. In complex III it functions along with cytochrome c.

Ubiquinone Q, also called Coenzyme Q, is a mobile electron and proton carrier. It is structurally and functionally analogous to plastoquinone of the thalkoid membranes of plant plastids. It can donate either electron or proton in steps. Ubiquinone can receive two electrons from complex I or succinate dehydrogenase and take up to protons from the matrix.

Major diseases caused by its malfunction or mutation are encephalopathy, hyperglycemia, Leber's disease, and myopathies.

Cytochrome c-O$_2$ or Complex IV is comprised of 10 nuclear and 3 mitochondrial subunits and it is the most hydrophobic enzyme complex containing 3 copper and 2 heme A protein molecules.

---

964   http://www.jbc.org/content/282/1/1.full.pdf
965   http://neuromuscular.wustl.edu/pathol/diagrams/mito.htm#complexII

Complex IV is directly involved in pumping two electrons. Its three dimensional structure is known but proton pumping path is not known yet [966]. One monomer is composed of thirteen subunits each different from one another. There are six METAL CENTERS, HEME A, HEME A3, CUA, CUB, MG AND ZN. This complex plays a regulator role in actions of cyclooxygenase (COX) that is blocked by antiinflammatory pain killers like aspirin and advil. **The binuclear center is the site of oxygen reduction.** Enzymes are vectorially arranged so as to transfer charge across the membrane as electrons are passed to O_2. The electrogenic process is contributed by vectorial electron transfer, and the uptake of H^+ on reduction of O_2. The protons are taken up for the reduction of O_2 and additional protons are transferred across the membrane, from matrix to intermediate space. Diseases due to its malfunction and mutation include Alexander's, ataxia, cardiomyopathy, Leber's, Leigh's, and myopathies in general.

5.19 B. F_1/F_0 ATP Synthase: The Molecular Motor of Life

ATP synthase in present in the inner membrane of the Mitochondria. It supports lives of all living organismas. All cells, including those in our brain, shall surely be useless and dead without this ATP producing organelle. Please review Table 5.19.01 for detailed calculations pertaining to works of ATP synthase.

This huge enzyme molecule has 2 mitochondrial DNA and 14 nuclear DNA encoded subunits: 10 subunits make F_0 and 4 subunits make globular F_1 that is encoded by nuclear DNA. The complex couples proton gradient and flow of protons from intermediate space back to the matrix. Much of the mechanical power of this enzyme complex depends on conformational and shape changes.

ATP synthase of the inner mitochondrial membrane is the oldest enzyme on earth that powers our existence. Acting as proton pump, it can also generate proton motive force by hydrolyzing ATP.

This sub nano-scale molecular motor make our life possible inside and outside of our cells. Examples are sperm's flagellum, endoplasmic reticulum, ribosome, myosin motors, heart muscles, antibodies, calcium pumps, and enzyme protein kinases. This wonder of mechanochemical chemistry is conserved in biological evolution. Without it, there will be no DNA and

---

966   http://www.rcsb.org/pdb/explore/explore.do?structureId=1OCC

protein synthesis, no muscle contraction, no nutrient transport, and no neuronal activity. Actually, there will be no harvesting of sun's energy during photosynthesis by the plants which make majority of nutrients humans depend on.

ATP synthase is two molecular motors in one designed to work in harmony in order to convert electromotive force into torque as a combination of rotor and stator [967], [968]. **The torque is 10 Pico Newtons nanometer or 40 x 10⁻¹² Newtons 10⁻⁹ meters.** *This 9 nanometer asymmetric structure of 500,000 Daltons using 8 subunit structures acts almost like a reversible rotor-stator setup for converting the energy of 10 protons (hydrogen ions) into chemical bond of ATP with 100% efficiency.* Visible under transmission electron microscope, the structure is ubiquitous in biology as the most wonderful example of molecular mechanics. It uses electrochemical gradient energy to make ATP's high energy bond by joining ADP and P_i (phosphorus) by using 3 protons per ATP molecule and another for moving it around.

The hydrophobic F_o unit is embedded in the inner mitochondrial membrane and is extended by a molecular shaft in the matrix that fastens through a large head piece called F_1. **F_o and F_1** are further connected by another anchoring shaft in order to avoid any drag (5.18.01 and 5.18.02).

The center rotates relative to surrounding structures and the motion is a consequence of geometry and conformation of proteins. Downhill flow of hydrogen ion causes the rotor to turn and transform energy mechanochemically to make ATP with high energy terminal phosphate bond. **Protons give energy away as they travel downhill through the enzyme molecule.** During ATP hydrolysis, F_o rotor reverse rotates as a proton pump. **F_1 as a chemical motor is ATP driven and F_o as a generator is proton driven.** Powered by different fuels, their direction of rotation are opposite: The electric (proton motive force conversion to torque) generator Fo is clockwise and chemical or ATP motor F1 is counterclockwise. When F_o dominates, the rotation is clockwise although both F_o and F_1 can operate in both directions. Nano-scientists in Japan demonstrate the mechanochemical transformation under magnetic tweezers [969]. **F_o uses proton energy and forces F_1 to make one ATP as 3-5 protons pass through.** The stator connecting the two is the most elusive design of a protein molecule.

Mitochondria make 100 ATP molecules per second and the molecular motors turn at 6000 rpm. Amino acid arginine hands down protons to

967   http://nature.berkeley.edu/~goster/pdfs/EMB.pdf
968   http://dipbsf.uninsubria.it/seminars/fotosint/yoshida.pdf
969   http://www.nature.com/nature/journal/v433/n7027/abs/nature03277.html

aspartic acid and the game continues as one motor turns the other making it into a generator.

Total ATP turn over in average human body is 63.4 Kg (Table 5.18.01). Most of it is recycled though. As a rule of thumb, we use our weight equivalent of ATP every day and there are 10 million ATP molecules in each cell of our body.

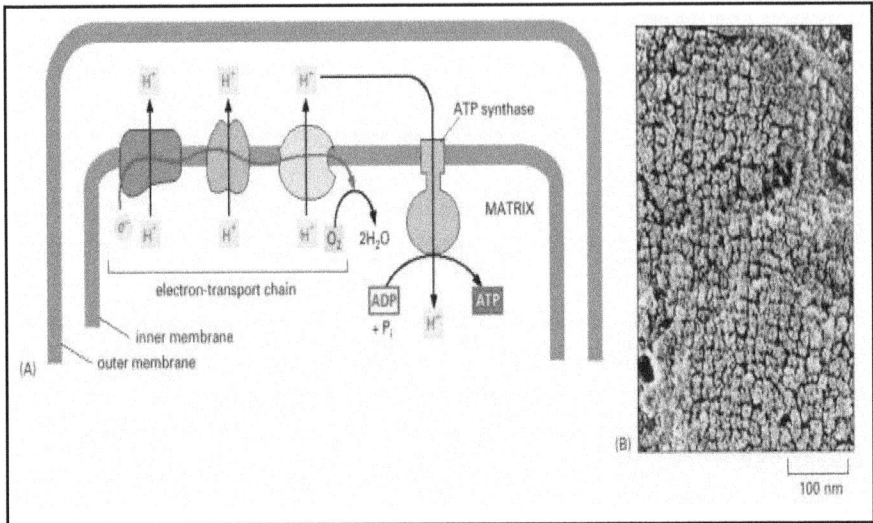

Fig. 5.19.01 ATP Synthase Embedded in Inner Mitochondrial Membrane with its Large Head protruding in the Matrix by a Shaft.

Source: National Institute of Health.

The following structure of this molecular motor and its details are universal in biology[970].

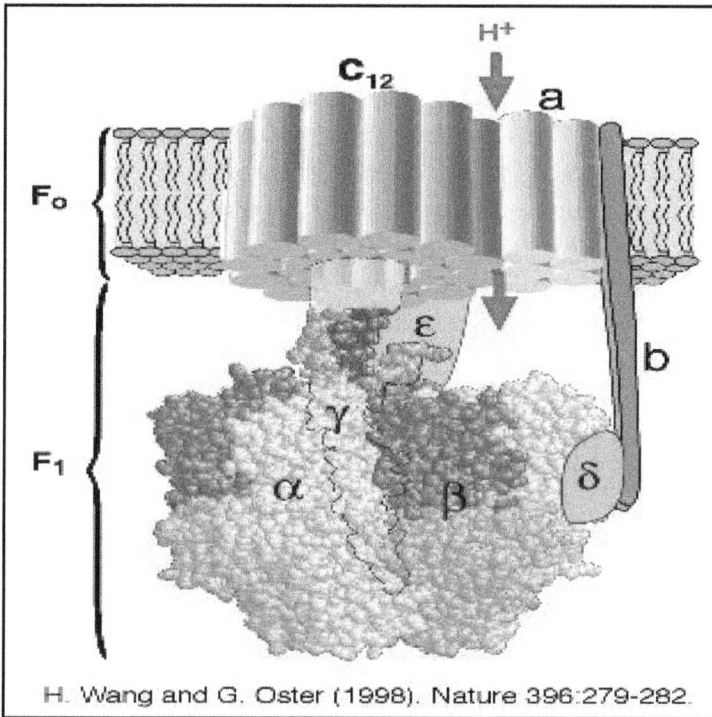

H. Wang and G. Oster (1998). Nature 396:279-282.

Fig. 5.19.02 Details of ATP Synthase

Source: National Institute of Health

The geometrical arrangements of protein units in ATP synthase of mitochondria and their ability of converting proton energy into high chemical energy of terminal phosphate bond in ATP, although not understood well, is quantum mechanical in nature[971],[972], [973]. Electrons tunnel through the electron transport chain, and protons are pushed out in the intermediate space and then conveyed into the matrix through ATP synthase for making ATP with 100% efficiency. This is now researched to be quantum mechanical. So seems to be ATP hydrolysis by F_1 involving proton tunneling [974]. It appears

970   http://twinkle_toes_engineering.home.comcast.net/~twinkle_toes_engineering/atp_synthase_tur-
        bine.jpg
971   http://www.ncbi.nlm.nih.gov/pubmed/20000803
972   http://www.ks.uiuc.edu/Research/quantum_biology/
973   http://pubs.acs.org/doi/abs/10.1021/bi901965c
974   http://www.ncbi.nlm.nih.gov/pubmed/23345443

that physics met biology a few million years ago. The evolution has afforded us and the rest of the living systems with a conserved molecular stator-motor system of proton pumping TWO-IN-ONE enzyme system and staying alive. The "how" of the system is not yet understood well.

We can stay healthy by avoiding manganese, copper, and zinc deficiencies and those of antioxidants superoxide dismutase, glutathione, and CoenzymeQ$_{10}$. This can be routinely done by a methylation diet consisting of snacks of pumpkin seed, sunflower seed, and mixed nuts by copious consumption of cabbage, broccoli, green pepper, kale, other green vegetables along with chaga mushrooms.

Many diseases result from inefficiency in ATP synthesis and decline of ATP concentration in our cells. Low efficiency causes lactic acidosis, chronic fatigue syndrome, tiredness, and vitality.

Table 5.19.04 Public Domain Statistics on ATP Utilization in Human Body
1. A person of 70 Kg weight uses 125 moles (63.40 Kg) of ATP per day.
2. Assume that the 70 Kg person consumes 2000 Kcalories per day.
3. For an illustration, assume all of it is glucose.
4. Since there are 4 Kcal/gram glucose, 2000 Kcal equates to 500 gram glucose
5. 500 gram glucose equate to 500/180.16 = 2.7753 Moles.
6. 2.7753 Moles accounts for 1.67×10^{24} molecules of glucose.
7. A 2000 Kcal (1.67×10^{24} molecules of glucose) can produce 6.01×10^{25} molecules of ATP
8. 1 ATP releases 8 Kcal and 2000 Kcal diet accounts for 250 Moles of ATP.
9. 250 Moles per day = 2.9×10^{-3} moles of ATP per second.
10. There are 10 million ATP molecules in every cell of our body.
11. Whereas electron energy converts at 90%, the proton energy converts at 100%
Note 1: one glucose molecule produces 36 molecules of ATP

> Note2: Molecular weight of glucose = 180.16; Molecular Weight of sucrose = 342.3, and Molecular weight of ATP is 507.18 grams; Number of molecules in moles/liter = 6.02 X 10^{23}.

Power of Mitochondrial Transplants and Gene Therapy

5.20 Mitochondrial Gene Therapy

We can now sequence 500 human genomes a day say the executives at Illumina, 23andMe, Pathway Genomics, Genewiz, and NantHealth. There are more than 30 companies dispersed all over industrialized countries and the cost is now below less than $100.00. This business is growing as fast as the business of blood testing, sweat testing, and big data analysis by programs common to National Random Rail used by NASA. **These developments will have a great impact on mitochondrial gene therapy and therapies of diseases controlled by single genes such as cystic fibrosis, sickle cell disease, Fragile X syndrome, muscular dystrophy, or Huntington disease.**

There are already clinical trials on ocular gene therapy for treatment of mutated mitochondrial gene [975]. Mutated genes can be selectively destroyed in case of optic neuropathy [976]. In other words a DNA can now be edited and rewritten. Neurodegenerative disorders in UK are clinically tried for gene therapy via third party oval DNA [977], [978]. The list of mitochondrial gene therapy includes Leber hereditary optic neuropathy and ND_4 gene injection, gene for fractaxin protein for iron-sulfur protein in electron transport chain, replacement of mitochondrial gene of ovum, gene product that blocks proton translocation at the F_o/F_1 ATPase, and treatments of aging, Parkinson's, and cancer.

---

975   http://med.miami.edu/news/clinical-trial-uses-gene-therapy-to-target-mutations-in-mitochon
976   http://med.miami.edu/news/breakthrough-dna-study-opens-door-to-potential-treatments-for-mito-chondrial
977   http://www.nature.com/news/uk-sets-sights-on-gene-therapy-in-eggs-1.9883
978   https://www.gov.uk/government/news/innovative-genetic-treatment-to-prevent-mitochondrial-dis-ease

Editas Medicine of Cambridge Massachussetts hopes to start a clinical trial in 2017 on CRISPR-Cas9 as a treatment for a rare genetic disease of blindness described earlier as Leber congenital amaurosis[979] .

Powers of Mitochondria

5.21 Mitochondrial Communication and Cross-Talk

Mitochondria talk to the nucleus and other cell organelles [980]. Such talks are necessary because a majority of enzymes for mitochondrial function are coded by the nuclear genes. Unfortunately, mitochondria are producers and also target of Reactive Oxygen Species (ROS) or free radicals. Let us always keep in mind that free radicals are not always bad. Mitochondria use them to maintain immune system and a balance of power in controlling cell death and aging [981].

Mitochondria talk to endoplasmic reticulum which works with Golgi apparatus of our cell to modify proteins and carbohydrates [982]. Lysosomes break down and destroy the cell and ribosomes make brand new control. All this is controlled with a kind of supervisory role by mitochondria[983], [984], [985], [986], [987]. Mitochondria are interactive during our 45 degree message sessions via maximum piezoelectricity from collagen, a strong dipolar molecule [988]. There is negative electron charge on collagen of around 10 mVolt in the tendons.

Collagen is a nanowire and water is a repository of solar radiation for our body. It reacts with IR radiation also. When exclusion zone of water grows, it squeezes mitochondria, creates large voltage, and thus controls H-Bond. Sunlight tightens collagen and transition metals in collagen increase electron flow. Massage stimulates fibroblasts and helps produce more collagen. Message reorients collagen and offers pain relife.

979   http://editasmedicine.com/documents/ASGCT%20PR%20-%20FINAL.pdf
980   http://www.sciencedirect.com/science/article/pii/S1568163709000166
981   http://www.hindawi.com/journals/jst/2012/329635/
982   http:/ http://www.nature.com/nm/journal/v6/n5/full/nm0500_513.html /www.jci.org/articles/
       view/36445
983   http://www.nature.com/nm/journal/v6/n5/full/nm0500_513.html
984   http://circres.ahajournals.org/content/111/9/1208.full
985   http://www.sciencedirect.com/science/article/pii/S0092867411012864
986   http://www.sciencedirect.com/science/article/pii/S0304416513004819
987   http://www.acupuncturehamilton.com/36/world-health-organizationacupuncture-proven-effec-
       tive-for/

988   http://onlinelibrary.wiley.com/doi/10.1002/jbm.b.33006/abstract

5.22 Mitochondrial Connection of Exercise and Yoga

Exercise and mobility is central enough to mitochondrial function to require added details beyond section 5.03.01. We need a high number of mitochondria in our active cells. We can resuscitate and double them by simple standing around and walking during the day or even night. Yoga exrcises do much more[989]. It increases mitochondria in number and optimizes their functions via electron transport chain by making complexes 2, 3, and 4 more efficient and productive[990], [991]. **High intensity exercise in particular is very effective by activating protein PGC1-Alpha, the master molecule that regulates production of mitochondria has gene PPARGC1.** Yoga and meditation have similar activating effect on this gene[992]. The fact of life and living is that there are mitochondria in our brain, in our heart, in the skeletal muscles, and down in our Achilles tendons. Exercise tones them all and it is specially good to cardiac muscles and the brain. We need more energy when we exercise and to get more energy we need more mitochondria for appropriate response.

Twenty million Americans are now committed to Eastern practices exercise in motion of yoga, meditation, TiChi, and Qigong. The values come from vasodilator effect via nitric oxide [993]. Deep breathing practice of yoga is very helpful [994]. Let's take an account of all benefits from yoga.

- Yoga and meditation induce cross-talk between our brain and mitochondria.
- Practice of posture, meditation, and breathing in yoga can change our brain with respect to enlarged hippocampus that reduces stress, helps produce more grey matter and increases brain volume for a better mental map and relaxed mind, increases neuroplasticity, thickens frontal cortex, induces cognitive gene expression, and increased inhibitory neurotransmitters [995].
- Yoga reduces inflammation, increases C-Reactive protein, interlukin 6, Gamma Amino butyric Acid, serotonin, and dopamine and it boosts immune system [996], [997], [998], [999].

989 http://www.hindawi.com/journals/jar/2012/194821/
990 http://fitstar.com/high-intensity-exercise/
991 http://livehealthy.chron.com/happens-mitochondria-during-aerobic-exercise-5350.html
992 http://corescholar.libraries.wright.edu/cgi/viewcontent.cgi?article=1220&context=biology
993 http://www.ncbi.nlm.nih.gov/pubmed/14599231
994 http://www.sharecare.com/health/yoga/why-deep-yoga-breathing-beneficial
995 http://www.scientificamerican.com/article/how-yoga-changes-the-brain/
996 http://www.forbes.com/sites/alicegwalton/2011/06/16/penetrating-postures-the-science-of-yoga/
997 http://www.psychologytoday.com/blog/evolutionary-psychiatry/201303/yoga-ba-gaba
998 file:///C:/Users/Owner/Downloads/0fcfd509449ef22d72000000.pdf
999 http://evolutionarypsychiatry.blogspot.com/2010/08/yoga-ba-gaba.html

- Yoga has healing power[1000] and regulates nervous system, parasympathetic in particular. Actually, toning of the vagus, the largest cranial nerve that controls breathing, heart rate, and digestion is conditioned by yoga.
- It is claimed by National Center for Complementary Medicine and Dr. Herbert Bensons' relaxation response center that practice of yoga makes one mindful by self regulation and controlling of flow of thoughts[1001]. **Nobel Prize winner Dr. Elizabeth Blackburn of University of California, Loss Angeles finds that yoga increases telomerase activity and Dr. John Denninger of Harvard says that yoga can switch genes "on" and "off". Yoga can definitely rearrange collagen in our body and facilitate body and mind connectivity electronically.**

Yoga intervenes and allocates functional activity of mitochondria [1002]. *We are beginning to learn from research at Harvard, Benson-Henry Institute of Body mind Medicine and Beth Israel Deaconess Medical Center that genes of energy metabolism and of enzyme proteins of electron transfer complexes in mitochondria are affected by yoga and practice of mindfulness* [1003], [1004]. High intensity exercise and physical posturing in yoga simply makes mitochondria happy. **Harvard scientists say that yoga can arrest aging by improving mitochondrial function [1005]. Qigong and TiChi seem to have similar effects[1006]** . More immediate epigenetic factors like daily food, stress, and emotions affect mitochondria and our health [1007]. Meditation boosts genes that promote good health[1008]. *Three effects are noteworthy.*

Meditation improves ATP production.
- **Meditation promotes insulin production.**
- **Meditation prevents the depletion of telomeres, the caps on chromosomes.**

1000 http://news.nationalgeographic.com/news/2014/02/140207-yoga-cancer-inflammation-stress/
1001 http://www.forbes.com/sites/alicegwalton/2011/06/22/penetrating-postures-part-ii-the-psycholo-gy-of-yoga/
1002 http://www.ncbi.nlm.nih.gov/pmc/articles/PMC3573548/
1003 http://hms.harvard.edu/news/genetics/mind-body-genomics-5-1-13
1004 http://www.plosone.org/article/info%3Adoi%2F10.1371%2Fjournal.pone.0062817
1005 http://healthland.time.com/2013/12/19/reversing-aging-not-as-crazy-as-you-think/
1006 http://www.qigonginstitute.org/html/epigenetics.php
1007 htt ww.newscientist.com/article/dn23480-meditation-boosts-genes-that-promote-good-health.html#.VGkhSPnzuIYp://www.qigonginstitute.org/html/epigenetics.php
1008 http://www.newscientist.com/article/dn23480-meditation-boosts-genes-that-promote-good-health.html#.VGkkG_nzuIY

Behind these activities are NF-Kappa genes that reduce activity of inflammatory genes. There is strong reason to believe that meditation improves mitochondrial efficiency and resiliency [1009]. Even more important is the effect of meditation on neuroplasticity, that is, making of new neurons and new circuits. *In other words yoga, meditation, Ti-Chi, and Qigong help make more extensive neural networks.* Relaxation response, just the opposite of stress response and in a way meditation, can improve energy production by mitochondria via a group of genes that control cell signaling [1010], [1011]. It is all about mind control. We can call it by different names of mindfulness or my *Akaagrata of early childhood*, meditative concentration, intense introspection, and self-control. A rare technical advance of last 20 years, mind control is now well known to modulate mitochondrial function and the genes behind such functions. **It says in nut shell that "you" can be a better "you" by deliberate control of your mind.** The mind begins to relate to your mitochondria and the critical physiology that it controls. There are well established scientific grounds to believe that yoga is a means to induce cross-talk between the brain and mitochondria everywhere in the body. Concentration even for only for five minutes accounts.

Necessary downtime.

• Necessary mending our thought processes for relaxation response.

Necessary for the tune up of our consciousness [1012], [1013].

It appears that meditation determines what neurons can or can't do.

Therefore meditate and stay conscious by managing the electrical laboratory in mitochondria.

5.23 Needles of Acupuncture make Neurons Talk.

We have been told that chiropractic works by securing a connection between the spine and nervous system and that simple application of pressure during massage does help relieve pain. Exercise and physical therapy are usual prescriptions by our physicians and so are applications of hot and cold treatments. Herbal medicine, if they work, are very close to any other drug if found safe. But what about acupuncture?

1009 http://jonlieffmd.com/tag/meditation-helps-mitochondrial-resilience
1010 http://hms.harvard.edu/news/genetics/mind-body-genomics-5-1-13
1011 http://www.sciencedaily.com/releases/2013/05/130501193204.htm
1012 http://cephalove.southernfriedscience.com/?p=290
1013 http://www.neuroacoustic.com/cells.html

In view of excellent meta-analyses by Harvard University, Sloan Kettering Cancer Center, John Hopkins, Kaiser Permanente, University of Rochester, and National Institute of Health acupuncture works by its effects on our immune, stress hormone, neurotransmitter, and endogenous endomorphine systems. [1014],[1015],[1016],[1017],[1018],[1019] [1020]. National Institute of Health recommends it as a therapeutic intervention for treatment of various chronic pains. Let us explore further and a bit deeper.

There have been two reports by World Health Organization on the curative value of acupuncture, a 6000 year old Chinese practice [1021], [1022]. FDA has approved the needles used in acupuncture and National Health Institutes supports its validity [1023]. [1024]. John Hopkins medical center endorses it [1025]. There is a confirmatory work from China on mechanotransduction involved in acupuncture What follows is a summary of fundamental reasoning behind acupuncture.

It is true that living cells are electromagnetic units. Placement of a needle 1 to 2.5 inches below the skin has got to have electromagnetic intervention and modulation of impulses related to pain perception via not just one or but more than one neurons. *Both mast cells and fibroblast cells that produce collagen trigger production of ATP. ATP is degraded rather quickly once it gets above a threshold causing resulting adenosine to act as a neurotransmitter.* As a matter of fact, scientists now find that excited water is the source of superconducting protons for rapid intercommunication within the body (peripheral cell to nociceptor to mind) that may be associated with the acupuncture meridians[1026]. Acupuncture system may thus function through superconducting liquid crystalline collagen fibers and facilitate body wide communication with central nervous system by proton conduction via nanotubes of bound water to the collagen continuum [1027], [1028].

1014 http://archinte.jamanetwork.com/article.aspx?articleid=1357513
1015 http://www.ncbi.nlm.nih.gov/pubmed/24910530
1016 http://www.livescience.com/29494-acupuncture.html
1017 http://www.jpain.org/article/S1526-5900(12)00830-9/fulltext
1018 http://www.urmc.rochester.edu/labs/nedergaard-lab/projects/acupuncture
1019 http://www.the-scientist.com/?articles.view/articleNo/31107/title/Puncturing-the-Myth/
1020 http://newsinhealth.nih.gov/issue/Feb2011/Feature1
1021
1022
1023 http://newsinhealth.nih.gov/issue/Feb2011/Feature1
1024 http://www.ijbs.com/v10p0511.htm
1025 http://www.hopkinsmedicine.org/integrative_medicine_digestive_center/services/acupuncture.html
1026 http://www.mdpi.com/1099-4300/16/9/4874
1027 http://www.i-sis.org.uk/lcm.php
1028 http://www.i-sis.org.uk/acupunc.php

That mice lacking adenosine A1 receptor show no effect of acupuncture indicates that acupuncture does affect our neurobiology [1029]. In biochemical terms, it seems to affect Nerve Growth factors of sympathetic and sensory nervous system[1030]. There are very credible research works regarding adenosine and serotonin release by needle placements[1031], [1032]. **Adenosine can serve as an inhibitory neurotransmitter.** ATP release triggered by the needle may be modulating the hypothalamus-pituitary-adrenal system of nervous activity and signals. Like all drugs that we know of, the effect of acupuncture is found to be very individual. Purinergic signaling by adenosine and ATP via receptors that affect memory, learning, and feeding habit, is most likely the key to effects of acupuncture [1033], [1034].

Mitochondria make ATP in response to stimulation and it can be released by gentle mechanical stimulation by massage of the skin and mast cells [1035]. There are already meta-analyses done in China and Canada suggesting such effects [1036], [1037], [1038], [1039]. These works are based on modern day advanced functional magnetic resonance imaging and positron emission tomography[1040], [1041]. Scientists at Harvard note that it works beyond placebo [1042].

Sections 5.22 and 5.23 suggest that treatments like massage[1043], acupuncture [1044], electroaccupuncture [1045], transcutaneous electrical stimulation [1046], a good night sleep [1047], [1048], exercise, yoga, and mindful meditation that we subject our body to have their effects on the mitochondria through water-collagen channels. Although much of it has to be more accurately corroborated and approved by authorities in view of valid scientific experiments, we seem to be headed in the right direction. The leader in this area is U.K.

1029 http://www.hindawi.com/journals/ecam/2004/308536/abs/
1030 http://www.ncbi.nlm.nih.gov/pubmed/11058557
1031 http://www.sciencedaily.com/releases/2010/05/100530144021.htm
1032 http://www.ncbi.nlm.nih.gov/pubmed/16565594
1033 http://www.the-scientist.com/?articles.view/articleNo/31107/title/Puncturing-the-Myth/
1034 http://www.ucl.ac.uk/ani/GB's%20PDF%20file%20copies/CV1408.pdf
1035 http://www.hindawi.com/journals/ecam/2013/350949/
1036 http://www.ncbi.nlm.nih.gov/pubmed/22965186
1037 http://www.sciencebasedmedicine.org/an-acupuncture-meta-analysis/
1038 http://archinte.jamanetwork.com/article.aspx?articleid=1357513
1039 http://theness.com/neurologicablog/index.php/another-acupuncture-meta-analysis-low-back-pain/
1040 http://www.ncbi.nlm.nih.gov/pubmed/18562019
1041 http://www.ncbi.nlm.nih.gov/pubmed/18562019
1042 http://www.naturalnews.com/025057_acupuncture_placebo_changes.html
1043 http://www.lighthousenmt.com/massage-and-mitochondria-let-the-scientists-debate/
1044 http://link.springer.com/chapter/10.1007%2F978-3-540-79039-6_168#page-1
1045 http://www.ncbi.nlm.nih.gov/pubmed/16309089
1046 http://www.mitophysiology.org/fileadmin/user_upload/MiP2005/013_Session_1.pdf
1047 http://www.mitoaction.org/blog/sleep-disorders
1048 http://www.uphs.upenn.edu/news/News_Releases/2014/03/veasey/

5.24 Mother Earth Talks to Our Mitochondria

Our evolution simply didn't take place in defiance with the rhythms of earth, moon, and sun. We find mother earth to be a giant magnet with its electric field. The North and South poles attract each other and that is why the North end of the compass points to the South and vice versa. This routine fact aroused the child in Dr. Einstein to run after electromagnetism and come up with the Theory of Relativity. It appears that electromagnetism runs our lives.

The oscillations of earth's potential set up our chronobiology and circadian rhythm that control our daily physiology and homeostasis [1049]. The truth is that chronobiology of all life on earth is related to solar and lunar rhythms [1050]. Our diurnal rhythm is regulated endogenously, we have morning and evening people, and even our gene expressions oscillate with time of the day [1051]. Electrocardiogram that we are often subjected to at our physician's office is a proof of electricity doing its work in running our heart and Magnetic Resonance Imaging is possible only because our tissues have tiny magnets of protons. Also, our brain cells and synapses are busy firing currents every millisecond of our life. We get life energy ATP via electron transport chain in the mitochondria. In fact we are a negative being and much of our cellular communication happens by ions like calcium, potassium, and sodium. Iron-Sulfur clusters in enzyme complexes of electron transport chain in mitochondria produce infrared photons and free radicals. They are like a magnetic compass telling mitochondria what the environment is calling for. Mitochondria, the masters of managing electron spin, act as quantized heat pumps via use of electric and magnetic fields . Electric field of a human body is around 10 kV/meter with an a current of 250 nano-amperes per square centimeter. All this is true but how does mitochondrial function relate to earthing, a practice that is gaining world wide practice. Let's examine a few instructive facts about possible cross-talk of mitochondria with mother earth.

- We are beginning to understand that our retina can sense earth's magnetism [1052].
- NASA research tells us that gravity helps our body in normalizing muscle mass.

1049 http://www.crystalinks.com/biologicalclock.html
1050 https://www.princeton.edu/~achaney/tmve/wiki100k/docs/Chronobiology.html
1051 http://www.the-scientist.com/?articles.view/articleNo/41325/title/Circadian-Atlas-Chroni-cles-Gene-Expression/
1052 http://www.sciencedaily.com/releases/2011/06/110621121319.htm

- Surprisingly the oscillation frequency of atmospheric field is 10 Hz, same as the frequency of our brain's alpha wave.
- **Can earthing** that reportedly deals with behavior of electrons as they conduct from surface of earth through our sole to upper body really happen? The mode of electron transfer, we are told, can be either literally by grounding by wearing a bracelet connected by a cord to the ground hole on the wall socket or simply by walking barefoot on ground. We know that electrons do not move freely. They can have mass and position in spacetime (x,y,z,t) and a probability wave in dimension commensurate to Plank's constant ($6.62606957 \times 10^{-34}\,m^2\,kg\,/\,s$). However, the charges can move by capture and ionization because skin does have anions and cations. The electrons have to be anchored and transferred by a defined bio-energetically possible mechanism. This we do not know about yet but it is rather convincing that the forces of planet we are born to live on do dictate our day-to-day living. The vast supply of electrons on earth's surface can beneficially conduct through our body and serve as environmental medicine is a new area of research with numerous medicinal effects [1053]:

- Lowering of cortisol [1054].

- Better sleep, less chronic pain, blood thinning [1055].

- Prevention of chronic diseases [1056].

- Antioxidant power of electrons from the surface of earth [1057].

- Low inflammation, longevity and anti-aging effects.

No doubt ! Mitochondria are the electronic support system and charges regulate protein formation, enzyme transformations, and pH in our body[1058]. We know that a sixty microsecond 2 KV/cm pulse induces even cell fusion [1059]. We exist because of currents and action potentials in an ionic plasma of water in our body. and our health improves by negative ions around us [1060], [1061], [1062]. The electrons from earth's surface may flow through our body via water-Collagen network. Actually, it is rather natural and tied to human

1053 http://www.ncbi.nlm.nih.gov/pmc/articles/PMC3265077/
1054 http://www.ncbi.nlm.nih.gov/pubmed/15650465
1055 http://www.ncbi.nlm.nih.gov/pmc/articles/PMC3576907/
1056 http://www.ncbi.nlm.nih.gov/pmc/articles/PMC3151462/
1057 http://www.ncbi.nlm.nih.gov/pubmed/18047442
1058 http://www.i-sis.org.uk/Cancer_a_Redox_Disease.php
1059 http://www.ncbi.nlm.nih.gov/pmc/articles/PMC3843160/
1060 http://www.inspiredliving.com/surround-air-ionizers/benefits-negative-ions.htm
1061 http://advanced-water-ionizers.com/Health-Benefits-of-Negative-Ions.html
1062 http://www.ncbi.nlm.nih.gov/pubmed/11198431

evolutionary biology [1063]. "Running barefoot is good for health" proposes Scientific American [1064]

Let us get a good grasp of certain fundamentals about earth. Its surface potential is considered as a reference point of zero. Electric field on the earth's surface is 300 V/meter directed inward rather radialy with a density of 20 electrons per cubic centimeter. Earth on its surface has negative charge. When we make contact with the ground barefoot we end up making an equi-potential surface. Air being a poor conductor, the current is very small with a density of 10 micro micro amperes/square meter. How do electrons from earth then beneficially affet our cercadian rhythm, meridian systems, sweat glands, bloodstream, and autonomic nervous system ?

The air around us has more positive ions than negative ions. Modern office space has 150 negative ions compared to 200 positive ions per cubic centimeter. **The negative ions are more mobile and more healthful.** Easy to believe fact in all this is that our wet skin unlike dry and calloused skin is conductive,. The electrons can get in and transport themselves through the collagen underneath the skin [1065]. The Body Electric: Electromagnetism And The Foundation of Life by Robert O. Becker and Gary Selden is a good read on this subject. How do electrons get to various tissues and organs is not understood well.

It is said that Pastor Sebastian Kneipp started it all in Bavaria in late nineteenth century and today there are barefoot walk trails and parks in Trentham estates in U.K, St. Ulrich and Soll in Austria, Dornstetten and all over black forest in Germany, Rodekro in Denmark, Orbey in France, Gonten and Zurich in Switzerland, Seoul Grand Park in South Korea, and NARA in Kyoto, Japan. Barefoot walking is a matter of healthful tourism in Switzerland. The first championship in barefoot walking took place in Canberra, Australia. To me bearfoot walking on grass with morning dew is not new. As a child in India I repeatedly heard that walking barefoot on a dew laden grassy ground early in the morning is very healthful. Of late, the Institute of Medical Sciences at Banaras Hindu University in Varanasi, India conducted barefoot walking trial on 58 people with prescription eye glasses. Barefoot walking helped improve vision and eliminated need for eye glasses in more than half of the participants. Miraculously, the 6000 year old Ayurvedic environmental medicine worked. How did these beliefs in far apart places on the globe

---

1063 http://www.fas.harvard.edu/~skeleton/danlhome.html
1064 http://blogs.scientificamerican.com/observations/2010/01/27/running-barefoot-is-better-research-ers-find/
1065 http://www.ncbi.nlm.nih.gov/pmc/articles/PMC2763825/

came to be? May be simply because earth's magnetism and electricity have not only have a lot to do with our daily living but undoubtedly with our evolution itself. People learned by being part of the earth and time became their teacher. I should tell the skeptics that barefoot waking as **an exercise** is good for functions of mitochondria. A 15 minute walking barefoot is a good exercise in movement that can help blood pressure control, balance, strength, and posture. It definitely helps secure a good dose of vitamin D, the gift from the morning sun.

Epigenetic Power of Daily Food

5.25 Power of Food for Our Nerves and Neurons

Our nerve cells depend for their survival on mitochondrial dynamics (trafficking, dividing, fusing, dying) controlled by special proteins on its surface[1066] and neurotransmission via membrane excitability depends on highly dynamic mitochondria in the cell bodies of neurons[1067]. They are directed to stay stationary or committed to specified movements for nerve functions[1068]. Comparative mitochondrial dynamics of electrically active neurons and those at rest is not well understood though and neither is mitochondrial dynamics [1069]. *Key neurotransmitters like serotonin, melatonin, dopamine, and inhibitory gamma amino butyric acid are all food dependent.* Whereas serotonin and melatonin help manage our daily sleep and circadian rhythm, dopamine for which good proteins, beets, fruits, nuts, seeds, and wheat germ are necessary in our diet is a cell to cell neurotransmitter. Human body, being a reduction-oxidation based electrical impulse system, is critically based on $NAD^+/NADH$ ratio. Sufficiency of vitamins niacin and riboflavin is necessary for maintaining an optimum ratio of $NAD^+/NADH$ critical to regulation of key enzyme proteins like sirtuins that prevent aging.

Brain function simply means cell to cell electrical conduction. Electricity is behind opening the eye lids, eyes telling our brain what they saw, and heart pumping blood on demand. We now know that human brain grows

---

1066 http://cshperspectives.cshlp.org/content/5/6/a011304.full
1067 http://www.ncbi.nlm.nih.gov/pubmed/17092996
1068 http://www.nature.com/nrn/journal/v13/n2/full/nrn3156.html
1069 http://www.plosbiology.org/article/info%3Adoi%2F10.1371%2Fjournal.pbio.1001755

and matures with tiny neurons every day. *They are so tiny that 30,000 of them fit on a pin head.* Higher activity of neurons- thinking, learning, moving, and experiencing- uses an electrical network. In the network a single neuron may connect to 10,000 to 100,000 synapses permitting impulse flow at a speed of 400 miles an hour. The human neuron at rest is at 70 milliVolt and action potentials of impulses can reach up to 200 milliVolt. Myelin, the insulating sheath around neurons, controls speed of impulse conduction. All this is critically nutrient dependent. *Choline from egg yolk is a necessary nutrient for building myelin. As part of lecithin, choline comes from soybeans and wheat germ. Vitamin B$_{12}$ from eggs, meat, and poultry is essential for making myelin.* Calorie restriction promotes making more mitochondria and mitigates DNA and protein damage and other deleterious effects of aging [1070].

Consider vitamins and minerals are building blocks for the brain. Vitamins C, B$_1$, B12, B$_6$ are memory vitamins, antioxidants protect our brain, omega-3 fatty acids build our brain, high quality proteins with essential amino acids tryptophan and tyrosine can spark our brain by creating serotonin like neurotransmitters, fiber helps the brain function better by controlling glucose supply, and magnesium prevents memory loss. Most important of all is the fact that the brain must stay well hydrated all the time with a daily intake of around two liters of water.

It must be re-emphasized even at the risk of repetition that apples supply quercetin, Brazil nut supplies selenium, blackberries supply polyphenols, brown rice supplies tryptophan for making serotonin, chocolate supplies polyphenols and flavonoids, curry powder supplies cucurmin from turmeric, olive oil supplies hydroxytyrisol, and oleocanthal, salmon supplies omega-3 fatty acids, cinnamon supplies proanthocyanindins, coffee supplies many antioxidants, tea supplies catechins, grape juice supplies resveratrol that repairs mitochondria, papaya and kiwi supply pyrroloquinoline quinone, and spinach supplies vitamins folic acid, E and K. All such foods are integral to methylation diet.

Nutrition serves as an epigenetics switch for health and wellness. Punctuality in eating keeps circadian rhythm in balance. *Almost 75% myelin is made of fats, omega-3 fatty acids and phospholipids literally negating the idea of fat-free diet.* Sufficiency of vitamins niacin and riboflavin is necessary for maintaining and optimum ratio of NAD$^+$/NADH critical to regulation of key enzyme proteins like sirtuins that prevent aging. Beyond

---

1070 http://www.ncbi.nlm.nih.gov/pubmed/23217257

proper nutrition which is necessary for producing myelin, we need to learn something new every day for forced building of more myelin. The brain improves only by building more myelin and the more of it is made the more difficult it is to build new myelin.

GABA, gamma amino butyric Acid is an inhibitory neurotransmitter and consumption of high GABA foods such as tea, fermented foods of yogurt, kimchi, sour kraut, whole grains of oat and brown rice, germinated brown rice, broccoli, lentils, wheat and rice bran, almond, and walnut calms us down [1071], [1072],[1073]. Probiotic foods and sprouts in general should be part of a well designed methylation diet.

5.26 Hallucinating Foods

Nutrition has been a more dominant reason for use of psychodelics in most cultures on earth. For example mushrooms have been used for flavor, vitamins, and nutrients in general before their psychodelic effects would have been ever recognized. Psychedelic mushrooms of genera psilocybin containing psilocybin are known to bend and expand our mind with a dream like effect on emotion, memory, psychological health, and arousal. This may have served even as a needful antidepressant[1074],[1075]. Today it is schedule 1 drug and prohibited from use under US law.

Rye bread with ergot fungus containing ergotamine used for making LSD or lysergic acid, myristicin from spice nutmeg and mace, hallucinogen ichthyoallyeinotoxism from atlantic fish head, high tryptophan stilton cheese, mulberries, poppy seed with small amounts of codeine and morphine, and caffeine from our morning coffee are other examples of their primary flavor and nutrition values before they got recognized as mind stimulating and mood changing foods. Other common kitchen food item such as Chile pepper, potato and tobacco like nightshade plants, parsnips, saffron, various teas can be a hallucinogens responsible for endomorphin rush. An ordinary banana peel with serotonin and norepinephrin can bring out the same effect.

Myristein, a powerful narcotic, can quickly accentuate the fun of pumpkin pie on a Thanksgiving day specially when followed by excessive

1071 http://www.vitalityandwellness.com.au/health-blog/low-gaba-levels-increase-gaba-naturally
1072 http://www.balancingbrainchemistry.co.uk/33/GABA-Deficient-Anxiety.html
1073 http://www.jphysiolanthropol.com/content/33/1/2
1074 http://www.pnas.org/content/109/6/2138.abstract
1075 http://science.howstuffworks.com/magic-mushroom5.htm

coffee. Centuries old drinks of absinthe, laudanum (alcohol, herbs, and opium), poppy tea, ayahuasca vine extract, and salamander brandy have been known to have mind bending effects. Although psychedelic berry or miracle fruit and coleslaw can pretty much rewire our brains their, consumption is legal in USA.

The key point to be made here is the cross-talks in our brain when we consume excess of common foods and drinks. What happens on a Thanksgiving night when one consume five cups of strong coffee after a high capsaicin spicy dinner followed by a load of pumpkin pie containing nutmeg? Then comes Christmas promoting multicolored cookies, rainbow cakes and crispy treats, marshmallow men, and pistachio fudge. A few months later we go after color crazy Easter eggs and Easter egg cakes. Our food intake in a way is punctuated with ingestion of psychedelic foods but there is very little research on such potentially dangerous hallucinogens used singly or in combination. What do they do to routine mitochondrial function and its DNA. Where does psychedelic science stand in terms of deciphering brain chemistry and function [1076]?

Even more urgent question is effect of permitted psychedelics in human food chain by way of culture, religion, or pure faddism. Salvia divinorum plant used by the Shamans contains diterpinoid salvinorin A, a potent opioid. Other plant psychedelics used in religious ceremonies around the world include heavenly morning glory containing ergoline alkaloid, fly agaric mushroom containing ibotenic acid, magic mushroom containing psilocybin talked about earlier, Jimson weed containing atropine, wormwood containing thujone, kava containing kavalactone, ayahuasca containing beta-carboline, peyote cactus containing mescaline, and now famous cannabis containing tetrahydrocannabinol. All these plant chemicals talk to our brain via their effects on mitochondria no matter what the cultural norms are and what the old or contemporary politics is[1077], [1078], .

5.27 The Methylation Diet

Can nutrients act as epigenetic switch? We know that pyruvate, the product of glucose splitting, transfer to mitochondria is central to energy production and now a mitochondrial pyruvate carrier (MPC) has been discovered giving

1076 http://reason.com/archives/2014/11/02/psychedelic-science

1077 http://www.plosone.org/article/info%3Adoi%2F10.1371%2Fjournal.pone.0106533

1078 http://users.rcn.com/jkimball.ma.ultranet/BiologyPages/D/Drugs.html

us hope to control energy production [1079]. We know that ketogenic diets of high medium chain triglyceride and adequate protein-low carbohydrate diet, bypass complex I and go to complex II and pretty much change the energy production schemes and both Type I or Type II diabetics lose weight by such diet programs [1080]. *It appears that mitochondria have a way of controlling electrons coming from glucose via anaerobic fermentation and β-oxidation of fatty acids from high fat diet* [1081].

When we consume foods of carbohydrates, proteins, and fats we dump electrons and ions in the proton rich body fluids. The foods are initially digested into units of small molecules before going to our blood stream but the final digestion really occurs in electron extracting mitochondria for production of vital energy ATP. We know in general terms that foods we eat do somehow control this conversion but a true health maintenance protocol requires knowledge of specifics of nutrients interactions in daily metabolism, interactions that deal with Coenzyme Q_{10}, PQQ, and lipoic acid and genes behind their utilization pattern in cells in our body.

Nutrition as a dominant epigenetic factor may reveal as to how our cells know about how to stay alive and conscious. Look at the life of a cell, a living unit that is 1000 times smaller than what we can see and yet what we eat influences the workings of molecules that the cell is made of and that it makes. Cell in our organs albeit crowded and congested can extract order out of chaos. This true of our brain cells also. Organelles like flagellum of sperm, antibodies, ribosome, mitochondria, calcium pump, protein kinase, ATP synthase, and myosin are molecular machines that do the job of extracting and exacting. The cell's walls and various organelles within including mitochondria work at molecular speeds that defy gravity but only as modified by water. An average protein in the mitochondria is 1000 times smaller its size just so it can travel at a speed of 5 meters per second. That is molecular execution even under crowded and congested conditions.

Yes! We can program our nutrition and our gut bacteria. And yes! we can program our cells and the DNA, RNA, proteins, and key metabolites in it by nutrition. Thus we can program our health. Reprogramming, however, should begin early during mom's pregnancy to be and then continue to be of value for the baby who becomes an adult. A methylation diet will do the job of reprogramming[1082]. Our daily diet, we are beginning to learn,

1079 http://www.med.upenn.edu/timm/documents/Lazar_Background1_Science2013.pdf
1080 http://jackkruse.com/quantum-biology-4-metabolic-syndrome/
1081 http://www.ncbi.nlm.nih.gov/pmc/articles/PMC2633313/
1082 http://www.eufic.org/article/en/artid/Nutritional-programming/

can program the fetus and the new born but depending on the individuals though because of their genetic and epigenetic differences. Programming can happen by way of inhibiting or activating DNA methylation enzymes and altering substrates for them for gene expression.

Nutrients that are key DNA methylation are folic acid, choline, methionine, B vitamins, B_{12} in particular, betaine, and transition metal micronutrients like selenium, iron, copper, and sulfur. For practical purposesMediterranean, DASH, REDOX, and Mind diets are close to each other. We need to design a complete blend of major and minor nutrients. These are methyl donating nutrients. They are the epigenetic switch by affecting DNA methylation and DNA sheet chromatin modification by acetylation. Such nutrients manage gene expression. What follows is a list of observed epigenetic effects of nutrients.

1. Aerobic exercise is a natural need for mitochondrial health.
2. A methylation diet is is a blend of DASH, Mediterranean, Redox, and so called Mind diets. Examine them carefully and you will find that they are close to being identical.
3. Methylation diet must contain sources of high quality protein and antioxidants. Nutrition can modify G protein receptors. Long chain polyunsaturated omega-3 fatty acids improve heart health [1083] by affecting mitochondrial membrane composition and organization [1084].
4. Methylation diets help maintain intracellular communication, improve brain health, and prevent onset of Alzheimer's and Parkinson's diseases. Methylation nutrients act as epigenetic targets against cancer cells; they are anti-angiogenic and prevent blood supply to cancer cells? The answer is yes with high antioxidant methylation diet.
5. Fifteen percent calorie restriction diets reduce expression of inflammatory genes and cucurmin from turmeric has similar effects. Too much eating is cause of obesity in case of grand children.
6. Bioactive polyphenols, soybean Genistein, and isothiocyanates reduce hypermethylation of DNA and help prevent cancer.
7. The protein of DNA sheath chromatin is modified by sulforafanes, anthocyanins, diallyl sulfides and all such bioactive nutrients are anticarcinogenic by their DNA decoding effects.
8. Resveratrol affects histone acetylation and suppresses Cox 2 enzymes that cause inflammation. It improves mitochondrial biogenesis. Flavan-

1083 ht http://advances.nutrition.org/content/1/1/8.full
1084 http://www.ncbi.nlm.nih.gov/pubmed/24396061

3-ols from chocolate have positive impact on mitochondrial function and health improvement [1085].

9.   Quercetin, the *natural antihistamine*, must be part of our daily foods of tea, apple, onion, beans, and sprouts.

It is our personal responsibility to maintain structure and function of mitochondria. Purely for this purpose I add the chart below as a matrix of nature's color coded antioxidants that can act as epigenetic switch for reprogramming.

Color	Antioxidants	Routine Food Sources
Coenzyme Q_{10}, Vitamin E, Gamma Amino Butyric Acid, and creatine are suggested supplements for nutritional intervention in cases of Alzheimer's, Parkinson's and Huntington's diseases.		
Red	Lycopene	Tomato, grape fruit, watermelon
Purple/Red	Anthocyanins Polyphenols	Beans, grape, wine, and prune
Orange	Beta-Carotene	Carrots, mango, and pumpkin
Yellow	Beta-cryptoxanthin Flavonoids	Cantelope, Peaches, Papaya, nectarine
Green	Lutein, Zeaxanthine	Spinach, avocado, collard, and turnip greens.
Green	Sulforaphanes, indols	Cabbage, broccoli, brussels sprout, cauliflower
White Green	Allyl sulfides	Leek, onion, garlic

Nanotechnology rules the cell and the mitochondria within it. ATP synthase like molecular machines of 40,000 atoms work in mitochondria and do their job flawlessly. Other enzyme proteins in mitochondria provide 1000 types of surfaces and sizes. *No more than 2 nanometer thick lipid bilayers of outer and inner mitochondrial membranes have more operating mechanisms than any modern production plant we know of.* Hydrogen bonds rule the

---

1085 http://biohacksblog.com/flavan-3-ols-red-wine-chocolate-fruit-enhanced-mitochondrial-bioenergetics/

worlds of mitochondrial DNA, messenger RNA ,transfer RNA, and many key proteins and our daily nutrients rule the world of hydrogen bonds.

The mystery of immortal mitochondria in our cells is understood today only a little but that they program our life and health and much of our being is an undeniable fact in biology. Mitochondria can be transplanted in the egg of a female just like any other organ [1086] and mitochondrial genome can be edited (by insertion, deletion, and breakage of DNA on purpose) by special enzymes. It can even be repaired by our cell's endogenous mechanism [1087]. Disease causing somatic mutations, i.e., mutations in our life time as we grow, can be best prevented by daily nutrition by way of methylation diet. Future of medicine may lie more in what and when we eat than what drugs we consume because nutrients dictate the workings, quality control, and cross-talk of mitochondria with all cells in our body and extracellular environment around.

5.28 Immuno Therapy

Cancer cells skillfully co-opt the checkpoint pathways of immune system and use them for their uninhibited growth. Immunotherapy is about preventing high-jacking of immune system by blocking the checkpoint pathways by monoclonal antibodies, T-cell therapy, and even vaccines. The success of antibodies such as Keytruda by Merck and Opdivo by Bristol Meyers may the most significant development in cancer therapy.

5.29 Food Allergies: Immune system's Inappropriate Response

Allergy is a case of hypersensitivity of the immune system. Allergies are inappropriate responses by our immune system to harmless molecules it regards as bacteria like hostile antigen surfaces [1088]. Certain allergens damage various enzyme complexes of the electron transport chain in mitochondria. Exposure of airway epithelial cells to ragweed pollen extract (RWE) induces the oxidative modifications to NADH dehydrogenase (ubiquinone) Fe-S protein (NDUFS) 1 and NDUFS2 in mitochondrial respiratory complex I, as

1086 http://www.ncbi.nlm.nih.gov/pubmed/23080556
1087 https://www.biotech.wisc.edu/tgef
1088 http://www.embriahealth.com/resources/healthlifestyle_reports/

well as ubiquinol-cytochrome c reductase core protein I (UQCRC1) and II (UQCRC2) in complex III. Respiratory chain-associated proteins, the 75-kDa glucose-regulated protein, heat shock protein 70, heat shock protein 60, citrate synthase and voltage-dependent anion selective channel 1 have also been found damaged significantly [1089],[1090], [1091].

Close to 5% children in US suffer from food allergies from milk, eggs, peanuts, tree nuts, fish, shell-fish, soybeans, sesame and mustard seeds, and wheat. The answer to food allergy may be in allergen containing anti-allergy patches like the one DBV Technologies of France has come up with against peanut. This appears to be a very practical remedy to a devastating health problem. For instance, L-arginine has been found to be a good remedy to asthma patients [1092]. Only future research will indicate if rewriting of genes and genome wide editing may be a better and for sure answer to specific problems.

5.30 Our Life Under Bobardment of Nutrino Radiation

Whereas day light radiation is good for activating vitamin D and we can treat cancer with radioactive Cobalt [60], UV, X-ray, and γ-ray radiation can damage our DNA and cause cancer. Now we find that billions of nutrinos travelling at a speed faster than light pass through our body every second [1093], [1094]. They can convert chlorine [37] to Argon[37], an isotope that can cause cancer [1095]. These nutrinos are the smallest, fastest, and ghostliest of all particles. Our life evolved with radiation and it can end with it [1096]. Good news is that a boron nutrino may even treat breast cancer [1097]. Biocassette-Telebiological-Microscopy (BTM) can be used to watch cancer formation [1098] So nutrinos from radiation even give us hope for renewed life.

More than 65 billion nutrinos pass through every square centimeter of earth from one side to the other every second. Human body is no

1089 http://www.nature.com/cddis/journal/v5/n10/full/cddis2014460a.html
1090 http://www.ncbi.nlm.nih.gov/pmc/articles/PMC3028535/
1091 http://www.ncbi.nlm.nih.gov/pubmed/19786549
1092 http://thorax.bmj.com/content/54/11/1033.long
1093 http://timeblimp.com/?page_id=1033
1094 http://spie.org/Publications/Proceedings/Paper/10.1117/12.438188
1095 http://adsabs.harvard.edu/abs/2001SPIE.4378...90M
1096 http://research.duke.edu/five-questions-catching-ghost-particles-kate-scholberg
1097 http://www.medicaldaily.com/new-type-cancer-radiation-therapy-hopes-eliminate-side-effects-244889
1098 http://spie.org/Publications/Proceedings/Paper/10.1117/12.438188

impediment to nutrino travel. BTM technology may be of help for monitoring and helping design cancer cure therapy.

5.31 The Mitochondria, The Organelle of Health, Life, and Death

We live by synergies of our immune, digestive system including the microbiome, and the mitochondrial function. Whereas the digestive system is largely catabolic or breaking down of big molecules major nutrients making of new molecules on demand uses redox reactions. We do all this *by Free Energy* which equalls the redox system's energy minus chaos called entropy amplified by temperature: Enthalpy - Entropy multiplied by temperature. Our cells spend a lot of energy maintaining order and we die when disorder prevails.

Our life and death is linked to mitochondria whose function determines of our life span because the very basis of multicellular design of our specialized cells, organs, organ systems, and thus the body is mitochondria [1099]. We knew very little about it just a decade ago and even today the biology of mitochondria, an organelle of our cells that knows how to create and kill itself, is not fully understood. May be Google's Calico (California Life Company) will come up with better answers in the areas of biology of aging and disease monitoring by indigestible magnetic nano-particles capable of patrolling the human body. Other nano-science companies involved in this area are Nanosphere, Inc., Aurasense Therapeutics LLC, and Bind Therapeutics, Inc. We are told that we can measure disease processes in four dimensions. Electron and light microscopes can be used to make structural and temporal 3-D measurements of molecules, molecular machines, tissues, and organs. Angstrom to centimeter size diseased and virgin assemblies can be compared within nanoseconds to minutes and in length scale of Angstroms to centimeters. In case of cancer, we should be able to measure mutation, the speed at which cancer cell is growing, probability of spread, and the best likely treatment option. We are beginning to understand that most parts of molecular machines of protein complexes are pre-fabricated and kept in stock [1100]. A few crucial and critical parts are made when the molecular machine is needed. This is a kind of just in time production

---

1099 http://www.ncbi.nlm.nih.gov/pmc/articles/PMC2801852/
1100 http://www.sciencedaily.com/releases/2005/02/050204214435.htm

designed to avoid any mistakes. The time element in human chronobiology is very critical.

Scientists have identified close to 1,100 proteins in mitochondria to date but the interaction among genes that express them is still a mystery. Mitochondrial medicine for chronic diseases of cancer, cardiovascular system, diabetes, and neurological disorders is a clear-cut possibility as we perfect learning about mitochondrial functions of storing charged calcium ions, making iron proteins for oxygen transport, and making steroid hormones. On the other hand, learning how mitochondria make too many free radicals, create conditions of undue stress, and select and kill underproductive cells is equally important for discovering new drugs. The bad news is that we know not enough. Research continues and at the top of the list is research on why mitochondrial function of producing energy (ATP) declines as we age. New streams of knowledge on quantum mechanics of mitochondrial function coming in every day is the good news. The potential is rather obvious in view of routine use of quantum machines like smart phone, digital camera, fluorescent light, and fiber optic communications.

This book familiarizes us with particles like electrons, protons, and ions, their positions and spins, molecules of proteins and molecular machines that transfer electrons and translocate protons and energy. Although evolution as we know it today has been a constant struggle between entropy, it has perfected signaling and communication as mitochondrial function by electromagnetic molecules of receptors and neurotransmitters and receptors on top of producing the life energy as ATP. *They are an organelle to be recognized as superbly controlled motors of consciousness* [1101]. *A good example is 15- 20 Hz frequency of revolution of ATP synthase, the molecular motor that makes energy, processing a proton at every 30 degrees and releasing an ATP at every 120 degrees. These are the frequencies that determine firing of miraculous neurons.* Although most miraculous is the case of mitochondria of neurons but mitochondrial miracles are common to the cells of all our vital organs- heart, lungs, liver, eyes, and stomach. The process is dictated by a mitochondrial gene.

Computers help us think faster and digest volumes of data in a hurry but can a teacher communicate a mathematical model to a stuednt? Can a medical student learn surgery from his mentor at the first pass? In other words can we engineer human brain? Claustrum or the grey matter below the neocortex that allows us to see, hear, reason, think, and connect right

---

1101 http://www.bio.net/mm/mol-evol/2000-November/007082.html

and left hemispheres of our brain may be the foundation of consciousness said Francis Crick. He is the Noble Laureate who along with James watson discovered the double helix of DNA. Much hinges though on the proteins in the claustrum cells and nutrients that upgrade or downgrade consciouness. How does exercise train our brain? How does it correct brain's metabolism and dementia by countering gene APOE e$_4$? How do resilient bacteria that cause diseases deploy molecular cameflauge and sucessfully deceive our immune system, a system that is superbly designe to tack the seniority of the antigens from these bacteria? These questions are unfathomable today.

Origin of thought in brain can be contextualized in terms of biological relativity [1102], a phenomenon like Einstein's theory of relativity. Many scientists believe that our consciousness is a quantum state, a notion that I run away from as an overly abstract and esoteric fundamental in physics. But what compels me to explore as deep as possible is the fact that our consciousness can decipher worldly realities better than the reality of its own origin. Is mitochondria then behind consciousness and biological relativity? Just look at case histories of dementia and Alzheimer's patients with their brain cells and mitochondria gone faulty. We are already investigating nucleotides that code and regulate DNA methylation for a methylation diet that helps maintain healthy and stable mitochondria for a long life span[1103].

We can create artificial organism and we already know how to quickly sequence a patient's genome. The big step may be to extend life span by rewriting the genes but without the problems of obesity and cancer. "How will the big data in nutrigenomics help us and how much?" is the question of the day. There may be nutrients capable of remaking receptors for flawless memory that we simply don't understant today. Research is emerging in the areas of Magnetic Erasure Therapy [1104], Ultrasound healing [1105], and bone healing in particular [1106]. What we don't know is the significance of nutrients in routin brain bionics. There is much to learn.

We know for sure that nutrients fuel health by building our immune system, our white blood cells, and hemoglobin. The next frontier is to understand effects of daily food on the time-woven basis of perception and consciousness. Let us hope that you and I will soon have techniques in our hand to highjack our own cells and make them do thing we want them to do by simple choice of our daily food. We fight diseases and upgrade our

1102 http://www.amazon.com/Consciousness-Four-Dimensions-Biological-Relativity/dp/0071354999
1103 http://pritchardlab.stanford.edu/publications/pdfs/Bell11.pdf
1104 http://www.technologyreview.com/news/408238/erasing-memories/
1105 http://medicaledu.com/ultrasnd.htm
1106 http://www.bioventusglobal.com/products/ultrasound-bone-healing

brain by our daily food. The proof is in Okinawans living long, people with KL-VS variant of KLOTHO gene living longer without fears of Alzheimer's diseases, and various degree of mitochondrial gene mutations among various populations. Our life and health will be very predictable if we could design a gene that signals lack of any key methylation nutrient and poor expression of a good gene. In final analysis our genes run our life.

Afterall we put synthetic gene in E. coli and made insulin. We now have CRISPR-cas (Clustered Regulatory Interspersed Short Paliondronic Repeats) technology of a nuclease enzyme along with RNA as molecular search for DNA editing and repair [1107]. We can use microfluidics technology in order to transiently break cell membranes and make intracellular delivery of quantum dots, nanotubes, and proteins [1108], and we can make 1 microwatt battery from mitochondria in saliva [1109]. These are great innovations for fighting disease and improving health.

Cancer cell initiation, progression, and metastasis begin with mitochondria[1110], [1111],[1112], the biosynthetic factory of cell gone cancerous. Aerobic oxidation of glucose may be switched to glycolysis, excessive production of reactive oxygen soecies may damage DNA and alter cell signaling, and programed apoptosis may be compromised. This is exactly why cancer cell mitochondrial aberrations are targets for drug and phytochemical treatments. DNA can be alkylated to a patient's benefit and even abnormal gene expressions can be stopped.

A lot of questions still remain to be answered. Do mitochondria assist our minds decipher space, time, mass, and energy? Are electrons and protons involved in telling mind how to know itself? How does claustrum work as on-off switch as it deals with the cerebral cortex? Cerebellum seems to have nothing to do with conciousness, says Giulio Tononi at the University of Wisconsin in Madison. Life and living in biochemical terms revolves around 45 nutrients we consume regularly. Glucose as the only energy source for mitochondria in our body makes us tick. Actually, electrons from carbohydrate, protein, and fat are the real energy source for mitochondria. So our life is electronic and its control is electronic. Press the skin and piezoelectricity runs through the collagen network. Making sense of 300 million meters per second light as it falls on our retina, of 340 meter per

1107 https://www.addgene.org/CRISPR/guide/
1108 http://newsoffice.mit.edu/2013/putting-the-squeeze-on-cells-0123
1109 http://www.nanowerk.com/spotlight/spotid=34901.php
1110 http://www.ncbi.nlm.nih.gov/pmc/articles/PMC3336361/
1111 http://www.ncbi.nlm.nih.gov/pmc/articles/PMC149412/
1112 http://www.nature.com/onc/journal/v25/n34/full/1209589a.html

second as it falls on our ear drum, and vibration speeds of flavorful foods for smell is possible only by joint works of mitochondria respectively in the eye, ear, and the nose. We need to visualise this superphysical integration critical to our daily health and long-term longevity. We need to replace pseudoscience in food and nutrition with robust science. The next decade may do us more good than we have witnessed during the last fifty years and much of it will be about mitochondria.

Major Research Institutions

lso, included below is the list of major research institutions that our readers can consult for timely research on clinical and routine therapeutics.

University of California at Davis and San Francisco

Shibaura Institute of Technology

Centre de Recherche Paul Pascal, Université de Bordeaux, UPR8641

Avenue Albert Schweitzer, 33600 Pessac, France;

Bhabha Atomic Research Center in Mumbai, India;

Chinese Academy of Sciences, 5625 Renmin Street, Jilin 130022, China; Université Paris Diderot, Sorbonne Paris Cité, 15 rue Jean-Antoine de Baïf, F-75205 Paris Cedex 13,France

Duke University

Italian Proteomic Association.

Emotive of Australia

Mayo Clinic, Rochester, MN, USA

University of Washington, Seattle, WA

Welcome trust, New Castle Medical School, UK

University of California, San Diego, CA

Center for Genomic and Mitochondrial Medicine, Irvine, CA

The UT Mitochondrial Center of Excellence, Houston, TX, USA

Center for Mitochondrial and Epigenetic Medicine, Philadelphia

Glossary and Definitions

Aerobic implies oxygenated conditions for respiration and mitochondrial function.

Alpha-Lipoic Acid is an antioxidant molecule used in mitochondria for energy production.

Anaerobic implies ATP production under non oxygenated conditions in muscle cells without mitochondria.

Antioxidants is a reducing chemical found in natural foods that can capture and quench free radicals before it damages DNA, proteins, and lipids in our cells.

Aspartame is a dipeptide sweetener sold by NutraSweet that is capable of increasing neurotransmitter levels and create toxic conditions. ATP Synthase: As a multi-protein F_0F_1 complex, it catalyzes ATP synthesis as protons flow back through the inner membrane down their electrochemical proton gradient. F_0 is a transmembrane complex that forms a regulated H^+ channel. F_1 is tightly bound to F_0 and protrudes into the matrix; it contains three β subunits that are the sites of ATP synthesis (see Figure 16-28). This is complex V of the electron transport chain which uses energy of protons flowing back into the matrix to attach phosphorus atoms to ADP molecules and thus produce ATP which exits through the adenosine nucleotide translocase (ANT) channel where ATP is exchanged for ADP.

Autoimmune Encephalitis is a model of multiple sclerosis used to study cause and cure of multiple sclerosis.

Axon is connection between brain cells or neurons.

Beta endomorphin is a pain killer generated in brain by exercise. It is a relaxant and an antiinflammatory molecule produced naturally.

BDNF (Brain Derived Neurotrophic Factor) is a molecule generated by exercise; it stimulates growth of brain cells.

Brown fat: Inner <u>membrane</u> of brown fat mitochondria contains thermogenin, a proton transport <u>protein</u> that converts the <u>proton-motive force</u> into heat. Certain chemicals (e.g., DNP) have the same effect, uncoupling <u>oxidative phosphorylation</u> from <u>electron transport</u>.

Note that the transmembrane electric potential that contributes to the <u>proton-motive force</u> and the resting electric potential across the <u>plasma membrane</u>, discussed in Chapter 15, are generated by fundamentally different mechanisms. The first results from the transport of H$^+$ ions *against* their concentration gradient powered by <u>electron transport</u>; the second results primarily from the movement of K$^+$ ions from the <u>cytosol</u> to the cell exterior, *down* their concentration gradient, through open potassium channels.

Note that the transmembrane electric potential that contributes to the <u>proton-motive force</u> and the resting electric potential across the <u>plasma membrane</u>, discussed in Chapter 15, are generated by fundamentally different mechanisms. The first results from the transport of H$^+$ ions *against* their concentration gradient powered by <u>electron transport</u>; the second results primarily from the movement of K$^+$ ions from the <u>cytosol</u> to the cell exterior, *down* their concentration gradient, through open potassium channels.

Cas9 is a protein that acts like molecular scissor. It can recognize the structure made by CRISPR RNA binding site on DNA and cuts precisely that point in sequence.

Celiac Disease is wheat gluten protein allergy characterized by damage to small intestine. It causes mal-absorption of nutrients and neurological disorders.

Coenzyme Q$_{10}$ is analogous to ubiquinone used in transporting electrons as part of electron transport chain for final production of ATP.

Coherence: An ideal property of waves that enables stationary (temporary but spatially constant) interference. Quantum coherence refers to a pure state where particles and their behavior cohere. In living systems water molecules oscillate between ground and excited states close to ionization potential of water, a plasma of free electrons for redox reactions. Coherent domains, stabilized by high surface area cellular or mitochondrial membrane, trap electromagnetic frequencies for biochemical reaction, eg., precise regulation of gene functions.

Collagen: A protein of triple helix in our skins, tendons, and all over in our body. With water it is responsible for signaling and communication.

Components of **electron transport** chain: four inner <u>membrane</u> multi-protein complexes: succinate-CoQ reductase, NADH-CoQ reductase, CoQH$_2$ – cytochrome c reductase, and cytochrome c oxidase. The last complex transfers electrons to O$_2$ to form H$_2$O.

CoenzymeQ: Is a <u>lipid</u>-soluble carrier of electrons and protons across the inner <u>membrane</u>. The Q cycle allows additional protons to be translocated per pair of electrons moving to cytochrome c.

Creatine is an amino acid.

CRISPR or Clustered regularly interspersed short paliandropmic repeats, a feature in the genome of bacteria used for fighting viruses.

Cristae: Peninsular extensions of inner membrane of mitochondria that add tremendous surface area for electron transfer.

Cruciferacea represents family of vegetables that include broccoli, cabbage, cauliflower, collards, kale, kohlrabi, and radish.

Cytokines molecules that are behind inflammations.

Decoherence : Loss of quantum coherence or order of phase angles between the components of a system in a quantum superposition.

Dendrites are connections between brain cells or neurons.

Depolarization is electronic process that brain cells use in order to transmit signals along the length of the nerve.

DHA (Docosahexanoic Acid) is an omega-3 fatty acid necessary for nerve cell structure, in particular, the myelin insulation. This is an old molecule in our evolution.

Electron Tunneling : ability of electron particle to tunnel through an energy barrier in inner membrane of mitochondria. This is managed by adjusting distances of REDOX cofactors in a range of 10-14 Angstroms.

EPA (Eicosapentanoic Acid) is an omega-3 fatty acid necessary for nerve cell structure, in particular, the myelin insulation.

Electron Transfer Chain is a reversible reduction and oxidation of iron-sulfur clusters, ubiquinone (CoQ), cytochromes, and copper ions. Each electron carrier accepts an electron or electron pair from a carrier with a less positive reduction potential and transfers the electron(s) to a carrier with a more positive reduction potential. Thus the reduction potentials of electron carriers favor unidirectional electron flow from NADH and FAD_{H2} to O_2 (Oxygen). Also called respiratory chain, five enzyme complexes use the energy from electron to pump hydrogen ions (protons) into the intermediate space of mitochondria for the sole purpose of harvesting energy as ATP. Various electron carriers are NADH, FADH, ubiquinone, and cytochrome C.

Entanglement: A quantum state described for s system of particles which cannot be described independently for pairs or groups of particles. Multiple particles are liked and as such can affect each other over long distances. DNA is kept from breaking apart by entanglement.

Excito-Toxicity is too much uncontrolled transmission causing stress and death of nerve cells.

FAD (Flavin Adenosine Dinucleotide) is a riboflavin or vitamin B$_2$ derived electron carrier molecule used by mitochondria.

Free Radicals are very reactive molecules like super oxide and hydrogen peroxide with unpaired electron (always looking around for an extra electron that they can steel) that damage DNA, proteins, and lipids in the cell. They are by products of the process of ATP production and also produced by white blood cells to kill bacteria and viruses. Also they are very useful in cellular signaling and communication. Antioxidants quench or sequester them.

GABA (gamma Amino Butyric Acid) is an inhibitory neurotransmitter that counters glutamic acid transmission and helps calm the brain.

Glial Growth Factor is a protein molecule produced in brain cells. It helps make myelin, the lining of the nerve cells.

Glutamic Acid is the most abundant neurotransmitter necessary for learning. It is found under conditions of chronic pain, muscle spasm, and neurodegenerative diseases like muscular d=sclerosis. It is toxic when present in excess.

Glutathione is a molecule of amino acids glutamic, cysteine, and glycine. It is a powerful antioxidant. Also it is involved in production of GABA.

Glycolysis breaks down glucose to two pyruvate molecules. It happens in the cytoplasm of the cell producing 4 ATP and 2 NADH. Since two ATP are invested in the process, the net gain is only two ATP.

Health depends on cellular signaling.

Impulse is often comprised of molecules of oxygen, water, and food based nutrient chemicals.

Inner Mitochondrial Membrane: A very complex protein-phospholipid rather impervious membrane where large molecules move by active transport. In all likely hood, inner membrane is the site of quantum operations.

Intermediate Space: The space between outer and inner mitochondrial membranes containing ATP synthase.

Insulin Like Growth Factor is an exercise induced molecule produced in brain cells that stimulates growth of brain cells.

Kelp is iodine containing seaweed used in Japanese food preparations.

Krebs cycle or citric acid cycle breaks down pyruvate (a product of glucose metabolism) and beta oxidation product acetyl CoA from fatty acids and produce electron carrier molecules NADH and $FADH_2$ from NAD^+ and FAD.

L-carnitine is a compound made from methionine and lysine. It is used for transporting fatty acids for eventual burning in mitochondria.

Matrix: Is the inner core space within two membranes where Krebs cycle and ribosome operates take place with many enzyme proteins.

Melatonin is hormone secreted by brain cells for sleep during darkness.

Metastability: A state of long life in stable energy configuration ant transient excitation notwithstanding.

Mitochondria is an organelle of bacterial origin present in our cells for energy production by processing electrons and protons.

MSG (Monosodium Glutamate) is sodium salt of glutamic acid. When present in excess, it causes headache, weakness, and even neurological disorders.

Myelin is fatty insulation axons and dendrites that connect brain cells.

NAD (Niacin amide Adenosine Dinucleotide) is the key high energy electron carrier used in mitochondria for production of ATP.

N-Acetylcysteine is a sulfur containing amino acid necessary for the production of GABA or gamma amino butyric acid.

Negentropy: Negative entropy in our cellular systems is that they export to keep they entropy low and stay ordered.

Neurotransmitter are molecules used by brain cells to communicate to each other. Examples include serotonin, glutamic acid, and gamma amino butyric acid.

NGF (Nerve Growth Factor) is an exercise induced molecule produced in brain. It promotes growth of brain cells.

Niacin amide or Niacin (B$_3$) is a water soluble B vitamin critical to function of mitochondria.

Norepinephrine is a neurotransmitter involved in anxiety, attention deficit disorder, and hyperactivity.

Outer Mitochondrial Membrane: a permeable phospholipid membrane with pores for passage of proteins and other large molecules.

Omega-3 Fatty Acids are essential fatty acids that are part of myelin structure,. They decrease inflammation when present in high amount.

Omega-6 Fatty Acids are essential fatty acids. They increase inflammation when present in excess.

Organic Sulfur compounds are amino acid antioxidants good for health of mitochondria. They are necessary for producing gamma amino butyric acid.

Oxidative Stress is a condition of poor mitochondrial function and low ATP production for lack of B vitamins and antioxidants.

Qbit is an unit of two-state quantum information analogous to bit used in computor processing.

Parkinson's Disease is a case of brain's inability to make enough dopamine leading to muscle stiffness, tremors, and even dementia.

Phonon: a quantum of energy or a quasi-particle associated with a compressional wave such as sound or a vibration of a crystal lattice.

Piezoelectricity: Production of electric current bu mechanical force like massage of skin.

Polyphenols are plant based antioxidants including flavones, isoflavones, carotene, leutin, lignans, lycopene, and quinones.

Proton-motive force: a combination of a proton concentration (pH) gradient generated across the inner mitochondrial membrane, chloroplast thalkoid membrane, and bacterial plasma membrane. It is the energy source for ATP synthesis by the F_0F_1 ATP synthase complexes located in these membranes. The proton-motive force also powers the uptake of inorganic phosphate (P_i) and ADP from the cytosol in exchange for mitochondrial ATP and OH⁻(see Figure 16-32). Import of ADP and P_i to the mitochondrion and the export of ATP from it coordinate and limit the rate of ATP synthesis to meet the cell's needs.

Proton Translocation: Electrons flow from NADH and $FADH_2$, they are couple to uphill transport of protons from matrix of inner membrane to intermediate space between inner and outer membrane. Coupling of flow of electrons from NADH and $FADH_2$ to O_2 to the uphill transport of protons from the matrix across the inner membrane to the intermembrane space for generation of proton-motive force (pmf), 10 H^+ ions for each pair of electrons. Proton movement occurs at three points: the NADH-CoQ reductase (four H^+), $CoQH_2$ – cytochrome c reductase (four H^+), and cytochrome c oxidase (two H^+). Proton translocation through F_0 powers the rotation of the γ subunit of F_1, leading to changes in the conformation of the nucleotide-binding sites in the F_1 β subunits. By means of this binding-driven mechanism, the F_0F_1 complex harnesses the proton-motive force to power ATP synthesis. The F_0F_1 complexes in bacterial plasma membranes and chloroplast thalkoid membranes are very similar in structure to the mitochondrial F_0F_1 complex.

Proton Tunneling : Proton tunneling is proton transfer against an energy barrier in view of Heisenberg Uncertainty Principle and wave particle duality. Proton tunneling in hydrogen bonds of DNA is a great example in case of DNA mutations.

Oxidation of NADH: Mitochondrial <u>oxidation</u> of NADH and the <u>reduction</u> of O_2 to water continue to proceed only if sufficient ADP is present. This constitutes a major respiratory control of ATP synthesis.

Resonance: All vibrations and waves have this property of storing energy called resonance including sinusoidal waves, covalent bond vibrations in case of delocalized electrons, and resonance of electron spin. It is a vibration of large amplitude in response to small periodic stimulus like a vibration of same frequency.

Resveratrol is an antioxidant molecule found in dark purple or black fruits like grapes. It enhances longevity.

Riboflavin or vitamin B$_2$ is a water soluble vitamin necessary for function of mitochondria.

Serotonin is a neurotransmitter involved in depression and mania.

SNP (Single Nucleotide Polymorphism) is a change in DNA by change of a base pair or nucleotide causing mutation and eventual poor or no synthesis of proteins and enzymes.

Sodium Channels are special proteins as part of nerve cell membrane permitting transfer and movement of sodium ions.

Superposition : it is about an electron or protons ability to occupy all their possible states simultaneously. This property may make biomolecules tunable and life possible.

Taurine is a sulfur containing amino acid used in making gamma amino butyric acid.

Theanine is an amino acid that reduces norepinephrinine and thus improves attention and focus.

Ubiquinone is structurally similar to B vitamin. This molecule is part of the electron transport chain in mitochondria.

REFERENCES
FOR ADDITIONAL READING

Chapter 1: Introduction

Adachi M, Liu Y, Fujii K, Calderwood SK, Nakai A, Imai K, Shinomura Y. (2009). Oxidative stress impairs the heat stress response and delays unfolded protein recovery. *PLoS One*, 4:e7719.

Alberts B, Johnson A, Lewis J, et al. (2002). Molecular Biology of the Cell. 4th edition. New York: Garland Science, Electron-Transport Chains and Their Proton Pumps.

Ali-Khalili, Jim and Johnjoe Mcfadden (2014). Life on the Edhe; The coming of Age of Quantum Biology, Bantam Press,/Random House group, New York, N. Y.

Audesirk, Teresa and Audesirk, Gerald. (1999). Biology, Life on Earth, 5th Ed., Prentice-Hall.

Azqueta A, Shaposhnikov S, Collins AR. (2009). DNA oxidation: investigating its key role in environmental mutagenesis with the comet assay. *Mutat Res*, 674:1-8.

Becker, W.M. and Deamer, D.W. (1991). In *The World of the Cell,* 2nd ed., The Benjamin/Cummings Publishing Co., Inc.: Redwood City, CA, pp. 291-307.

Berg, J., Tymoczko, J.L., and stryer, L. (2011). Biochemistry, 7th Edition, Pulgrave Mcmillan.

Borman,Stu (2007). "Protein Factory Reveals Its Secrets", Chem & Eng News: 85(8) February 19, , p13-16.

Cohen, Bruce M. and Gold Deborah R. (2001). Mitochondrial cytopathies in adults: What we know so far, Cleveland Clinic J Medicine, 68(7); 625-642.

Enger, Eldon D. and Ross, Frederick C.(2003). Concepts in Biology, 10th Ed., McGraw-Hill.

Evans, Joseph, L. (2009). Secret Life of of Mitochondria, P & N Development, St Louis, MO

Garrett, H., Reginald and Charles Grisham. (2008). Biochemistry. Boston: Twayne Publishers.

Goodsell, Davis, S. (2009). The Machinery of Life, Springer Verag, New York

Grauer, Ken. (1992). A Practical Guide to ECG Interpretation, Mosby Year Book.

Guyton, Arthur C. (1971). Basic Human Physiology, W. B. Saunders Company.

Hevitt, John (2014). Better Living Through Mitochondria Derived Vesicles, Medical Press, http://medicalxpress.com/news/2014-08-mitochondrial-derived-vesicles.html

Hickman, Cleveland P., Roberts, Larry S., and Larson, Allan. (1995). Integrated Principles of Zoology, 9th. Ed., Wm C. Brown.

Karp, Gerald. (2008). Cell and Molecular Biology, 5th Ed., Wiley.

Kendrew, John (1966). British Broadcasting Corporations Television Series on Thred of Life.

Kim, Y., Coppey, M., Grossman, R., Ajuria, L., Jimenez, G., Paroush, S., Shvartsman, S. (2010). Current Biology: 20, 3/9/2010, p1-6.

Know, Lee (2014). Life: The Epic Story of Mitochondria, Friesen Press, Victoria, British Colombia, Canada.

Lane, Nick (2006). Power, Sex, and Suicide: Mitochondria and meaning of life, Oxford University Press, Cary, North Carolina, USA

Levy, Charles K., (1982). Elements of Biology, Addison-Wesley.

Lodish; Harvey with Berk, Matsudaira, Kaiser, Krieger, Scott, Zipursky and Darnell. (2004). Molecular Cell Biology, 5th edn, W.H. Freeman and Company.

Munn, E.A (1974). Structure of Mitochondria, Academic Press, Inc., New York.

Nave, C. R. and Nave, B. C. (1985). Physics for the Health Sciences, 3rd Ed., W. B. Saunders.

Nelson, Philip. (2004). Biological Physics, W. H. Freeman.

Peterson, B.M., Johnson, D.L., and Revussin, E (2012). Skeletal muscle cell mitochondria and aging, J. Aging Research, 19: 1155

Raven, Peter. (2005). Biology. Boston: Twayne Publishers.

Sceffler, Imma (2007). Mitochondria, second edition, Wiley, New Yok.

Shier, David, Butler, Jackie and Lewis, Ricki, Hole (2007). Human Anatomy and Physiology, 11th Edition, McGraw-Hill..

Thibodeau, Gary & Patton, Kevin,. (1996). Anatomy and Physiology, 3rd Ed., Mosby. Wohls,

Tuszynski, J. A. and Dixon, J. M. (2002). Biomedical Applications of Introductory Physics, Wiley.

Urbani, A., et al. (2013) "The mitochondrial Italian Human Proteome Project initiative (mt-HPP)," Molecular BioSystems, 9, pp 1984-1992.

Wahls, Terry, L. (2014). Minding My Mitochondria, TZ Press LLC, Iowa City, IA, USA

Yockey, Hubert. (2005). "Information Theory, Evolution, and the Origin of Life", Cambridge University Press, N.Y.

Zubay, G. (1983). *Biochemistry,* 3rd. ed., Wm. C. Brown Publishers: Dubuque, IA, p. 42.

Chapter 2: Food for Mitochondrial Health

Ahmed F: (1999). The role of oxidative stress in environmental carcinogenesis. *Journal Environmental Science and Health*, 17:111-142.

Al-Tahan, J. Gonzalez-Gross, M/, and Pietrzik, K. (2006). B vitamins status and intake of European adolescents. A rev of the literature, Nutrition in Hospitals, 21(4): 452-465.

Balk, E., Chung, M., and Raman G. etal. (2006). B vitamins and berries and age related neurodegenerative disorders, Evid Rep Technol Assess, 134: 1-161.

Bartley, J. (2008). Prevalance of vitamin D deficiency among patients attending a multidisciplinary tertiary pain clinic, N. Z. Med J., 121 (1286): 57-62.

Barreto G, Schäfer A, Marhold J, Stach D, Swaminathan SK, Handa V, Döderlein G, Maltry N, Wu W, Lyko F, Niehrs C (2007). Gadd45a promotes epigenetic gene activation by repair-mediated DNA demethylation. *Nature*, 445:1-5.

Baschetti, R. (1997). Paleolithic nutrition, Eur J Clin Nutr, 51(10): 715-716.

Beal, M.F. (2002). Coenzyme Q_{10} as a possible treatment for neurodegenerative diseases, Free radical Research., 36(4): 455-460.

Berger, J.L., Kayo, T., and Vann J.M. etal. (2008). A low dose of dietary resveratrol partially mimics calorie restriction and retards aging parameters in mice, PLos ONE, 3(6): e2264.

Bergquist, A.G., Chee, C.M., and Lutchka, L. etal. (2003). Selenium deficiency associated with cardiomyopathy: a compilation of the ketogenic diet, Epilepsia, 44(4): 618-620.

Bhagavan HN, Chopra RK (2007). Plasma coenzyme Q10 response to oral ingestion of coenzyme Q10 formulations. *Mitochondrion*, 7(Suppl):S78–S88.

Bhutani N, Burns DM, Blau HM (2011). DNA demethylation dynamics. *Cell* 2011, 146:866-872.

Borchert A, Wilichowski E, Hanefeld F. (1999). Supplementation

---

with creatine monohydrate in children with mitochondrial encephalomyopathies. *Muscle Nerve*, 22:1299–1300.

Bottiglieri, T. (1996). Folate, vitamin B$_{12}$, and neuropsychiatric disorders, Ntrition Review, 54(12): 382-390.

Bough KJ, Wetherington J, Hassel B, et al. (2006). Mitochondrial

biogenesis in the anticonvulsant mechanism of the ketogenic diet. *Annals of Neurology*, 60:223–235.

Brown TP[1], Rumsby PC, Capleton AC, Rushton L, Levy LS.. (2006). Pesticides and Parkinson's disease- Is there a link, Environtal Health Perspect 114(2): 156-164.

Bugiani M, Lamantea E, Invernizzi F, et al. (2006). Effects of

ribolavin in children with complex II deficiency. *Brain Development*, 28:576–581.

Bhusari SS, Dobosy JR, Fu V, Almassi N, Oberley T, Jarrard DF. (2010). Superoxide dismutase 1 knockdown induces oxidative stress and DNA methylation loss in the prostate. *Epigenetics*, 5:18.

Cedar H, Bergman Y. (2009). Linking DNA methylation and histone modification: patterns and paradigms. *Naure Review of Genetics*, 10:1-10.

Calabrese, V.,B Giufrida, Stella A.M., and Calvini M. etal. (2006). Acetylcarnitine and cellular stress response: role in nutritional redox homeostasis and regulation of longevity genes, Journal of Nutritional Biochemistry, 17(2): 73-88

Cantorna, M.T., Mahon, B.D. (2004). Mounting evidence for vitamin D as an environmental factor affecting autoimmune disease prevalance, Expt Biol Med (Maywood), 229(11): 1136-1142.

Cantorna, M.T., Mahon, B.D. (2006). Vitamin D and its role in in immunology: multiple sclerosis and inflammatory bowel disease syndrome., Progress in Biophysics and Molecular Biology, 92(1): 60-64

Chang CL, Marra G, Chauhan DP, Ha HT, Chang DK, Ricciardiello L, Randolph A, Carethers JM, Boland CR. (2002). Oxidative stress inactivates the human DNA mismatch repair system. *American Journal of Cell Physiol*, 283:1-8.

Chou, H.S., Kim, seung, Lee, S.K., Park, J.A, Kim, S.J.,and Chum, H.S.. (2008). Protective effect of the green tea component I-Theanine on environmental toxins-induced neuronal cell death, neurotoxicity, 29(4): 656-662.

Clark, A.J., Massholder, S., and Gates, R. (1987). Folacin status in adolescent females, American Journal of Clinical Nutrition, 46(2): 302-306.

Collins AR, Azqueta A, Langie SA . (2012). Effects of micronutrients on DNA repair. *European Journal of Nutrition*, 51:261-279.

Cotman, C.W. and Berchtold, N.C. (2002). Exercise: a behavioral intervention to enhance brain health and plasticity, Trends Neuroscience, 25(6): 2950- 301.

Davis. D.L (1987). Paleilithic diet, evolution, and carcinogens, Science 238(4834): 1633-1634.

Delmas, D., Jennin, B. and Latruffe N. (2005). Reveratrol: preventing properties against vascular alterations and aging, Molecular Nutrition Research, 49(5): 377-395.

Dermakova, E.V., Korobov, V.P., and Lemkina, L.M. (2003). Determination of gammaaminobutyric acid concentration and activity of glutamate decarboxylase in blood serum of patients with multiple sclerosis, Clinical Laboratory Diagnostics, 4(: 15-17.

Eaton, S.B., and Koner, M. (1985). Paleilithic nutrition: A consideration of its nature and current implications, New England Journal of Medicine, 312(5): 283-289.

Eaton, S.B., Eaton, S.B. III, and Konner, J. (1997). Paleolithic nutrition revisited: a twelve year retrospective on its nature and implications, European Journal of Clinical Nutrition, 51(4): 207-216.

Eaton, S.B., Eaton III, S.B., Sinclairb, A.J., and Cordainc, L.(1998). Dietary intake of long-chain polyunsaturated fatty acids during the paliolithic world, Review Nutrition and Dietetics, 83: 12-23.

Furukawa S, Fujita T, Shimabukuro M, Iwaki M, Yamada Y, Nakajima Y, Nakayama O, Makishima M, Matsuda M, Shimomura I (2004). Increased oxidative stress in obesity and its impact on metabolic syndrome. *Journal of Clinical Investigations*, 114:1-10.

Goshima, M., Murakami, T, and Nakagaki, H. etal. (2008). Iron, zinc, manganese, and copper intakes in Japanese children ages 3-5 years, J ournal ofNtritional Science Viaminology (Tokyo), 54(6): 475-482.

Ghoshal K, Li X, Datta J, Bai S, Pogribny I, Pogribny M, Huang Y, Young D, Jacob ST (2006). A folate- and methyl-deficient diet alters the expression of DNA methyltransferases and methyl CpG binding proteins involved in epigenetic gene silencing in livers of F344 rats. *Journal of Nutrition*, 136:1522-1527.

Haas RH. (2007). : The evidence basis for coenzyme Q therapy in oxidative phosphorylation disease. *Mitochondrion*, 7(Suppl):S136–S145.

Han CY, Umemoto T, Omer M, den Hartigh LJ, Chiba T, LeBoeuf R, Buller CL, Sweet IR, Pennathur S, Abel ED, Chait A. (2012). NADPH oxidase-derived reactive oxygen species increases expression of monocyte chemotactic factor genes in cultured adipocytes. *Journal of Biological Chemistry* , 287:10379-10393.

Hayes, C. E., Cantorna, M.T. and Deluca, H.F. (1997). Vitamin D and Multiple sclerosis, Proceedings of Society of Experimentat Biology and Medicine, 216(1): 21-27

Igisu, H., Matsuoka, M., and Iryo, Y. (1995). Protection of the brain by carnitine, Sangyo Eiseigako Zassi, 37(2): 75-82.

Ingrosso D, Cimmino A, Perna AF, Masella L, de Santo NG, de Bonis ML, Vacca M, D'Esposito M, D'Urso M, Galletti P, Zappia V (2003). Folate treatment and unbalanced methylation and changes of allelic expression induced by hyperhomocysteinaemia in patients with uraemia. *Lancet*, 361:1-7.

Kow YW (2002). Repair of deaminated bases in DNA. *Free Radic Biology and Medicine* , 33:1-8.

Krystal JH, Sanacora G, Blumberg H, Anand A, Charney DS, Marek G, Epperson CN, Goddard A, Mason GF. (2002). Glutamate and GABA systems as targets for novel antidepressant and mood-stabilizing treatment, Molecular Psychiatry, 7 Supp 1, S71-S80.

Lim GP, Chu T, Yang F, Beech W, Frautschy SA, Cole GM. (2001). "The Curry Spice Curcumin Reduces Oxidative Damage and Amyloid Pathology in an Alzheimer Transgenic Mouse". *The Journal of Neuroscience* 21 (21): 8370–7.

Linnane AW, Kios M, Vitetta L. (2007). Coenzyme Q(10)—its role as a prooxidant in the formation of superoxide anion/hydrogen peroxide and the regulation of the metabolome, *Mitochondrion*, 7(S):S51–S61.

López-Lluch G[1], Irusta PM, Navas P, de Cabo R. (2008). Mitochondrial biogenesis and healthy aging, Expeimental Gerontology, 43(9): 813-819.

Jeppesen TD[1], Schwartz M, Olsen DB, Wibrand F, Krag T, Dunø M, Hauerslev S, Vissing J. (2006). Aerobic training is safe and improves exercise capacity in patients with mitochondrial myopathy. *Brain*, 129:3402–3412.

Kendell, S.F., Krystal, J.H., and Sanacora, G. (2005). GABA and glutamate systems as therapeutic targets in depression and mood disorders, Expert Opin Ther Targets, 9(1): 153-168.

Koga Y, Akita Y, Nishioka J, Yatsuga S, Povalko N, Tanabe Y, Fujimoto S, Matsuishi T.. (2005). L-arginine improves the symptoms of strokelike episodes in MELAS. *Neurology*, 64:710–712.

Koga Y, Ishibashi M, Ueki I, et al. (2002). Effects of L-arginine on the acute phase of strokes in three patients with MELAS. *Neurology*, 58:827–828.

Kovacic P, Pozos RS, Somanathan R, Shangarin,N/, and O'Brien, P.J.. (2005). Mechanism of mitochondrial uncouplers, inhibitors, and toxins: focus on electron transfer, free radicals, and structure-activity relationships. *Current Medicinal Chemistry*, 12:2601–2623.

Lakhan, S.E., and Vieira, K.F. (2008). Nutritional therapies for mental disorders, Nutr J 7:2

Liu, Y.; Dargusch, R.; Maher, P.; Schubert, D. (2008). "A broadly neuroprotective derivative of curcumin". *Journal of Neurochemistry* 105 (4): 1336–1345.

McGarvey KM, Fahrner JA, Greene E, Martens J, Jenuwein T, Baylin SB. (2006). Silenced tumor suppressor genes reactivated by DNA demethylation do not return to a fully euchromatic chromatin state. *Cancer Research*, 66:3541-3549.

Mohr, S.B. (2009). A brief history of vitamin D and cancer prevention, Ann Epidemiol 19(2): 79-83.

Marriage BJ, Clandinin MT, Macdonald IM, et al. (2004). Cofactor treatment improves ATP synthetic capacity in patients with oxidative phosphorylation disorders. *Molecular Genetics and Metabolism*, 81:263–272.

Milagro FI, Campión J, García-Díaz DF, Goyenechea E, Paternain L, Martínez JA (2009). High fat diet-induced obesity modifies the methylation pattern of leptin promoter in rats. *Journal of Physioogy andl Biochemistry*, 65:1-9.

Nencini, C. Giorgi, L. and Micheli L. (2007). Protective effect of silymarin (flavonolignan) on oxidative stress in rat brain, Phytomedicine, 14(2-3)_: 129- 135.

Niture SK, Velu CS, Smith QR, Bhat GJ, Srivenugopal KS. (2007). Increased expression of the MGMT repair protein mediated by cysteine prodrugs and chemopreventative natural products in human lymphocytes and tumor cell lines. *Carcinogenesis*, 28:378-389.

Meeusen, R. (2005). Exercise and the Brain: Insight in new tharapeutic modalities, Annals of Transplant, 10(4): 49-51.

Miller, A., Korem, M., Almong, R. etal. (2005). Vitamin B_{12} , demethylation remethylation and repair in mulriple sclerosis, Journal of Neurological Science., 233(1-2): 93-97

Morava E, van den Heuvel L, Hol F, de Vries MC, Hogeveen M, Rodenburg RJ, Smeitink JA. (2006). Mitochondrial disease criteria: diagnostic applications in children. *Neurology*, 67:1823–1826.

Morava E[1], Rodenburg R, van Essen HZ, De Vries M, Smeitink J. (2006). Dietary intervention and oxidative phosphorylation capacity. *Journal of Inheritable Metabolic Diseases*, 29:589.

Nakamura S, Takamura T, Matsuzawa-Nagata N, Takayama H, Misu H, Noda H, Nabemoto S, Kurita S, Ota T, Ando H, Miyamoto K, Kaneko S. (2009). Palmitate induces insulin resistance in H4IIEC3 hepatocytes through reactive oxygen species produced by mitochondria. *Journal of Bioogical Chemistry*, 284:14809-14818.

Newsholme P, Haber EP, Hirabara SM, Rebelato EL, Procopio J, Morgan D, Oliveira-Emilio HC, Carpinelli AR, Curi R. (2007). Diabetes associated cell stress and dysfunction: role of mitochondrial and non-mitochondrial ROS production and activity. *Journal of Physiol*, 583:1-16.

Pari, L. and Murugan P. (2007). Tetrahydrocucurmin prevents brain lipid peroxidation in streptozotocin-induced diabetic rats, J Med Food 10(2): 323-329

Paroush Z, Keshet I, Yisraeli J, Cedar H. (1990). Dynamics of demethylation and activation of the alpha-actin gene in myoblasts. *Cell*, 63:1229-1237.

Perry, T.L., Yong, V.W., and Bergeron, C., Hansen, S., and Jones, K. (1987). Amino acids, glutathione, and glutathione transferase activity in the brains of patients with Alzheiner's disease, Annals of Neurology, 21(4): 331-336.

Patavino, T. and Brady M. (2001). Natural medicine and nutritional therapy as an alternative treatment in systemic lupus erythematosus, Alternative Medicine Reviews, 6(5): 460-471.

Pescosolido, N. , Imperatrice, B., and Karavitis, P. (2008). The aging eye and the role of L-carnitine and its derivatives, Drugs R D, 9(supp 1): 3-14

Quadri, P., fragiacomo, C., and Pezzati, R. etal. (2005). Homocysteine and B vitamins in mild cognitive impairment and dementia, Clinical Chemistry and Laboratory Medicine, 43(10): 1096-1100.

Renolds, E. (2006). Folate, Vitamin B_{12}, and nervous system, Lancet Neurology, 5(11): 949-960.

Rosenberg, I.H., (2001). B vitamins, homocysteine, and neurocognitive function, Ntritional Review, 59(2): s69-s73.

Rossi L, Mazzitelli S, Arciello M, Capo CR, Rotilio G.. (2008). Benefits from dietary polyphenols for brain aging and Alzheimer's disease, Neurochemical Research, 33(12); 2390-2400.

Saiko P, Szakmary A, Jaeger W, Szekeres T. (2008). Resveratrol and its analogs: defense against cancer, coronary disease and neurodegenerative maladies or just a fad? *Mutation Research*,658:68–94.

Saltman, P.D., and Strause, G. (1993). The role of trace minerals in osteoporosis, Journal American College of Nutrition, 12(14): 384-389.

Savolainen, K.M., Loikhanen, J., and Eerikainen, S. etal. (1998). Glutamate stimulated ROS production in neuronal cultures: Interactions with lead and the chlorinergic system, Neurotoxicology, 19)4-5): 669-674.

Silva MF, Aires CC, Luis PB, et al.(2008). Valproic acid metabolism and its effects on mitochondrial fatty acid oxidation: a review. *Journal of Inheritable Metabolic Diseases*, 31:205–216.

Shults CW, Flint Beal M, Song D, et al. (2004). Pilot trial of high dosages of coenzyme Q10 in patients with Parkinson's disease. *Experimental Neurology*, 188:491–494.

Shekelle P, Morton S, Hardy M. (2003). Effect of Supplemental Antioxidants Vitamin C, Vitamin E, and Coenzyme Q10 for the Prevention and Treatment of Cardiovascular Disease . Evidence

Shukla, T. P. (2014). Our Gene Our Food Our Lifestyle, Penguin Press, N.Y.

Shukla, T.P. (2014). Our Genes Our Food Our Lifestyle, Penguin Press, New York (in press).

Simopoulos, A.P. (1991). Omega-3 fatty acids in health and disease and in growth and development, American Journal Clinical Nutrition 54(3): 438-463.

Simopoulos, A.P. (1998). Human requirements for N-3 polyunsaturated fatty acids, Poult Sci., 97(7): 961-970.

Simopoulos, A.P. (1999). Evolutionary aspects of omega-3 fatty acids in the food supply: postglandins, leukotrienes, and Essent Fatty Acids, 60(5-6): 421-429.

Spiller HA, Sawyer TS. (2006). Toxicology of oral antidiabetic medications. *American Journal of Health System Pharmacology*, 63:929–938.

Sinatra ST. (2009). Metabolic cardiology: an integrative strategy in the treatment of congestive heart failure. Alternative Therapeutic and Health Medicine , 15(3):44-52.

Srivastava, K.C.; Bordia, A.; Verma, S.K. (1995). "Curcumin, a major component of food spice turmeric (Curcuma longa) inhibits aggregation and alters eicosanoid metabolism in human blood platelets". *Prostaglandins, Leukotrienes and Essential Fatty Acids* 52 (4): 223.

Taivassalo T, Haller RG. (2005). Exercise and training in mitochondrial myopathies. *Medical Science for Sportsand Exercise*,37:2094–2101.

Tankova, T. Cherninkova, S., and Koeb, D. (2004). Alpha-lipoic acid in the treatment of autonomic diabetic neuropathy (controlled, randomized, open-label study), Rom J. Intern Med 42(20: 457-464.

Trasler J, Deng L, Melnyk S, Pogribny I, Hiou-Tim F, Sibani S, Oakes C, Li E, James SJ, Rozen R. (2003). Impact of Dnmt1 deficiency, with and without low folate diets, on tumor numbers and DNA methylation in Min mice. *Carcinogenesis*, 24:1-7

Tarnopolsky MA. (2009). Mitochondrial DNA shifting in older adults following resistance exercise training. *Applied Physiological Nutrition and Metabolism*, 34:348–354.

Tarnopolsky MA, Raha S. (2005). Mitochondrial myopathies: diagnosis, exercise intolerance, and treatment options, *Medical Sciencefor Sports and Exercise*, 37:2086–2093.

Tarnopolsky MA, Parise G (1997). Direct measurement of high-energy phosphate compounds in patients with neuromusculardisease. *Muscle Nerve*, 22:1228–1233.

Tarnopolsky MA, Roy BD, MacDonald JR (1997). A randomized, controlled trial of creatine monohydrate in patients with mitochondrial cytopathies. *Muscle Nerve*, 20:1502–1509.

Tatsch E, Bochi GV, Piva SJ, de Carvalho JA, Kober H, Torbitz VD, Duarte T, Signor C, Coelho AC, Duarte MM, Montagner GF, Da Cruz IB, Moresco RN. (2012). Association between DNA strand breakage and oxidative, inflammatory and endothelial biomarkers in type 2 diabetes. *Mutation Research*, 732:1-5.

Van Meetteren M.E., Teunissen, C.E., Dijkstra, C.D., and van Tol, E.A. (2005). Antioxidants and polyunsaturated fatty acids in multiple sclerosis, Euopean Journal of Clinical Nutrition. 59(12): 1347-1361.

Vogel, J.K., Bolling, S.F., and Costello R.B. (2005). American College of Cardiology Foundation Task Force on Clinical Expert Consensus Documents. Integrating complementary medicine into cardiovascular medicine. A report of the American College of Cardiology Foundation Task Force on Clinical Expert Consensus Documents (Writing Committee to Develop an Expert Consensus Document on Complementary and Integrative Medicine). Journal of American College of Cardiology, 46(1):184-221.

Wagner BK, Kitami T, Gilbert TJ, et al. (2008). Large-scale chemical dissection of mitochondrial function. *Natural Biotechnology*, 26:343–351.

Waris G, Ahsan H. (2006). Reactive oxygen species: role in the development of cancer and various chronic conditions. *Journal of carcinogenesis*, 5:1-8.

Wasson GR, etal. (2006). Global DNA and p53 region-specific hypomethylation in human colonic cells is induced by folate depletion and reversed by folate supplementation. *J Nutr*, 136:1-6.

Wei Q, Shen H, Wang L, Duphorne CM, Pillow PC, Guo Z, Qiao Y, Spitz MR (2003). Association between low dietary folate intake and suboptimal cellular DNA repair capacity, Cancer Epidemiol Biomarker Review., 12(10): 363-369

Weinstock-Guttman B[1], Baier M, Park Y, Feichter J, Lee-Kwen P, Gallagher E, Venkatraman J, Meksawan K, Deinehert S, Pendergast D,Awad AB, Ramanathan M, Munschauer

F, Rudick R. (2005). Low fat dietary intervention with omega-3 fatty acid supplementation in multiple sclerosis patients, Postglandins Leukot Essential Fatty Acids, 73(5): 397-404

Wortmann SB[1], Zweers-van Essen H, Rodenburg RJ, van den Heuvel LP, de Vries MC, Rasmussen-Conrad E, Smeitink JA, Morava E.. (2009).

Mitochondrial energy production correlates with the age related BMI (Body Mass Index), *Pediatric Research*, 65:103–108.

Yamada, T., Terashima, T, and Kawano S., Furuno,R., Okubo, T., Juneja, L.R., and Yokogoshi, H.I. (2009). Theanine, gammaglutamylethylamine, a unique amino acid in tea leaves, modulates neurotransmitter concentrations in the brain striatum interstitiium in concious rats, Amino Acids, 36(1): 21-27.

Yamori, Y. Liy, L., and Mori, M. etal. (2009). Taurine as the nutritional factor for the longevity of the Japanese revealed by a world-wide epidemiological survey, Advances in Experimental Medical Biology, 643: 95-103.

Chapter 3: Vital Signs and Vital Organs

Acres JC, Kryger MH. (1981). Clinical significance of pulmonary function tests: Upper airway obstruction. Chest, 80: 207-11.

Alexander C, Votruba M, Pesch UE, Thiselton DL, Mayer S, et al. (2000). OPA1, encoding a dynamin-related GTPase, is mutated in autosomal dominant optic atrophy linked to chromosome 3q28. Nature Genetics 26: 211–215.

Alveres, Alvito P. and Kappas Attallah (1975). How the liver metabolize foreign substances, Scientific American, 232(60, June issue.

American Heat Association (1980). Recommendations for human blood pressure determination by sphygmomanometers. American Heart Association Publication.

Ames A 3rd.(2000). CNS energy metabolism as related to function. *Brain Research*, 34: 42–68

Andrews JL, Badger TL. (1979). Lung sounds through the ages: From Hippocreates to Laennec to Osler. Jounal of American Medical Association, 241: 2625-30.

Andersson, S. G. et al.(2003). On the origin of mitochondria: A genomics perspective. *Philosophical Transactions of the Royal Society of London, Series B: Biological Sciences* **358**, 165–177.

Andreyev AY, Kushnareva YE, Starkov AA. (2005). Mitochondrial metabolism of reactive oxygen species. *Biochemistry,* 70: 200–14

Avery, Marry Ellen, Wang Nai San, and Taeusch, H. william Jr. (1973). The lung of the newborn infant, Scientific American, 228(4), April 1 issue.

Beck JF, Donini JC, Maneckjee A.(1983). The influence of sulfide and cyanide on axonal function. *Toxicology,* 26:37–45

Betts J, Lightowlers RN, Turnbull DM. (2004). Neuropathological aspects of mitochondrial DNA disease. *Neurochemistry Research,* 29: 505–11

Bianconi, E. Piovesin, A. et al. (2013). Annals of Human Biology, Nov–Dec; 40(6) 463-71

Bickley L. S. (1999). Bates' Guide to Physical Exam and History Taking. 7th edition, Philadelphia; Lippincott, 292-99.

Bilsland LG, Sahai E, Kelly G, Golding M, Greensmith L, et al. (2010) Deficits in axonal transport precede ALS symptoms in vivo. Proceedings of National Academy of Sciences, U S A 107: 20523–20528

Brickley K, Stephenson FA (2011) Trafficking kinesin protein (TRAK)-mediated transport of mitochondria in axons of hippocampal neurons. J Biological Chemistry 286: 18079–18092.

Bird L. (2012). Innate immunity: Linking mitochondria and microbes to inflammasomes. Nat Rev Immunol, Mar 9;12(4):229View Abstract

Bosley TM, Constantinescu CS, Tench CR, Abu-Amero KK. (2007). Mitochondrial changes in leukocytes of patients with optic neuritis. *Mol Vis,* **13**: 1516–28

Bowen J. (2006). Educational strategies to promote clinical diagnostic reasoning. New England Journal of Medicine, 355 (21): 2217-25.

Bristow EA, Griffiths PG, Andrews RM, Johnson MA,Turnbull DM.(2002). The distribution of mitochondrial activity in relation to optic nerve structure. *Archives of Ophthalmology*, 120: 791–6

Caldwell PC, Hodgkin AL, Keynes RD, Shaw TL. (1960). The effects of injecting 'energy-rich' phosphate compounds on the active transport of ions in the giant axons of Loligo. *Journal of Physiology,* 152: 561–90

Chan DC (2012). Fusion and fission: interlinked processes critical for mitochondrial health. Annual Review of Genetics 46: 265–287.

Cagalinec M, Safiulina D, Liiv M, Liiv J, Choubey V, et al. (2013). Principles of the mitochondrial fusion and fission cycle in neurons. Journal of Cell Science 126: 2187–2197.

Clark JB. (1998). N-acetyl aspartate: a marker for neuronal loss or mitochondrial dysfunction. *Dev Neurosci,* 20:271–6

Cleeter MW, Cooper JM, Darley-Usmar VM, Moncada S, Schapira AH. (1994). Reversible inhibition of cytochrome c oxidase, the terminal enzyme of the mitochondrial respiratory chain, by nitric oxide. Implications for neurodegenerative diseases. *Federation of Experimental Biologyu Letters,* 345: 50–4

Coles AJ, Wing MG, Molyneux P, Paolillo A, Davie CM,

Hale G, Miller D, Waldmann H, Compston A. (1999). Monoclonal antibody treatment exposes three mechanisms underlying the clinical course of multiple sclerosis. *Ann Neurol,* 46: 296–304

Criste G.A., Trapp B.D. (2006). N-acetyl-L-aspartate in multiple sclerosis. *Advances in Exeprimental Medical Biology*; 576: 199–214

Christophe M and Nicolas S. (2006). Mitochondria: A target for neuroprotective interventions in cerebral ischemiareperfusion.

Curruent Pharmaceutical Design, 12: 739–757

Day CP, James OF. Steatohepatitis (1998). : a tale of two "hits"? Gastroenterology, Apr;114(4):842-5

Dutta R, McDonough J, Yin X, Peterson J, Chang A, Torres T, Gudz T, Macklin WB, Lewis DA, Fox RJ, Rudick R, Mirnics K, Trapp BD.(2006). Mitochondrial dysfunction as a cause of axonal degeneration in multiple sclerosis patients. *Annals of Neurology,* 59: 478–89

Delettre C, Lenaers G, Griffoin JM, Gigarel N, Lorenzo C, Belenguer P, Pelloquin L, Grosgeorge J, Turc-Carel C, Perret E, Astarie-Dequeker C, Lasquellec L, Arnaud B, Ducommun B, Kaplan J, Hamel CP. (2000) Nuclear gene OPA1, encoding a mitochondrial dynamin-related protein, is mutated in dominant optic atrophy. Nature Genetics 26 (2): 207–210.

Dondas, A. etal. (2013). The Effects of Single Versus Subchronic Administration of Riboflavin on Orofacial Formalin-Induced Pain and Nociception, Cephalalgia, 2013, 33, 265

DiMauro S, Schon EA. (2003) Mitochondrial respiratory-chain diseases. *N Engl J Med* , 348: 2656–68

Feder, Martin E. (1987). *New directions in ecological physiology*. New York: Cambridge Univ. Press.

Fransson A, Ruusala A, Aspenström P (2003). Atypical Rho GTPases have roles in mitochondrial homeostasis and apoptosis. J Biol Chem 278: 6495–6502.

Giulivi C, Zhang YF, Omanska-Klusek A, Ross-Inta C, Wong S, Hertz-Picciotto I, Tassone F, Pessah IN. (2010). Mitochondrial dysfunction in autism. *Journal ofAmerican Medical Association*, 304(21):2389-96.

Gray, M. W., Burger, G. & Lang, B. F.(2001). The origin and early evolution of mitochondria. *Genome Biology*, **2**(6)http://genomebiology. com/2001/2/6/reviews/1018

Guthrie JF, Lin B-H, Frazao E. (2002). Role of food prepared away from home in the American diet, 1977–78 versus 1994–96: changes and consequences. J Nutrition Education and Behavior, 34:140–50.

Habuchi S, Tsutsui H, Kochaniak AB, Miyawaki A, van Oijen AM (2008). mKikGR, a monomeric photoswitchable fluorescent protein. PLoS One 3: e3944

Hanke J, Sabel BA. (2002). Anatomical correlations of intrinsic axon repair after partial optic nerve crush in rats, *Annals of Anatomy,* 184: 113–23

Henao-Mejia, J. *et al.*(2012). Inflammasome-mediated dysbiosis regulates progression of NAFLD and obesity, Nature, 482, 179–185

Hodgkin A.L.(1964). The ionic basis of nervous conduction, *Science*; 145: 1148–54

Iwasaki, A. & Medzhitov, R. (2010). Regulation of adaptive immunity by the innate immune system. *Science,* 327, 291–295.

Jabr, Ferris (2013). The reading brain in the digital age: The science of paper versus screens, Scientific American, April, 5 issue.

Jaros E, Mahad DJ, Hudson G, Birchall D, Sawcer SJ, Griffiths PG, Sunter J, Compston DA, Perry RH, Chinnery PF. (2007). Primary spinal cord neurodegeneration in Leber hereditary optic neuropathy. *Neurology* 69: 214–16

Katayama H, Kogure T, Mizushima N, Yoshimori T, Miyawaki A (2011). A sensitive and quantitative technique for detecting autophagic events based on lysosomal delivery. Chemical Biology 18: 1042–1052.

Klionsky DJ, Abdalla FC, Abeliovich H, Abraham RT, Acevedo-Arozena A, et al. (2012). Guidelines for the use and interpretation of assays for monitoring autophagy. Autophagy 8: 445–544.

Kovacs GG, Hoftberger R, Majtenyi K, Horvath R, Barsi P, Komoly S, Lassmann H, Budka H, Jakab G. (2005). Neuropathology of white matter disease in Leber's hereditary optic neuropathy. *Brain,* 128: 35–41

Korecka A, Arulampalam V. (2012). The gut microbiome: scourge, sentinel or spectator? Journal of Oral Microbiology. Vol 4 : 1, Feb 21.

Krusic P. J., Wasserman E, Keizer PN, Morton J.R., Preston K.F. (1991). Radical reactions of C60. *Science*; 254: 1183–5

Kubes P, Mehal WZ. (2012). Sterile inflammation in the liver, Gastroenterology, 143(5):1158-72.

Kutzelnigg A, Lucchinetti CF, Stadelmann C, Bruck W, Rauschka H, Bergmann M, Schmidbauer M, Parisi JE, Lassmann H. (2005). Cortical demyelination and diffuse white matter injury in multiple sclerosis. *Brain,* 128: 2705–12

Kassirer J. P. (1989). Diagnostic Reasoning. Annals of Internal Medicine, 110: 893-900.

Lassmann H. (1998). Neuropathology inmultiple sclerosis: new concepts. *Multiple Scleosis,r* 1998; 4: 93–8

Lin MT, Beal MF. (2006). Mitochondrial dysfunction and oxidative stress in neurodegenerative diseases. *Nature,* 443: 787–95

Lindenmeyer, C. Forsblom, W. Wu, J. H. Ix, T. Ideker, J. B. Kopp, S. K. Nigam, C. D. Cohen, P.-H. Groop, B. A. Barshop, L. Natarajan, W. L. Nyhan, R. K. Naviaux. (2013). Metabolomics Reveals Signature of Mitochondrial Dysfunction in Diabetic Kidney Disease. *Journal of the American Society of Nephrology,* October 10 issue, 10: 1681

Lu F, Selak M, O'Connor J, Croul S, Lorenzana C, Butunoi C, Kalman B. (2008). Oxidative damage to mitochondrial DNA and activity of mitochondrial enzymes in chronic active lesions of multiple sclerosis. *J Neuroogicall Science,* 131: 95–103 2008.

Mangione S, Nieman L. Z. (1997). Cardiac auscultatory skills of internal medicine and family practice trainees: A comparison of diagnostic proficiency. Journal AmericanMedical Association, 278: 717-22.

MacAskill AF, Rinholm JE, Twelvetrees AE, Arancibia-Carcamo IL, Muir J, et al. (2009). Miro1 is a calcium sensor for glutamate receptor-dependent localization of mitochondria at synapses. Neuron 61: 541–555.

Misgeld T, Kerschensteiner M, Bareyre FM, Burgess RW, Lichtman JW (2007). Imaging axonal transport of mitochondria in vivo. Nature Methods 4: 559–561.

Ohno N, Kidd GJ, Mahad D, Kiryu-Seo S, Avishai A, et al. (2011). Myelination and axonal electrical activity modulate the distribution and motility of mitochondria at Central Nervous System nodes of Ranvier. J Neuroscence. 31: 7249–7258

Mangione S, Nieman LZ, Gracely E, Kaye D. (1993). The teaching and practice of cardiac auscultation during internal medicine and cardiology training: nationwide survey. Annals of Internal Medicine , 119: 47-54.

Mahad D.J., Ransohoff R.M.. (2003). The role of MCP-1 (CCL2) and CCR2 in multiple sclerosis and experimental autoimmune encephalomyelitis (EAE), *Seminal Immunology*, 15: 23–32

Mahad, D. etal. (2008). Mitochondria and disease progression in Multiple Sclerosis, Neuropathalogy and Applied Neurobiology, 34: 577-589.

Matzinger, P. (1994). Tolerance, danger, and the extended family. *Annual Review of Immunology* 12, 991–1045.

Moore, Keith L., Dalley, Arthur F., Agur Anne M. R. (2010). *Moore's Clinically Oriented Anatomy*. Phildadelphia: Lippincott Williams & Wilkins. pp. 2–3.

Nardone, Lucan LM, Palac D. M. (1988). Physical examination: A revered skill under scrutiny, Southern Medical Journal, 81: 770-73.

Pathak D, Sepp KJ, Hollenbeck PJ (2010). Evidence that myosin activity opposes microtubule-based axonal transport of mitochondria. Journal of Neuroscience, 30: 8984–8992.

Perry VH, Cunningham C, Holmes C. (2007). Systemic infections and inflammation affect chronic neurodegeneration. *Nature Review of Immunoogyl*, 7: 161–7

Press C, Milbrandt J. Nmnat delays axonal degeneration caused by mitochondrial and oxidative stress. *J Neurosci* 2008; **28**: 4861–71

Qi X, Sun L, Lewin A.S., Hauswirth W.W., Guy J. (2007). Longterm suppression of neurodegeneration in chronic experimental optic neuritis: antioxidant gene therapy, *Invest Ophthalmol Vis Sci*; 48: 5360–70

Qi X, Lewin AS, Sun L, Hauswirth WW, Guy J. (2007). Suppression of mitochondrial oxidative stress provides longterm neuroprotection in experimental optic neuritis. *Invest Ophthalmol Vis Sci* ,48: 681–91

Sackett DL, Rennie D. (1992). The science of the art of the clinical examination, JAMA, 267: 2650-52.

Sackett DL, Richardson WS, Rosenberg W, Haynes R. B. (1998). Evidence-based Medicine: How to Practice and Teach EBM. 1st edition, Edinburgh; Churchill Livingstone.

Sapira J. D. (1989). Why perform a routine history and physical examination? Southern Medical Journal, 82: 364-65.

Sanyal AJ, Campbell-Sargent C, Mirshahi F, Rizzo WB, Contos MJ, Sterling RK, Luketic VA, Shiffman ML, Clore JN..*(2001)*. Nonalcoholic steatohepatitis: association of insulin resistance and mitochondrial abnormalities. Gastroenterology, 120 (5), 1183–1192

Sathornsumetee S, McGavern DB, Ure DR, Rodriguez M. (2000).

Quantitative ultrastructural analysis of a single spinal cord demyelinated lesion predicts total lesion load, axonal loss, and neurological dysfunction in a murine model of multiple sclerosis. *American Journalof Pathology,* 157:1365–76

Science Buddies (2012). Helping enzymes help you, Scientific American, May 8 issue.

Science Buddies (2014). Sweaty science: How does heart rate change with exercise, Scientific American, Jan 2, issue.

Smith KJ, Lassmann H. (2002). The role of nitric oxide in multiple sclerosis. *Lancet Neurol,* 1: 232–41

Smith KJ, Kapoor R, Hall SM, Davies M. (2001). Electrically active axons degenerate when exposed to nitric oxide. *Ann Neurol* , 49: 470–6

Stys PK,Waxman SG, Ransom BR. (1992). Ionic mechanisms of anoxic injury in mammalian Central Nervous System white matter: role of Na+ channels and Na(+)-Ca2+ exchanger, Journal of *Neuroscience,* 12: 430–9

Smith, Homer W. (1957). The Kidney, Scientific American, 188(1), January issue.

Stutz, Bruce (2009). Pumphead: Does the heart-lung machine have a dark side, Scientific American, Jan 9 issue..

Szeto H. H. (2006). Mitochondria-targeted peptide antioxidants: novel neuroprotective agents. *Americal Association of Pharmaceutical Scients' Journal,* 8: E521–31

Taylor RW, Turnbull DM. (2005). Mitochondrial DNA mutations in human disease. *Nauret Review,* 6: 389–402

Tien Peng, Ying Tian, Cornelis J. Boogerd, Min Min Lu, Rachel S. Kadzik, Kathleen M. Stewart, Sylvia M. Evans, Edward E. Morrisey. (2013). Coordination of heart and lung co-development by a multipotent cardiopulmonary progenitor. *Nature,* 500:589-592

Twig G[1], Elorza A, Molina AJ, Mohamed H, Wikstrom JD, Walzer G, Stiles L, Haigh SE, Katz S, Las G, Alroy J, Wu M, Py BF, Yuan J, Deeney JT, Corkey BE, Shirihai OS. (2008). Fission and selective fusion govern mitochondrial segregation and elimination by autophagy. European Molecular Biology Organization Journal, 27: 433–446.

Scorrano L (2013) Keeping mitochondria in shape: a matter of life and death. Eur Journal of Clinical Investigation, 43: 886–893.

Saotome M[1], Safiulina D, Szabadkai G, Das S, Fransson A, Aspenstrom P, Rizzuto R, Hajnóczky G.. (2008). Bidirectional Ca^{2+}-dependent control of mitochondrial dynamics by the Miro GTPase, Proceedings of National Academy of Sciences, USA, 105: 20728–20733.

Sterky FH, Lee S, Wibom R, Olson L, Larsson NG (2011). Impaired mitochondrial transport and Parkin-independent degeneration of respiratory chain-deficient dopamine neurons in vivo. Proceedings of National Academy of Sciences, U S A, 108: 12937–12942.

Sajic M, Mastrolia V, Lee CY, Trigo D, Sadeghian M, et al. (2013). Impulse conduction increases mitochondrial transport in adult mammalian peripheral nerves *in vivo.* Plos Biol 11: e1001754

Vyshkina T, Banisor I, Shugart YY, Leist TP, Kalman B.92005). Genetic variants of Complex I in multiple sclerosis, *Journal of Neurological Science,* 228: 55–64

Wang X, Schwarz TL (2009) The mechanism of Ca^{2+}-dependent regulation of kinesin-mediated mitochondrial motility. Cell 136: 163–174.

Wahls, Terry L. and Nelson, Tom (2010). Mind My Mitochondria, TZ Press LLC, Iowa City, IA, USA

Wanjek, Christopher (2013). Your liver may be "eating" your brain, scientific American, October 16 issue.

Waxman SG. (2008). Mechanisms of disease: sodium channels

and neuroprotection in multiple sclerosis-current status. *Nat Clin Pract,* 4: 159–64

Werner P, Pitt D, Raine CS. (2001). Multiple sclerosis: altered glutamate homeostasis in lesions correlates with oligodendrocyte and axonal damage. *Annals of Neurology* , 50: 169–80

Widmaier EP; Raff H, and Strang KT (2003). *Vander's Human Physiology* (11th ed.). McGraw-Hill

Wiener S, Nathanson M. (1976). Physical examination: Frequently observed errors. Journal American Medical Association, 2: 852-55.

Zhao C[1], Takita J, Tanaka Y, Setou M, Nakagawa T, Takeda S, Yang HW, Terada S, Nakata T, Takei Y, Saito M, Tsuji S, Hayashi Y, Hirokawa N. (2001). Charcot-Marie-Tooth disease type 2A caused by mutation in a microtubule motor KIF1Bbeta. Cell 105: 587–597.

Zimmer, Carl (2004). "Soul Made Flesh: The Discovery of the Brain – and How It Changed the World". *Journal of Clinical Investigations,* 114 (5): 604–604

Züchner S[1], Mersiyanova IV, Muglia M, Bissar-Tadmouri N, Rochelle J, Dadali EL, Zappia M, Nelis E, Patitucci A, Senderek J, Parman Y, Evgrafov O, Jonghe PD, Takahashi Y, Tsuji S, Pericak-Vance MA, Quattrone A, Battaloglu E, Polyakov AV, Timmerman V, Schröder JM, Vance JM. (2004). Mutations in the mitochondrial GTPase mitofusin 2 cause Charcot-Marie-Tooth neuropathy type 2A. Nature Genetics 36: 449–451. doi: 10.1038/ng1341

Zinsmaier KE, Babic M, Russo GJ (2009). Mitochondrial transport dynamics in axons and dendrites, Results and Problems in Cell Differentiatin, 48: 107–139.

Zhang CL, Ho PL, Kintner DB, Sun D, Chiu SY (2010). Activity-dependent regulation of mitochondrial motility by calcium and Na/K-ATPase at nodes of Ranvier of myelinated nerves. Journal of Neuroscience 30: 3555–3566

Chapter 4: Mitochondrial Diseases

Arpa J, Cruz-Martinez A, Campos Y, Gutierrez-Molina M, Garcia-Rio F, Perez-Conde C, Martin MA, Rubio JC, Del Hoyo P, Arpa-Fernandez A, Arenas J. (2003). Prevalence and progression of mitochondrial diseases: a study of 50 patients. Muscle Nerve, 28:690–5.

Barkhof F, Scheltens P. (2002). Imaging of white matter lesions. Cerebrovascular Diseases, 13 Suppl 2:21–30.

Barragan-Campos HM, Vallee JN, Lo D, Barrera-Ramirez CF, Argote-Greene M, Sanchez-Guerrero J, Estanol B, Guillevin R, Chiras J. (2005). Brain magnetic resonance imaging findings in patients with mitochondrial cytopathies. Archives of Neurology, 62:737–42.

Brownlee M (2001). Biochemistry and molecular cell biology of diabetic complications. *Nature*, 414:813-820.

Casari G, De Fusco M, Ciarmatori S, Zeviani M, Mora M, Fernandez P, De Michele G, Filla A, Cocozza S, Marconi R, Dürr A, Fontaine B, Ballabio A. (1998). Spastic paraplegia and OXPHOS impairment caused by mutations in paraplegin, a nuclear-encoded mitochondrial metalloprotease. Cell, 93:973–83.

Chinnery PF, Andrews RM, Turnbull DM, Howell NN. (2001). Leber hereditary optic neuropathy: Does heteroplasmy influence the inheritance and expression of the G11778A mitochondrial DNA mutation? American Journal of Medical Genetics, 98:235–43.

Chinnery PF, DiMauro S, Shanske S, Schon EA, Zeviani M, Mariotti C, Carrara F, Lombes A, Laforet P, Ogier H, Jaksch M, Lochmüller H, Horvath R, Deschauer M, Thorburn DR, Bindoff LA, Poulton J, Taylor RW, Matthews JN, Turnbull DM. (2004). Risk of developing a mitochondrial DNA deletion disorder. Lancet. 2004;364:592–6.

Chinnery PF, Howell N, Lightowlers RN, Turnbull DM. (1998). MELAS and MERRF. The relationship between maternal mutation load and the frequency of clinically affected offspring, Brain. 1998;121:1889–94.

Chinnery PF, Johnson MA, Wardell TM, Singh-Kler R, Hayes C, Brown DT, Taylor RW, Bindoff LA, Turnbull DM. (2000). The epidemiology of pathogenic mitochondrial DNA mutations, Annals of Neurology, 48:188–93.

Chinnery PF, Turnbull DM. (1997). Clinical features, investigation, and management of patients with defects of mitochondrial DNA. Journal of Neurology and Neurosurgical Psychiatry, 63:559–63.

Chinnery PF, Turnbull DM. (2001). Epidemiology and treatment of mitochondrial disorders. American Journal of Medical Genetics, 106:94–101.

Ciafaloni E, Santorelli FM, Shanske S, Deonna T, Roulet E, Janzer C, Pescia G, DiMauro S. (1993). Maternally inherited Leigh syndrome. Journal of Pediatrics, 122:419–22.

Craven L, Tuppen HA, Greggains GD, Harbottle SJ, Murphy JL, Cree LM, Murdoch AP, Chinnery PF, Taylor RW, Lightowlers RN, Herbert M, Turnbull DM. (2010). Pronuclear transfer in human embryos to prevent transmission of mitochondrial DNA disease. Nature, 465:82–5.

Darin N, Oldfors A, Moslemi AR, Holme E, Tulinius M. (2001). The incidence of mitochondrial encephalomyopathies in childhood: clinical features and morphological, biochemical, and DNA anbormalities. Annals of Neurology, 49:377–83.

DiMauro S, Schon EA. (1998). Nuclear power and mitochondrial disease. Nat Genet, 19:214–5.

DiMauro S, Schon EA. (2001). Mitochondrial DNA mutations in human disease. American Journal of Medical Genetics, 106:18–26.

DiMauro S, Hirano M, Schon EA. (2006). Approaches to the treatment of mitochondrial diseases. Muscle Nerve, 34:265–283.

Duthie SJ (2010). Folate and cancer: how DNA damage, repair and methylation impact on colon carcinogenesis. Journal of Inheritable Metabolic Diseases, 34:101-109.

Esteller M (2002). CpG island hypermethylation and tumor suppressor genes: a booming present, a brighter future. *Oncogene* 2002, 21:1-14.

Fahrner JA, Eguchi S, Herman JG, Baylin SB (2002). Dependence of histone modifications and gene expression on DNA hypermethylation in cancer. *Cancer Reearchs*, 62:7213-7218.

Finsterer, J. (2009). Mitochondrial disorders, cognitive impairment and dementia, J.\ournal of Neurological Sciences., 283(1-2): 143-148.

Finsterer, J. (2011). Inherited mitochondrial neuropathies, Journal of Neurological Science, 304(1-2): 9- 6.

Hammans SR, Sweeney MG, Brockington M, Lennox GG, Lawton NF, Kennedy CR, Morgan-Hughes JA, Harding AE. (1993). The mitochondrial DNA transfer RNA(Lys)A-->G(8344) mutation and the syndrome of myoclonic epilepsy with ragged red fibres (MERRF). Relationship of clinical phenotype to proportion of mutant mitochondrial DNA. Brain, 116:617–32.

Harding AE, Holt IJ, Sweeney MG, Brockington M, Davis MB. (1992). Prenatal diagnosis of mitochondrial DNA8993 T----G disease. American Journal of Human Genetics, 50:629–33.

Haas RH, Parikh S, Falk MJ, et al. (2007). Mitochondrial disease: a practical approach for primary care physicians. *Pediatrics*, 120:1326–1333.

Haas RH, Parikh S, Falk MJ, et al. (2008). The in-depth evaluation of suspected mitochondrial disease. *Moecular Genetic Metabolism*, 94:16–37.

Hirano M, Ricci E, Koenigsberger MR, Defendini R, Pavlakis SG, DeVivo DC, DiMauro S, Rowland LP. (1992). Melas: an original case and clinical criteria for diagnosis. Neuromuscl Disord, 2:125–35.

Holt IJ, Harding AE, Morgan-Hughes JA. (1988). Deletions of muscle mitochondrial DNA in patients with mitochondrial myopathies. Nature, 331:717–9.

Holt IJ, Harding AE, Petty RK, Morgan-Hughes JA. (1990). A new mitochondrial disease associated with mitochondrial DNA heteroplasmy. American Journal of Human Genetics, 46:428–33

Kane MF, Loda M, Gaida GM, Lipman J, Mishra R, Goldman H, Jessup JM, Kolodner R (1997). Methylation of the hMLH1 promoter correlates with lack of expression of hMLH1 in sporadic colon tumors and mismatch repair-defective human tumor cell lines. *Cancer Research* , 57:808-811.

Larsson NG, Clayton DA. (1995). Molecular genetic aspects of human mitochondrial disorders, Annual Review of Genetics, 29:151–78.

Leonard JV, Schapira AVH. (2000a). Mitochondrial respiratory chain disorders I: mitochondrial DNA defects. Lancet, 355:299–304.

Leonard JV, Schapira AVH. (2000b). Mitochondrial respiratory chain disorders II: neurodegenerative disorders and nuclear gene defects. Lancet, ;355:389–94.

Lutsenko S, Cooper MJ. (1998). Localization of the Wilson's disease protein product to mitochondria. Proceedings of National Academy of Sciences U S A, 95:6004–9.

Macmillan C, Lach B, Shoubridge EA. Variable distribution of mutant mitochondrial DNAs (tRNA(Leu(3243) in tissues of symptomatic relatives with MELAS: the role of mitotic segregation. Neurology. 1993;43:1586–90.

Majamaa K, Moilanen JS, Uimonen S, Remes AM, Salmela PI, Karppa M, Majamaa-Voltti KA, Rusanen H, Sorri M, Peuhkurinen KJ, Hassinen IE. Epidemiology of A3243G, the mutation for mitochondrial encephalomyopathy, lactic acidosis, and strokelike episodes: prevalence of the mutation in an adult population. American Journal of Human Genetics. 1998;63:447–54.

Moraes CT, DiMauro S, Zeviani M, Lombes A, Shanske S, Miranda AF, Nakase H, Bonilla E, Werneck LC, Servidei S, Nonaka I, Koga Y, Spiro AJ, Brownell AKW, Schmidt B, Schotland DL, Zupanc M, DeVivo DC, Schon EA, Rowland LP. (1989). Mitochondrial DNA deletions in progressive external ophthalmoplegia and Kearns-Sayre syndrome. New England Journal of Medicine, 320:1293–9.

Morgan PG, Hoppel CL, Sedensky MM. (2002). Mitochondrial defects and anesthetic sensitivity. *Anesthesiology*, 96:1268–1270.

Moroni I, Bugiani M, Bizzi A, Castelli G, Lamantea E, Uziel G. (2002). Cerebral white matter involvement in children with mitochondrial encephalopathies. Neuropediatrics, 33:79–85.

Munnich A, Rustin P. (2001). Clinical spectrum and diagnosis of mitochondrial disorders. American Journal of Medical Genetics, 106:4–17.

Nelson I, Hanna MG, Alsanjari N, Scaravilli F, Morgan-Hughes JA, Harding AE. (2000). A new mitochondrial DNA mutation associated with progressive dementia and chorea: a clinical, pathological, and molecular genetic study. Annals of Neurology, 37:400–3.

Poulton J, Macaulay V, Marchington DR. (1998). Mitochondrial genetics '98 is the bottleneck cracked? Am Journal Human Genetics, 62:752–7.

Prietsch V, Lindner M, Zschocke J, et al. (2002). Emergency management of inherited metabolic diseases. *Journal of Inherited Metabolic Diseases*, 25:531–546.

Ramaekers VT, Weis J, Sequeira JM, et al. (2007). Mitochondrial complex I encephalomyopathy and cerebral 5-methyltetrahydrofolate deficiency. *Neuropediatrics*, 38:184–187.

Rötig A, de Lonlay P, Chretien D, Foury F, Koenig M, Sidi D, Munnich A, Rustin P. (1997). Aconitase and mitochondrial iron-sulphur protein deficiency in Friedreich ataxia. Nat Genet. 1997;17:215–7.

Sarchielli P., Greco, L., Floridi A. etal. (2003). Excitatory amino acids and multiple sclerosis: evidence from cerebrospinal fluid, Archives of Neurology. 60(8): 1082-1088.

Scaglia F, Wong LJ, Vladutiu GD, Hunter JV. (2005). Predominant cerebellar volume loss as a neuroradiologic feature of pediatric respiratory chain defects. AJNR American Journal of Neuroradiology, 26:1675–80.

Schon EA, Bonilla E, DiMauro S. (1997). Mitochondrial DNA mutations and pathogenesis. Journal of Bioenergetics and Biomembranes, 29:131–49.

Shoubridge EA. (2001). Cytochrome c oxidase deficiency. American Journal of Medical Genetics, 106:46–52.

Skladal D, Halliday J, Thorburn DR. (2003). Minimum birth prevalence of mitochondrial respiratory chain disorders in children. Brain, 126:1905–12.

Sun H, Zhou X, Chen H, Li Q, Costa M. (2009). Modulation of histone methylation and MLH1 gene silencing by hexavalent chromium. *Toxicology and Applied Pharmacology* , 237:258-266.

Syburra, C., Passi, S. (1999). Oxidative stress in in patients with multiple sclerosis, Ukranian. Biokhemical Journal, 71(3): 112-115

Taivassalo T, Shoubridge EA, Chen J, Kennaway NG, DiMauro S, Arnold DL, Haller RG. (2001). Aerobic conditioning in patients with mitochondrial myopathies: physiological, biochemical, and genetic effects. Annals of Neurology, 50:133–41.

Tay SK, Shanske S, Kaplan P, DiMauro S. (2004). Association of mutations in SCO2, a cytochrome c oxidase assembly gene, with early fetal lethality. Archives of Neurology, 61:950–2.

Thorburn DR, Dahl HH. (2001). Mitochondrial disorders: genetics, counseling, prenatal diagnosis and reproductive options. American Journal of Medical Genetics, 106:102–14.

Thorburn DR, Sugiana C, Salemi R, Kirby DM, Worgan L, Ohtake A, Ryan MT. (2004). Biochemical and molecular diagnosis of mitochondrial respiratory chain disorders. Biochemical and Biophysical Acta, 1659:121–8.

Tiranti V, Viscomi C, Hildebrandt T, Di Meo I, Mineri R, Tiveron C, Levitt MD, Prelle A, Fagiolari G, Rimoldi M, Zeviani M. (2009). Loss of ETHE1, a mitochondrial dioxygenase, causes fatal sulfide toxicity in ethylmalonic encephalopathy. Nature Medicine, 15:200–5.

Uziel G, Moroni I, Lamantea E, Fratta GM, Ciceri E, Carrara F, Zeviani M. (1997). Mitochondrial disease associated with the T8993G mutation of the mitochondrial ATPase 6 gene: a clinical, biochemical, and molecular study in six families. Journal of Neurology and Neurosurgical Psychiatry., 63:16–22.

van den Ouweland JM, Lemkes HH, Ruitenbeek W, Sandkuijl LA, de Vijlder MF, Struyvenberg PA, van de Kamp JJ, Maassen JA. (1992). Mutation in mitochondrial tRNA(Leu)(UUR) gene in a large pedigree with maternally transmitted type II diabetes mellitus and deafness. Nat Genet., 1:368–71.

Vickers MH, Cupido C, Gluckman PD. (2007). Developmental programming of obesity and type 2 diabetes. *Fetal and Maternal Medicine Review*, 18:1-23.

Wallace DC. (1999). Mitochondrial diseases in man and mouse. Science, 283:1482–8.

White SL, Collins VR, Wolfe R, Cleary MA, Shanske S, DiMauro S, Dahl HH, Thorburn DR. (1999a). Genetic counseling and prenatal diagnosis for the mitochondrial DNA mutations at nucleotide 8993. American Journal of Human Genetics, 65:474–82.

White SL, Shanske S, McGill JJ, Mountain H, Geraghty MT, DiMauro S, Dahl HH, Thorburn DR. (1999b). Mitochondrial DNA mutations at nucleotide 8993 show a lack of tissue- or age-related variation. Journal of Inheritable Metabolic Diseases., 22:899–914.

Willington, K. and Jarvis, B. (2001). Silymarin ( ): A review of its clinical properties in the management of hepatic disorders, Biological Drugs 15(7): 465-489

Chapter 5: Summation

Alveraz, Bernard V and María Celeste Villa Abrille (2013). Mitochondrial NHE1: a newly identified target to prevent heart disease, Frontiers of Physiology. 10.3389.

Anderson, Mark (2013). Study bolsters quantum vibration of scent theory, Scientific American, January, 2013.

Arecherra, R.L., Waheed Abdul, Sly, W.S., and Minteer, S.D. (2011). Electrically wired mitochondrial electrodes for measuring mitochondrial function for drug screening, Analyst, 136: 3747

Attardi G, Schatz G. (1988). Biogenesis of mitochondria. Annu Rev Cell Biol, 4:289–333.

Angers B, Castonguay E, Massicotte R, (2010). Environmentally induced phenotypes and DNA methylation: How to deal with unpredictable conditions until the next generation and after. Molecular Ecology. 19: 1283–1295.

Babcock DF, Hille B. (1998). Mitochondrial oversight of cellular Ca2+ signaling. Current Opinion in Neurobiology, 8:398–404.

Bayona-Bafaluy MP, Muller S, Moraes CT.(2005). Fast adaptive coevolution of nuclear and mitochondrial subunits of ATP synthetase in orangutan. Molecular Biology and Evolution. 22: 716–724.

Beldade P, Mateus ARA, Keller RA, (2011). Evolution and molecular mechanisms of adaptive developmental plasticity. Molecular Ecology. 20: 1347–1363.

Bird A, (2002). DNA methylation patterns and epigenetic memory. Gene Development. 16: 6–21.

Brandon M, Baldi P, Wallace D C. (2000). Mitochondrial mutations in cancer. Oncogene, 25:4647–4662.

Carrol, Sean (2012). Quantum mechanics when you close your eyes, Science for the Curious Discoverer, May 25, 2012.

Chatterjee A, Mambo E, Sidransky D. (2006). Mitochondrial DNA mutations in human cancer. Oncogene, 25:4663–4674.

Chen JZ, Gokden N, Greene GF, Green B, Kadlubar FF. (2003). Simultaneous generation of multiple mitochondrial DNA mutations in human prostate tumors suggests mitochondrial hyper-mutagenesis. Carcinogenesis , 24:1481–1487.

Carchman E H, Whelan S, Loughran P, Mollen K, Stratamirovic S, Shiva S, Rosengart M R, Zuckerbraun B S (2013). Experimental sepsis-induced mitochondrial biogenesis is dependent on autophagy, TLR4, and TLR9 signaling in liver. Federation of American Society of Experimental Biology, J 27: 4703–4711, 2013.

Carré J E, OrbanJ C, ReL, Felsmann K, Iffert W, Bauer M, Suliman H B, Piantadosi C A, Mayhew T M, Breen P, Stotz M, Singer M (2010). Survival in critical illness is associated with early activation of mitochondrial biogenesis. American Journal of Respiratory Critical Care Medicine 182: 745–751.

Chinnery, Patrick F; Elliott, Hannah R; Hudson, Gavin; Samuels, David C; Relton, Caroline L.(2012). Epigenetics, epidemiology, and mitochondrial diseases, International Journal of Epigenetics, 41(1) 177-187.

Chen JZ, Gokden N, Greene GF, Mukunyadzi P, Kadlubar FF.(2002). Extensive somatic mitochondrial mutations in primary prostate cancer using laser capture microdissection. Cancer Research, 62:6470–6474.

Chen JZ, Kadlubar FF. (2004). Mitochondrial mutagenesis and oxidative stress in human prostate cancer. J Environ Sci Health C Environ Carcinog Ecotoxicology Review, 22:1–12.

Cruz C M, Rinna A, Forman H J, Ventura A L, Persechini P M, Ojcius D M (2007). ATP activates a reactive oxygen species-dependent oxidative stress response and secretion of proinflammatory cytokines in macrophages. Journalof BiolOgical Chemistry, 282: 2871–2879.

Dagda R K, Chu C T (2009). Mitochondrial quality control: insights on how Parkinson's disease related genes PINK1, parkin, and Omi/HtrA2 interact to maintain mitochondrial homeostasis. Journal of Bioenergy and Biomembrane, 41: 473–479, 2009.

Daggett, Valerie (2003). Advances in Protein Research Vol 66, Elsevier, Inc. N.Y.

Ji Gang Dai, Ying Bin Xiao, Jia Xin Min, Guo Qiang Zhang, Ke Yao, Ren Jie Zhou . (2006). Mitochondrial DNA 4977 BP deletion mutations in lung carcinoma. Indian Journal of Cancer, 43:20–25.

De Giusti VC[1], Caldiz CI, Ennis IL, Pérez NG, Cingolani HE, Aiello EA. (2013). Mitochondrial reactive oxygen species (ROS) as signaling molecules of intracellular pathways triggered by the cardiac renin-angiotensin II-aldosterone system (RAAS), Frontiers in Physiology. doi: 10.3389

DiMauro S, Schon E A. (2001). Mitochondrial DNA mutations in human disease. American Journal of Medical Genetics, 106:18–26.

Delsite R, Kachhap S, Anbazhagan R, Gabrielson E, Singh KK, (2002). Nuclear genes involved in mitochondria-to-nucleus communication in breast cancer cells. Molecular Cancer 1: 6.

Emine C Koc, Huseyin Cimen, Beril Kumcuoglu, Nadiah Abu, Gurler
Akpinar, Md Emdadul Haque, Linda L Spremulli and Hasan Koc.
(2013). Identification and characterization of CHCHD1, AURKAIP1,
and CRIF1 as new members of the mammalian mitochondrial
ribosome, Front. Physiol, 10.3389

El Meziane A, Lehtinen SK, Holt IJ, Jacobs HT. (1998). Mitochondrial
tRNALeu isoforms in lung carcinoma cybrid cells containing the np
3243 mtDNA mutation. Human Molecular Genetics, 7:2141–2147.

Forner F, Foster LJ, Campanaro S, Valle G, Mann M, (2006). Quantitative
proteomic comparison of rat mitochondria from muscle, heart,
and liver. Molecular. Cell Proteomics 5: 608–619.

Galley H F (2011). Oxidative stress and mitochondrial dysfunction in sepsis.
British Journal of Anaesthesiology 107: 57–64.

Gegg M E, Cooper J M, Schapira A H, Taanman J W (20090. Silencing
of PINK1 expression affects mitochondrial DNA and oxidative
phosphorylation in dopaminergic cells. PLoS One 4: e4756, 2009.

Guo XG, Guo QN. (2006). Mutations in the mitochondrial DNA D-Loop
region occur frequently in human osteosarcoma. Cancer Letter,
239:151–155.

Harrison, C.B. and Schulten, K (2012). Quantum and classical dynamics
simulations of ATP hydrolysis in solutions, Journal of chemical
Theory Computation, 8(7): 2328-2335

Hochhauser D. (2000). Relevance of mitochondrial DNA in cancer. Lancet,
356:181–182.

Ishikawa K[1], Takenaga K, Akimoto M, Koshikawa N, Yamaguchi A, Imanishi
H, Nakada K, Honma Y, Hayashi J. (2008). ROS-generating
mitochondrial DNA mutations can regulate tumor cell metastasis.
Science 2008; 320:661–664.

Hayashi, T. and Stuchenbrukenov, A.A. (2019). Electron tunnelling in the
respiratory complex, Proceedings if National Academy of Sciences,
USA 107(45): 19157-19162.

Huet O, Dupic L, Harrois A, Duranteau J (2011). Oxidative stress and
endothelial dysfunction during sepsis. Frontiers in Bioscience, 16:
1986–1995, 2011.

Kroemer G, Reed J C. (2000). Mitochondrial control of cell death. Nature Medicine, 6:513–519.

Jablonka E, Raz G, (2009). Transgenerational epigenetic inheritance: Prevalence, mechanisms, and implications for the study of heredity and evolution. Qurterly Review in Biology, 84: 131–176.

Jaenisch R, Bird A, (2003). Epigenetic regulation of gene expression: How the genome integrates intrinsic and environmental signals. Nature Genetics, 33: 245–254.

Jang S Y, Kang H T, Hwang E S (2012). Nicotinamide-induced mitophagy: event mediated by high NAD+/NADH ratio and SIRT1 protein activation. Journal Biological Chemistry 287: 19304–19314.

Judith Hagenbuchner and Michael J. Ausserlechner (2013). Mitochondria and FOXO3: breath or die, Frontiers in Physiology, 10.3389.

Kamata H, Hirata H.(1999). Redox regulation of cellular signalling. Cell, 11:1–14.

Khalili, Al and McFadden, Johnjoe (2014) The Life on Edge, Bantum Press, New York.

Klimova T, Chandel NS. (2008). Mitochondrial complex III regulates hypoxic activation of HIF. Cell Death Differ, 15:660–666.

King MP, Attardi G, (1989). Human cells lacking mtDNA: Repopulation with exogenous mitochondria by complementation. Science 246: 500–503.

Kluge M A, Fetterman J L, Vita J A (20130. Mitochondria and endothelial function. Circulation Research, 112: 1171–1188.

Kong J Y, Klassen S S, Rabkin S W (2005). Ceramide activates a mitochondrial p38 mitogen-activated protein kinase: a potential mechanism for loss of mitochondrial transmembrane potential and apoptosis. Molecular Cell Biochemistry, 278: 39–51.

Kucharski R, Maleszka J, Foret S, Maleszka R, (2008). Nutritional control of reproductive status in honeybees via DNA methylation. Science 319: 1827–1830.

Kuroda Y, MitsuiT, Kunishige M, Shono M, Akaike M, Azuma H, Matsumoto T (2006). Parkin enhances mitochondrial biogenesis in proliferating cells. Human Molecular Genetics 15: 883–895.

Liu VW[1], Shi HH, Cheung AN, Chiu PM, Leung TW, Nagley P, Wong LC, Ngan HY..(2001). High incidence of somatic mitochondrial DNA mutations in human ovarian carcinomas. Cancer Research, 61:5998–6001.

López-Ríos F[1], Sánchez-Aragó M, García-García E, Ortega AD, Berrendero JR, Pozo-Rodríguez F, López-Encuentra A, Ballestín C, Cuezva JM. (2007). Loss of the mitochondrial bioenergetic capacity underlies the glucose avidity of carcinomas. Cancer Research, 67:9013–9017.

Mambo E[1], Gao X, Cohen Y, Guo Z, Talalay P, Sidransky D. (2003). Electrophile and oxidant damage of mitochondrial DNA leading to rapid evolution of homoplasmic mutations. Proceedings of National Academy of Sciences, USA, 100:1838–1843

Lee HC[1], Yin PH, Lin JC, Wu CC, Chen CY, Wu CW, Chi CW, Tam TN, Wei YH.. (2005). Mitochondrial genome instability and mtDNA depletion in human cancers. Annals of New York Academy of Sciences, 1042:109–122.

Lee HC, Hsu LS, Yin PH, Lee LM, Chi CW. (20070. Heteroplasmic mutation of mitochondrial DNA D-loop and 4977-bp deletion in human cancer cells during mitochondrial DNA depletion. Mitochondrion, 7:157–163.

Leel H, Cao L, Mostoslavsky R, Lombard D B, Liu J, Bruns N E, Tsokos M, Alt F W, Finkel T (2008). A role for the NAD-dependent deacetylase Sirt1 in the regulation of autophagy. Proceedings of National Academy of Sciences USA 105: 3374–3379.

Lohrer HD, Hieber L, Zitzelsberger H. (2002). Differential mutation frequency in mitochondrial DNA from thyroid tumours. Carcinogenesis, 23:1577–1582.

Lombès A, Bories D, Girodon E, Frachon P, Ngo MM, Breton-Gorius J, Tulliez M, Goossens M. (1998). The first pathogenic mitochondrial methionine tRNA point mutation is discovered in splenic lymphoma. Hum Mutation Supplement 1:S175–S183.

Mayr JA, Meierhofer D, Zimmermann F, Feichtinger R, Kögler C, Ratschek M, Schmeller N, Sperl W, Kofler B. (2008). Loss of complex I due to mitochondrial DNA mutations in renal oncocytoma. Clinical Cancer Research, 14:2270–2275.

Nishikawa M[1], Nishiguchi S, Shiomi S, Tamori A, Koh N, Takeda T, Kubo S, Hirohashi K, Kinoshita H, Sato E, Inoue M. (2001). Somatic mutation of mitochondrial DNA in cancerous and noncancerous liver tissue in individuals with hepatocellular carcinoma. Cancer Research, 61:1843–1845.

Pedersen P L. (1978). Tumor mitochondria and the bioenergetics of cancer cells. Prog Experimental Tumor Research, 22:190–274.

Penta JS, Johnson FM, Wachsman JT, Copeland WC. (2001). Mitochondrial DNA in human malignancy. Mutation Research, 488:119–133.

Plas DR, Thompson CB. (2005). Akt-dependent transformation: there is more to growth than just surviving. Oncogene, 24:7435–7442.

Polyak K, Li Y, Zhu H, et al. (1998). Somatic mutations of the mitochondrial genome in human colorectal tumours. Nat Genet, 20:291–293

Preston TJ, Abadi A, Wilson L, Singh G. (2001). Mitochondrial contributions to cancer cell physiology: potential for drug development. Advances in Drug Delivery Review, 49:45–61.

Massicotte R, Whitelaw E, Angers B, (201). DNA methylation: A source of random variation in natural populations. Epigenetics 6: 421–427.

Minocherhomji S[1], Tollefsbol TO, Singh KK. (2012). Mitochondrial regulation of epigenetics and its role in human diseases, Epigenetics, 7(4) 326-334

Mukhopadhyay P, Rajesh M, Yoshihiro K, Haskó G, Pacher P (2007). Simple quantitative detection of mitochondrial superoxide production in live cells. Biochem Biophys Research Communications, 358: 203–208.

Narendra D P, Jin S M, Tanaka A, Suen D F, Gautier C A, Shen J, Cookson M R, Youle R J (2010). PINK1 is selectively stabilized on impaired mitochondria to activate Parkin. PLoS Biology 8: e1000298, 2010.

Nemoto S, Fergusson M M, Finkel T (2005). SIRT1 functionally interacts with the metabolic regulator and transcriptional coactivator PGC-1α. J Biol Chem 280: 16456–16460.

Ober Clinton and Sinatra, tephen, T. (2014). Earthing, second Edition, basic Health Publications, Inc., Laguna Beach, CA, USA

Park JS, Sharma LK, Li H, Xiang R, Holstein D, Wu J, Lechleiter J, Naylor SL, Deng JJ, Lu J, Bai Y. (2006). A heteroplasmic, not homoplasmic, mitochondrial DNA mutation promotes tumorigenesis via alteration in reactive oxygen species generation and apoptosis. Human Molecular Genetics, 18:1578–1589.

Pagano G. (2002). Redox-modulated xenobiotic action and ROS formation: a mirror or a window? Human Experimental Toxicology, 21:77–81.

Oenrose, Roger (1990). The Emeror's New Mind, Oxford University Press, New York.

Petros JA, Baumann AK, Ruiz-Pesini E, Amin MB, Sun CQ, Hall J, Lim S, Issa MM, Flanders WD, Hosseini SH, Marshall FF, Wallace DC. (2005). mtDNA mutations increase tumorigenicity in prostate cancer. Proceedings of National Academy of Sciences USA, 102:719–724.

Piquereau J, Godin R, Deschênes S, Bessi V L, Mofarrahi M, Hussain S N, Burelle Y. (2013). Protective role of PARK2/Parkin in sepsis-induced cardiac contractile and mitochondrial dysfunction. Autophagy 9: 1837–1851, 2013.

Price N L, Gomes A P, Ling A J, Duarte F V, Martin-Montalvo A, North B J, Agarwal B, YeL, Ramadori G, Teodoro J S, Hubbard B P, Varela A T, Davis J G, Varamini B, Hafner A, Moaddel R, Rolo A P, Coppari R, Palmeira C M, de Cabo R, Baur J A, Sinclair D A (2012). SIRT1 is required for AMPK activation and the beneficial effects of resveratrol on mitochondrial function. Cell Metab 15: 675–690, 2012.

Pyo J O, Yoo S M, Ahn H H, Nah J, Hong S H, Kam T I, Jung S, Jung Y K (2013). Overexpression of Atg5 in mice activates autophagy and extends lifespan. Nature Communications 4: 2300.

Reeve AK, Krishnan KJ, Turnbull D. (2008). Mitochondrial DNA mutations in disease, aging, and neurodegeneration. Annals of New Y ork Acad of Sciences, 1147:21–29.

Rizzuto R, Bernardi P, Pozzan T. (2000). Mitochondria as all-round players of the calcium game. Journal of Physiology, 529 Pt 1:37–47.

Rustin P. (2002). Mitochondria, from cell death to proliferation. Nature Genetics, 30:352–353.

Raha S, Robinson BH. (2001). Mitochondria, oxygen free radicals, and apoptosis. American Journal of Medical Genetics, 106:62–70.

Rodgers J T, Lerin C, Haas W, Gygi S P, Spiegelman BM, Puigserver P (2005). Nutrient control of glucose homeostasis through a complex of PGC-1alpha and SIRT1. Nature 434: 113–118.

Sabzali Javadov and Andrey V. Kuznetsov. (2013). Mitochondria: the cell powerhouse and nexus of stress, Frontiers in Physiology, 10.3389

Salas A, Yao YG, Macaulay V, McCauley, V., Vega, A., Carracedo, A., and Bendelt, H.J.. (2005). A critical reassessment of the role of mitochondria in tumorigenesis. PLoS Medicine, 2:e296.

Sureshbabu Angara and Vineet Bhandari (2013). Targeting mitochondrial dysfunction in lung diseases: emphasis on mitophagy, Frontiers in Physioogyl, 10.3389

Smiraglia DJ, Kulawiec M, Bistulfi GL, Gupta SG, Singh K. K. (2008). A novel role for mitochondria in regulating epigenetic modification in the nucleus. Cancer Biol. Ther. 7: 1182–1190.

Sangkhathat S[1], Kusafuka T, Yoneda A, Kuroda S, Tanaka Y, Sakai N, Fukuzawa M. (2005). Renal cell carcinoma in a pediatric patient with an inherited mitochondrial mutation. Pediatric Surgury International, 21:745–748

Schapira AHV. (2006). Mitochondrial disease. Lancet 368: 70–82.

ShinJ H, Ko H S, Kang H, Lee Y, Lee Y I, Pletinkova O, Troconso J C, Dawson V L, DawsonTM (2011). PARIS (ZNF746) repression of PGC-1α contributes to neurodegeneration in Parkinson's disease. Cell 144: 689–702.

Lisa S. Shocka, Prashant V. Thakkara, Erica J. Petersona, Richard G. Moranb, and Shirley M. Taylora. *(2011).* DNA methyltransferase 1, cytosine methylation, and cytosine hydroxymethylation in mammalian mitochondria. *Proceedings of. Nationall. Academy of Scencesi. USA 108, 3630-3635.*

Stein S, Schäfer N, Breitenstein A, Besler C, Winnik S, Lohmann C, Heinrich K, Brokopp C E, Handschin C, Landmesser U, Tanner F C, Lüscher T F, Matter C M (2010). SIRT1 reduces endothelial activation without affecting vascular function in ApoE−/− mice. Aging,2: 353–360.

Suzuki M[1], Toyooka S, Miyajima K, Iizasa T, Fujisawa T, Bekele NB, Gazdar AF. (2003). Alterations in the mitochondrial displacement loop in lung cancers, Clinical Cancer Research, 9:5636–5641.

Tamori A[1], Nishiguchi S, Nishikawa M, Kubo S, Koh N, Hirohashi K, Shiomi S, Inoue M. (2004). Correlation between clinical characteristics and mitochondrial D-loop DNA mutations in hepatocellular carcinoma. Journal of Gastroenterology, 39:1063–1068.

Tamura G[1], Nishizuka S, Maesawa C, Suzuki Y, Iwaya T, Sakata K, Endoh Y, Motoyama T. (1999). Mutations in mitochondrial control region DNA in gastric tumours of Japanese patients. European Journal of Cancer, 35:316–319.

Takasugi M, Yagi S, Hirabayashi K, Shiota K. (2010). DNA methylation status of nuclear-encoded mitochondrial genes underlies the tissue-dependent mitochondrial functions. Biomed Central Genomics, 11: 481.

Tang M, Baez S, Pruyas M, Diaz, A., Calvo, A., Riguelme, E., and Wistuba, I.I. (2004). Mitochondrial DNA mutation at the D310 (displacement loop) mononucleotide sequence in the pathogenesis of gallbladder carcinoma. Clinical Cancer Research, 10:1041–1046.

Tuuli Kaambre, Vladimir Chekulayev, Igor Shevchuk, Kersti Tepp, Natalja Timohhina, Minna Varikmaa, Rafaela Bagur, Aleksandr Klepinin, Tiia Anmann, Andre Koit, Andrus Kaldma, Rita Guzun, Vahur Valvere and Valdur Saks (2013). Metabolic control analysis of respiration in human cancer tissue, Frontiers of Physiology, 10.3389

Urbani A, De Canio M, Palmieri F, Sechi S, Bini L, Castagnola M, Fasano M, Modesti A, Roncada P, Timperio AM, Bonizzi L, Brunori M, Cutruzzolà F, De Pinto V, Di Ilio C, Federici G, Folli F, Foti S, Gelfi C, Lauro D, Lucacchini A, Magni F, Messana I, Pandolfi PP, Papa S, Pucci P, Sacchetta P (2013) "The mitochondrial Italian Human Proteome Project initiative (mt-HPP)," Molecular BioSystems., 9, (pp 1984-1992)

Valle I, Alvarez-Barrientos A, Arza E, Lamas S, Monsalve M (2005). PGC-1alpha regulates the mitochondrial antioxidant defense system in vascular endothelial cells. Cardiovascular Research 66: 562–573.

Van Trappen PO, Cullup T, Troke R, et al. (2007). Somatic mitochondrial DNA mutations in primary and metastatic ovarian cancer. Gynecol Oncol, 104:129–133.

Wallace DC. (1997). Mitochondrial DNA in aging and disease, Scientific American, 277: 40–47.

Wallace D C. (2001). A mitochondrial paradigm for degenerative diseases and ageing. Novartis Foundation Symposium, 235:247–263; discussion 263–246.

Wang Y, Xue WC, Liu VW, Ngan HY.(2007). Detection of mosaic pattern of mitochondrial DNA alterations in different populations of cells from the same endometrial tumor. Mitochondrion, 7:171–175.

Wang X. 2000. The expanding role of mitochondria in apoptosis, Genes and Development, 15(22):2922–2933.

Wardell TM, Ferguson E, Chinnery PF, Borthwick, G.M., Taylor, R.W., Jackson, G., Craft, A., Lightwler, R.N., Howel, N., and Tumbull, D.M. (2003). Changes in the human mitochondrial genome after treatment of malignant disease. Mutaion Research, 525:19–27.

Weaver I.C.G., Cervoni N, Champagne, F.A., D'Alessio, A.C., and Sharma (2004). Epigenetic programming by maternal behavior. Nature Neuroscience. 7: 847–854.

West A P, Shadel G S, and Ghosh S (2011). Mitochondria in innate immune responses. Nature Review Immunology 11: 389–402.

West, A. P., Brodsky, I. E., Rahner, C., Woo, D. K., Erdjument-Bromage, H., Tempst, P., Walsh, M. C., Choi, Y., Shadel, G. S., Ghosh, S. (2011). TLR signalling augments macrophage bactericidal activity through mitochondrial ROS. Nature 472: 476–480.

Wenz T (2013). Regulation of mitochondrial biogenesis and PGC-1α under cellular stress. Mitochondrion 13: 134–142.

Wittenberg, J. B. and Wittenberg, B. A. (2007). Myoglobin-enhanced oxygen delivery to isolated cardiac mitochondria. Journal of Experimental Biology. 210,2082-2090.

Wu, Z., Puigserver, P., Andersson, U., Zhang, C., Adelmant, G., Mootha, V., Troy, A., Cinti, S., Lowell, B., Scarpulla, R. C., Spiegelman B. M. (1999). Mechanisms controlling mitochondrial biogenesis and respiration through the thermogenic coactivator PGC-1. Cell 98: 115–124.

Wu, C.W., Yin, P.H., Hung, W.Y., Li, A.F., Li, S.H., Chi, C.W., Wei, Y.H., and Lee, H.C. (2005). Mitochondrial DNA mutations and mitochondrial DNA depletion in gastric cancer. Genes Chromosomes and Cancer, 44(1):19–28.

Warburg O. (1956). On the origin of cancer cell. Science, 123:309–314.

Wu M, Neilson A, Swift AL, Moran, R., Tamagnine, J., Parslow, D., Armstead, S., Lemire, K., Orrell, J., Tisch, J., Chomics S., and Ferrick, D.A. (2007). Multiparameter metabolic analysis reveals a close link between attenuated mitochondrial bioenergetic function and enhanced glycolysis dependency in human tumor cells. American Journal of Physiology Cell Physiol, 292(1):C125–C136.

Yin, P.H., Lee, H.C., Chau G.Y. Wy, Y.T., Li, S.H., Lui, W.Y., Wei, Y.H., Liu T.Y., and Chi, C.W. (2004). Alteration of the copy number and deletion of mitochondrial DNA in human hepatocellular carcinoma. British Journal of Cancer, 90:2390–2396.

Zhao ZQ.(2004). Oxidative stress-elicited myocardial apoptosis during reperfusion. Current Opinion in Pharmacology, 4:159–165

Zhao YB, Yang HY, Zhang XW, and Chen GY. (2005). Mutation in D-loop region of mitochondrial DNA in gastric cancer and its significance. World Journal of Gastroenterology, 11:3304–3306.

Xu L, Hu Y, Chen B, Tang, W., Han, X., Yu H., and Xiao, C., (2006). Mitochondrial polymorphisms as risk factors for endometrial cancer in southwest China. International Journal of Gynecology and Cancer, 16:1661–1667.

Yoneyama H, Hara T, Kato Y, et al. (2005). Nucleotide sequence variation is frequent in the mitochondrial DNA displacement loop region of individual human tumor cells. Molecular Cancer Research, 3:14–20.

Youle R. J. and Narendra D. P. (2011). Mechanisms of mitophagy, Nature Review Molecular Cell Biology 12: 9–14.

Yousefi S, GoldJ A, Andina N, Lee J J, Kelly A M, Kozlowski E, Schmidl, Straumann A, Reichenbach J, Gleich G J, Simon H U (2008). Catapult-like release of mitochondrial DNA by eosinophils contributes to antibacterial defense. Nature Medicine 14: 949–953.

Yousefi S, Mihalache C, Kozlowski E, Schmidl, Simon H U (2009). Viable neutrophils release mitochondrial DNA to form neutrophil extracellular traps. Cell Death and Differentiation, 16: 1438–1444.

Zhang Q, Raoof M, Chen Y, Sumi Y, Sursal T, Junger W, Brohi K, Itagaki K, Hauser C J (2010). Circulating mitochondrial DAMPs cause inflammatory responses to injury. Nature 464: 104–107.

Zhang X, Shan P, Alam J, Davis R J, Flavell R A, Lee P J (2003). Carbon monoxide modulates Fas/Fas ligand, caspases, and Bcl-2 family proteins via the p38 alpha mitogen-activated protein kinase pathway during ischemia-reperfusion lung injury. J Biological Chemistry 278: 22061–22070.

Zhang X, Shan P, Jiang G, Cohn L, Lee P J (2006). Toll-like receptor 4 deficiency causes pulmonary emphysema. J Clinical Investigations 116: 3050–3059.

ZhangY, , Jiang G, , Sauler M, and Lee P J (2013). Lung endothelial HO-1 targeting in vivo using lentiviral miRNA regulates apoptosis and autophagy during oxidant injury. Federation of American Society of Experimental Biologt Journal 27: 4041–4058.

INDEX

Cytochrome c Oxidase
Creatine
Cruciferacea
Cytokines
Decoherence
Dendrites
Depolarization
Docosahexanoic acid
Earthing
Electron tunnelling
EPA (Eicosapentanoic Acid)
Entanglement
Eugenol
Excito-toxicity
Exercise
Flavin Adenine Dinucleotide (FAD)
Ferulic acid
Free radicals
Fucaxanthin
GABA (gamma amino butyric acid)
Genestein
Geraneol
Glial Growth Factor
Glutathione
Glutathione Peroxidase
Glycirrhyzin
HCTZ (hydrochlorothiazide)
Immunotherapy
Insulin like growth factor
Irisin
Kelp
Krebs cycle
L-carnitine
Carnosin, an alanine-histidine dipeptide
Linatol
Lentinan
Lipoic Acid
Leteolin
Manganese Superoxide Dismutase

Melatonin
Menaquinone
Metastability
Micronutrients
Mitochondria
Mitophagy
Mobiletin
Monosodium glutamate
Myelin
N-Acetylcysteine
NADH-Ubiquinone oxidoreductase
Nattokinase
Negentropy
Nerve Growth Factor
Neurotransmitter
Nicotinamide Adenine Dinucleotide (NAD)
Norepinephrine
Oleocanthal
Omega-3 Fatty Acid
Omega-6 Fatty Acid
Oxidative Stress
Parkinson's Disease
Peperine
Perluxan
Piezoelectricity
Plasticity
Polarity
Polyphenols
Proton Motive Force
Proton Tunnelling
Psychodelic foods
Pterostilbene
Pycogenol
resonance
Resveratrol
Riboflavin
Rutin
Salicin
SAM-e (S Adenosyl Methionine)

Serotonin

Single Nucleotide Polymorphism (SNP)

Sodium Channel

Sccinate dehydrogenase

Superposition

Sylimarin

Taurine

L-taurine

Theanine

Theobromine

Thermogenin

Thread of Life

Ubiquinone

Umbelliferone

Withanolides (of Ashvagandha)

Zeaxanthine

APPENDICES

Appendix I

The Story of Human Mitochondroa

URL CITATIONS	Number
http://www.lef.org/magazine/mag2010/ss2010_Rejuvenate-Your-Cells-Growing-New-Mitochondria_01.htm http://www.sciencedaily.com/releases/2011/05/110510074433.htm	
20 % of all nuclear genes work and assist mitochondria 25,000 X 0.2	5000
Total power of mitochondria in Human body, BTU/hour	1800 Max
Human body with 10 trillion cells may have on average total mitochondria of number in trillions of	5000-10,000
Liver cell Mitochondria occupie 20 % of volume of cell volume	Up to 2000
Muscle cells have maximum number of mitochondria per cell	1500
Diameter of mitochondria, micrometer	0.5 to 1.0
Number of mitochondria per cell (average of 500)	2-2500
Percent damage at age 90 year	95

Low number and poor function of mitochondria causes cancer, heat diseases, kidney problems, and fast aging with impaired cognition	
Genome stability depends on the absence of certain proteins in mitochondroa	
Consume restricted calorie methylation diet, exercise, and live a mindful life for well functioning mitochondria	
Consume a lot of antioxidant; PQQ per day that helps, mg; others are lipoic acid, acetyl-L-carnitine, and coenzyme Q_{10}, Total daily intake	Up to 30 mg

Appendix II

Human Body Cells and Their Mitochondria

Our body has 10-to 100 trillion cells. I have elected to use the number to be 10 trillion. Some 30 billion nerve cells have the power to control the power and the function of the rest of cells and their mitochondria.

Appropriate URL Citations http://www.fountainmagazine.com/Issue/detail/The-Human-Being-in-Numbers-Last-Lesson-for-Peter http://rspb.royalsocietypublishing.org/content/early/2012/07/13/rspb.2012.1129.full http://www.disabled-world.com/artman/publish/brain-facts.shtml http://www.pnas.org/content/104/11/4718.full	
Information stores in human genome, 150 X 1021 bytes or in ettabytes	150
Number of cells in human retina, million	127
Number of values of same color we can see	200
Shades of light that we can perceive, number	500
Number of cells that die each day, million	50

Number of cells that are born each day, million	50
Number of cell type	200
Number of cells in human body, trillion	10
Number of red blood cells in 5 liter of blood, trillion	2.50
Surface area of red blood cells, meter2	1000
Number of white blood cells, billion	40
Lifespan of red blood cells, days	120
Number of RBS generated per second, million	2.50
Number of time RBS travels in blood in its life time	300
Number of nerve cells, billion	30
Number of mitochondria in nervecells	1000
Total number of capillaries, billion	30
Size of human sperm, micrometer	35
Diameter of human egg, micrometer	110
Length of liver cell, micrometer	40
Number of alveoli in Lungs, million	400
Lifespan of intestinal mucous cell, days	1.5
Life span of stomach entrance mucous cells, days	9.10
Lifespan of stomach exit cells (pylorus), days	1.80
Lifespan of Ling alveolar cells, days	8.1
Total air intake, liters	10
Air we breath in 75 years, million liter	285
Lifespan of colon mucous cells, days	10
Lifespan of upper skin cells, days	19.2
Lifespan of bladder epithelia, days	66.5
Lifespan of nutrophiles, days	45
Lifespan of eosinophiles, days	10
Lifespan of lymphocytes, days (can be i yr)	5
Lifespan of a liver cell, days	220
Lifespan of kidney cells	286
Length of nephrons in kidney, kilometer	50
Length of glomerlus cappilaries in kidney, kilometer	25
Total surface area of kidney channels, square meter	20

Total filtration area of kidner, square meter	1
Number of ribosomes created in liver cells per second	180
Total length of DNA in a cell, meter	2
Number of muscles in human body	600
Number of muscles that work when you smile	15
Number of muscles that work when you frown	43
Daily work of our muscles, Newtons (6 ton lift over 50 M)	3.1
Number of nerve fibers in Skin, kilometer	80
Number of sweat glands, million	2
Weight of dead keratin skin cells that fall of each day, gm	10
Total length of capillaries i Sq cm of skin, meter	1
Total surface area of Skin, m2	1.6
Total skin weight, kg	11.5
Number of sebaceous glands in skin	120,000
Number of cells in skin, billion	100
Number of sensory receptos in skin, million	60
Daily sweat amount, liter	0.80
Maximum daily sweat amout, liter	18

Appendix III

Human Body Statistics

Source: Center for Disease Control, An excerpt from July 14th, 2014

The human body is the entire structure of a human being and comprises a head, neck, trunk (which includes the thorax and abdomen), two arms and hands and two legs and feet. Every part of the body is composed of various types of cell. At maturity, the estimated number of cells in the body is given as 37.2 trillion. This number is stated to be of partial data and to be used as a starting point for further calculations. The number given is arrived at by totaling the cell numbers of all the organs of the body and cell types. The composition of the human body shows it to be composed of a number of certain elements in different proportions. The study of the human body involves anatomy and physiology. The human body can show anatomical non-pathological anomalies which need to be able to be recognized. Physiology focuses on the systems and their organs of the human body and their functions. Many systems and mechanisms interact in order to maintain homeostasis.

Average Human Body Measurements	Data
Men's Average Height	69.4 inches
Men's Average Weight	194.7 lbs
Men's Average Waist Circumference	39.7 inches
Women's Average Height	63.8 inches
Women's Average Weight	164.7 lbs
Women's Average Waist Circumference	37 inches
Body Fluid Statistics	
Average amount of water in the human body	40 litres
Average percent of body weight made up of water	57%
Amount of body fluid that is Intracellular fluid	25 litres
Amount of body fluid that is Extracellular fluid	15 litres
Amount of Extracellular fluid that is Plasma fluid	3 litres
Amount of Extracellular fluid that is Interstitial fluid	12 litres

Amount of Extracellular fluid that is Transcellular fluid	minute
Human Heart Statistics	
Average human heart beats per day	100,000
Average human heart beats per year	35 Million
Average human heart beats per lifetime	3 Billion
Gallons of blood pumped by the heart in a lifetime	48 Million
Human Lung Statistics	
Lung breathes per day	23,000
Gallons of air produced per year	80 Million
Kidney Statistics	
Urine produced each day by kidneys	1.5 Quarts
Urine produced in a lifetime by kidneys	10,000 Gallons
Blood processed each minute by kidneys	1 Quart
Blood processed each day by kidneys	423 Gallons
Blood processed in a lifetime by kidneys	13 Million Gallons
Food Composition	
Amount of food consumed each day by average human	3.5 pounds
Amount of food consumed in a lifetime by average human	53 Tons
Saliva produced in a lifetime	10,000 gallons
Average time it takes food to travel from mouth to stomach	7 Seconds
Body Makeup Statistics	
Number of cells that compose the body	100 Trillion
Number of cells that die and are replaced every minute	300 Million
Blood cells that die every minute	15 Million
Muscles in the human body	650
Bones in the human body	206
Square feet of skin in the human body	20 Square ft

Miles of blood vessels in the human body	60,000
Number of scents detected by the nose	50,000
Number of eye blinks each year	6 Million
Number of diseases that affect the human body	20,000

Author Biography

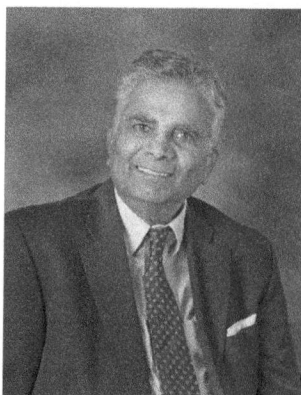

Triveni P. Shukla is a food technologist of international repute. His engagements in food product design, food process deployment, and food marketing have spanned to twenty countries on the globe.
He holds B.S. and M.Sc. degrees from India and Ph.D. from University of Illinois, Urbana-Champaign, IL

He has been critical of the adverse impacts of retail foods and beverages on public health all along his 40 years long professional carrier. The reason, he gives, is excessive consumption foods with careless disregard to frequency and time of eating. He has been even more critical of food industry's influence, albeit unplanned, on America's culture of "Nutritionally Empty" foods.

He made his prime food industry carrier during the period when all major US food laws on public education as to nutrition and nutrients were in making including later laws on health claims and food supplements during nineties. During his retirement years he devote his time to therapeutics against chronic diseases by daily nutrition via "Synbiotic and Engineered Probiotic Foods".

He sensed decades ago that food marketing overrules regulatory public health concerns and that the *"health maintenance and education"*, the basic intent of US laws, never gets reduced to practice in terms of public health promotion. This is true in the United States of America where a majority of processed food developed after World War II and also in other twenty countries where he practiced arts food science and technology.

This book springs from his concern about the impact of daily food on the health of mitochondria in our cells; foods that modulate and repair both mitochondrial and nuclear DNA and foods that promote health of human gastro-intestinal tract by interfacing with bacteria in the colon. His meta-analysis of works from centers of repute and his critical examination of commercial diet programs has convinced him of whole sale deception and misrepresentation of our daily foods. The mitochondria and our body cells live by proper foods and they die by bad foods. Our daily foods, he believes, must keep mitochondrial and nuclear DNA stable and gene expressions timely and to the target. He calls such foods "methylation Diet" typified by DASH, Okinawa, and Mediterranean diets. Neurotransmission and plasticity of our nerve cells depends on functions of the mitochondria in them. We must eat right foods for living long and well, he says.

Lightning Source UK Ltd.
Milton Keynes UK
UKHW010632260221
379439UK00001B/13

9 781643 988283